Current Topics in Microbiology

127 and Immunology

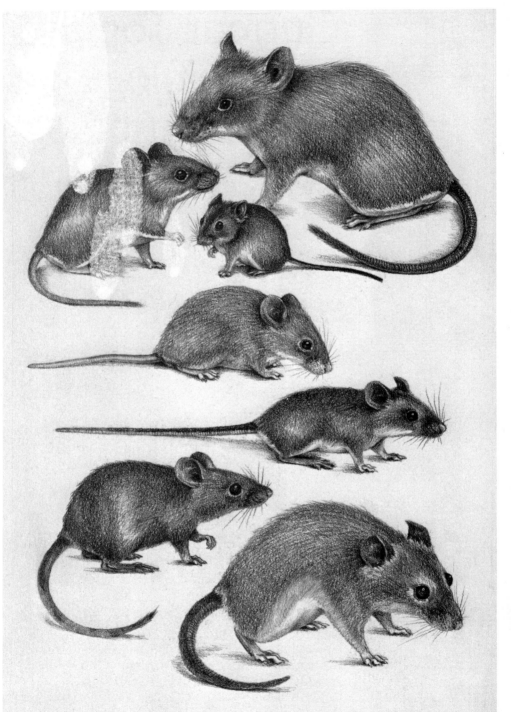

Saroff

The Wild Mouse in Immunology

Edited by M. Potter, J.H. Nadeau,
and M.P. Cancro

With 119 Figures

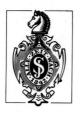

Springer-Verlag
Berlin Heidelberg NewYork Tokyo

MICHAEL POTTER, M.D.
Laboratory of Genetics, National Institutes of Health,
National Cancer Institute, Bethesda, MD 20205, USA

JOSEPH H. NADEAU, Ph.D.
The Jackson Laboratory, Bar Harbor, ME 04609, USA

MICHAEL P. CANCRO, Ph.D.
University of Pennsylvania, School of Medicine,
Department of Pathology,
36th Street and Hamilton Walk, Philadelphia, PA 19104, USA

Frontispiece

Drawings to scale; from top to bottom, left to right: *M. pahari*, *M. spretus*, *M. minutoides*, *M. cervicolor*, *M. caroli*, *M. castaneus*, *M. saxicola*; from the NCI colony, maintained at Hazleton Laboratories. The drawings of the mice were made by Phyllis Saroff. The sizes of the mice are drawn to scale in reference to each other.

ISBN 3-540-16657-2 Springer-Verlag Berlin Heidelberg New York Tokyo
ISBN 0-387-16657-2 Springer-Verlag New York Heidelberg Berlin Tokyo

© by Springer-Verlag Berlin Heidelberg 1986
Library of Congress Catalog Card Number 15-12910
Printed in Germany.

Printing: Beltz Offsetdruck, Hemsbach/Bergstr.
Bookbinding: Universitätsdruckerei H. Stürtz AG, Würzburg
2123/3130-543210

Preface

The present volume of "Current Topics in Microbiology and Immunology"
is a series of papers on subjects that are relevant to the growing
use of 'wild mice' in immunological, microbiological and genetical
research. 'Wild mice' is a jargonistic term that is used chiefly in
the laboratory to refer to the naturally living forms of house mice
(Mus musculus) and also other species closely related to M. musculus.
This group of species is designated by systematists as the genus
Mus. Immunologists began 20 years ago to study the polymorphisms of
immunoglobulins and major histocompatibility complex antigens in
wild mice. An extrordinary extension of the highly polymorphic
array of phenotypes known in inbred mice was encountered. Breeding
stocks of wild mice were brought into the laboratory. This included
not only M. musculus but also many of the available species in the
genus Mus from Southeast Asia and Europe. This availability led to
other comparisons of 'wild' and inbred mice and the discovery of
other new and interesting phenotypes and genotypes. It became
apparent that inbred strains of mice provided only a limited window
for viewing the genetic diversity of Mus musculus.

The papers in this book cover a broad range of topics: systematics
of the genus Mus; special populations of M. musculus such as island
populations and the mice in hybrid zones which offer intriguing
opportunities for population geneticists; polymorphisms in wild mice
of specialized genes of the immune system as well as several other
systems, such as the t-complex and retroviral insertions. Also,
there are papers on genes that determine susceptibility and resistance to viral, bacterial and protozoal infections.

The last chapter in the book is the first listing of available
stocks of wild mice, inbred strains derived from them and inbred-
wild mouse congenics. Included is a brief discussion of the current
status of the genus Mus.

The composition of the genus Mus is not clearly settled. It is
changing from a classification based on morphology to one based
more directly on genetical grounds. Molecular genetics will greatly
facilitate this development.

The classification of the genus Mus proposed by J. T. Marshall, Jr.,
has had wide influence and is the basis for many of the studies in
this book. Much of the current work focuses on M. musculus and the
other living species that are close relatives. This, of course, is
influenced by the vast amount of genetical, physiological and
pathological data that has been amassed in inbred strains of M.
musculus. There exist today species in the genus Mus, such as M.
spretus, that have been genetically isolated from M. musculus for
over a million years. During this time the two species have
diverged extensively but remarkably can be mated in the laboratory
to produce fertile hybrids (see Guenet, this book). A large part
of the genomes of M. spretus and M. musculus have drifted apart and
now have accumulated many new restriction enzyme sites, mutations

and differences in the gene copy numbers. This makes it possible
to find polymorphic forms of many genes in M. musculus and will
lead in the next few years to a detailed mapping of the mouse
genome.

The authors of these papers participated in a workshop on this
subject in Bethesda, Maryland, November 4-6, 1985, that was spon-
sored by the National Cancer Institute and the Jackson Laboratory.
The workshop brought together workers with a wide diversity of
interests. Remarkable enthusiasm was generated, not only because
of the realization that the genus Mus offers such a great potential
for extending our knowledge about the biology of the immune system
and the ways in which the mammalian organism defends itself against
microorganisms of diverse types, but also because it is now becoming
possible to understand the structure and function of the genome of a
single mammalian species Mus musculus. Understanding the chromosomal segments that govern specialized immune functions is becoming
more dependent on the concept of the complex genetical system of
which which they are but a part.

We are very grateful to Professor Dietrich Goetze, Ms. Anna Deus
and the staff of Springer-Verlag for their assistance in publishing
this book. Their willingness to rapidly publish the collections of
of papers in this developing field makes it possible for many to
assimilate the work and thoughts of the contributors. The pace of
development in modern genetics is so extensive this type of summary
becomes an invaluable aid to progress. We thank the National Cancer
Institute and Dr. Alan S. Rabson for sponsoring and encouraging the
workshop that brought most of the authors of this book together.
Most of all we acknowledge with appreciation the efforts of Ms.
Victoria Rogers of the Laboratory of Genetics, NCI, in organizing
and preparing the manuscripts in this book.

Michael Potter
National Cancer Institute

Joseph H. Nadeau
Jackson Laboratory

Michael P. Cancro
University of Pennsylvania

Table of Contents

IX

Retroviral Genes

List of Wild Mouse Stocks and Sources

Indexed in Current Contents

List of Contributors

ACKLIN, M., Institute for Immunology and Virology, University of Zürich, Gloriastrasse 30, CH-8028 Zürich

BERRY, R.J., Department of Zoology, University College London, London WC1E 6BT, United Kingdom

BLACKWELL, J.M., Department of Tropical Hygiene, London School of Hygiene and Tropical Medicine, Keppel Street, London WC1E 7HT, United Kingdom

BONHOMME, F., USTL, Institut des Sciences de l'Evolution, Université de Montpellier II, Place Eugène Bataillon, F-34060 Montpellier Cedex

BOYD, R.T., Department of Microbiology, University of Texas at Austin, Austin, TX 78712, USA

BRODEUR, P., Medical Biology Institute, 11077 North Torrey Pines Road, La Jolla, CA 92037, USA

BUDIMIR, O., Max-Planck-Institut für Biologie, Abteilung Immungenetik, Corrensstrasse 42, D-7400 Tübingen

BULLER, R.M.L., Laboratory of Viral Diseases, National Institute of Allergy and Infectious Diseases, Bethesda, MD 20205, USA

BUTLER, S., Department of Chemistry, University of Maryland, College Park, MD 20742, USA

CALLAHAN, R., Laboratories of Tumor Immunology and Biology, National Cancer Institute, National Institutes of Health, Bethesda, MD 20892, USA

CANCRO, M.P., Department of Pathology and Laboratory Medicine, University of Pennsylvania, Philadelphia, PA 19104, USA

CARDIFF, R., Department of Pathology, School of Medicine, University of California, Davis, CA 95616, USA

CAZENAVE, P.-A., Unité d'Immunochimie Analytique, Institut Pasteur, 25 Rue du Dr. Roux, F-75724 Paris Cedex 15

CHAPMAN, V.M., Department of Molecular Biology, Roswell Park Memorial Institute, 666 Elm Street, Buffalo, NY 14263, USA

CHEONG, N., Cytogenetics Laboratory, Department of Zoology, Banaras Hindu University, Varanasi-221005, India

CHO, W.S., Department of Biochemistry, Saitmana Cancer Center Research Institute, Kita-Adachi-gun, Saitama 362, Japan (HY, OG, YT)

CUDDIHY, A., Department of Chemistry, University of Maryland, College Park, MD 20742, USA

DANDEKAR, S., Department of Pathology, School of Medicine, University of California, Davis, CA 95616, USA

D'HOOSTELAERE, L.A., Laboratory of Genetics, National Cancer Institute, National Institute of Health, Bethesda, MD 20892, USA

ELLIOTT, B.W. Jr., Department of Biology, Massachusetts Institute of Technology, Cambridge, MA 02139, USA

ELLIOTT, R.W., Department of Molecular Biology, Roswell Park Memorial Institute, 666 Elm Street, Buffalo, NY 14263, USA

ESCOT, C., Laboratory of Tumor Immunology and Biology, National Cancer Institute, National Institutes of Health, Bethesda, MD 20892, USA

FIGUEROA, F., Max-Planck-Institut für Biologie, Abteilung Immungenetik, Corrensstrasse 42, D-7400 Tübingen

FISCHER LINDAHL, K., Basel Institute for Immunology, Grenzacher Strasse 487, CH-4058 Basel and Howard Hughes Medical Institute, UTHSCD, 5323 Harry Hines Blvd., Dallas, TX 75235, USA

GALLAHAN, D., Laboratory of Tumor Immunology and Biology, National Cancer Institute, National Institutes of Health, Bethesda, MD 20892, USA

GARDNER, M., Department of Pathology, School of Medicine, University of California, Davis, CA 95616, USA

GOLDE, T.E., Department of Biology, Amherst College, Laboratory of Genetics, NCI, NIH, Bethesda, MD, USA

GOLDRICK, M.M., Department of Microbiology, University of Texas, Austin, TX 78712, USA

GOLUBIĆ, M., Max-Planck-Institut für Biologie, Abteilung Immungenetik, Corrensstrasse 42, D-7400 Tübingen

GOTOH, O., Department of Biochemistry, Saitama Cancer Center Research Institute, Kita-Adachi-gun, Saitama, 362, Japan (HY, OG, YT)

GOTTLIEB, P.D., Department of Microbiology, University of Texas at Austin, Austin, TX 78712, USA

GUÉNET, J.L., Unité d'Immunochimie Analytique, Institut Pasteur, 25 Rue du Dr. Roux, F-75724 Paris Cedex 15

HALLER, O., Institute for Immunology and Virology, University of Zürich, Gloriastrasse 30, CH-8028 Zürich

HÄMMERLING, U., Division of Pathology, Sloan-Kettering Institute for Cancer Research, New York, NY 10021, USA

HANSEN, J.N., Department of Chemistry, University of Maryland, College Park, MD 20742, USA

HARDIES, S.C., Department of Biochemistry, University of Texas
   Health Science Center, 7703 Floyd Curl Drive, San Antonio,
   TX 78284, USA

HARTMAN, A.B., Laboratory of Genetics, National Cancer Institute,
   National Institutes of Health, Bethesda, MD 20892, USA.
   Present address: Laboratory of Oral Medicine, National Institutes
   of Dental Research, National Institutes of Health, Bethesda,
   MD 20892, USA

HELD, W.A., Department of Cell and Tumor Biology, Roswell Park
   Memorial Institute, 666 Elm Street, Buffalo, NY 14263, USA

HELLER, M., Laboratory of Genetics, National Cancer Institute,
   National Institutes of Health, Bethesda, MD 20892, USA

HILBERT, D.M., Department of Pathology and Laboratory Medicine,
   University of Pennsylvania, Philadelphia, PA 19104, USA

HOGG, E., Hazleton Laboratories America, Inc., 1330-B Piccard Drive,
   Rockville, MD 20850, USA

HUPPI, K., Laboratory of Genetics, National Cancer Institute,
   National Institutes of Health, Bethesda, MD 20892, USA

JOUVIN-MARCHE, E., Laboratory of Genetics, National Cancer Institute,
   National Institutes of Health, Bethesda, MD 20892, USA

JUY, D., Unité d'Immunochimie Analytique, Institut Pasteur,
   25 Rue du Dr. Roux, F-75724 Paris Cedex 15

KASAHARA, M., Max-Planck-Institut für Biologie, Abteilung Immungenetik,
   Corrensstrasse 42, D-7400 Tübingen

KINDT, T.J., Laboratory of Immunogenetics, NIAID, NIH, Building 5,
   Room B1-04, Bethesda, MD 20892, USA

KLEIN, J., Max-Planck-Institut für Biologie, Abteilung Immungenetik,
   Corrensstrasse 42, D-7400 Tübingen

KOZAK, C.A., Laboratory of Molecular Microbiology, National Institute
   of Allergy and Infectious Diseases, National Institutes of Health,
   Bethesda, MD 20892, USA

KURIHARA, Y., Department of Cell Genetics, National Institute of
   Genetics, Mishima, Shizuoka-ken, 411, Japan

MARSHALL, J.T., Biological Survey Section, Fish and Wildlife Service,
   National Museum of Natural History, Washington, DC 20560, USA

MATSUSHIMA, Y., Department of Biochemistry, Saitama Cancer Center
   Research Institute, Kita-Adachi-gun, Saitama, 362, Japan (HY, OG, YT)

McCONNELL, T.J., Laboratory of Molecular Biology, Department of
   Pathology, University of Florida, Gainesville, FL 32610, USA

McINDOE, R.A., Laboratory of Molecular Biology, Department of
   Pathology, University of Florida, Gainesville, FL 32610, USA

McKENZIE, I., Department of Pathology, University of Melbourne,
   Parkville, Victoria 3052, Australia

MILLER, D.R., Department of Molecular Biology, Roswell Park Memorial
Institute, 666 Elm Street, Buffalo, NY 14263, USA

MILLER BAKER, A.E., Department of Zoology and Department of Animal
Science, Colorado State University, Fort Collins, CO 80523, USA

MIYASHITA, N., Department of Cell Genetics, National Institute of
Genetics, Mishima, Shizuoka-ken, 411, Japan

MORIWAKI, K., Department of Biochemistry, Saitama Cancer Center
Research Institute, Kita-Adachi-gun, Saitama, 362, Japan (HY, OG, YT)

NADEAU, J.H., The Jackson Laboratory, Bar Harbor, ME 04609, USA

NOVAK, E., Department of Molecular Biology, Roswell Park Memorial
Institute, 666 Elm Street, Buffalo, NY 14263, USA

O'BRIEN, A.D., Department of Microbiology, F. Edward Hébert School
of Medicine, Uniformed Services University of the Health Sciences,
Bethesda, MD 20814-4799, USA

O'NEILL, R.R., Laboratory of Molecular Microbiology, National
Institute of Allergy and Infectious Diseases, National Institutes
of Health, Bethesda, MD 20892, USA

OSBORNE, B.A., Department of Biology, Amherst College, Amherst, MA.
and Laboratory of Genetics, NCI, NIH, Bethesda, MD 20892, USA.
Present address: Department of Veterinary and Animal Sciences,
University of Massachusetts, Amherst, MA, USA

PLANT, J.E., Department of Tropical Hygiene, London School of Hygiene
and Tropical Medicine, Keppel Street, London WC1E 7HT, United Kingdom.
Present address: Leicester House, Front Street Burnham Market,
Norfolk, United Kingdom

PONATH, P.D., Department of Microbiology, University of Texas at
Austin, Austin, TX 78712, USA

POTTER, M., Laboratory of Genetics, National Cancer Institute,
National Institutes of Health, Bethesda, MD 20892, USA

REIDL, L.S., Department of Biology, Massachusetts Institute of
Technology, Cambridge, MA 02139, USA

RIBLET, R., Immunology Graduate Group, University of Pennsylvania,
Philadelphia, PA 19104, USA

ROGERS, M.J., Laboratory of Genetics, National Cancer Institute,
National Institutes of Health, Bethesda, MD 20892, USA

RUDIKOFF, S., Laboratory of Genetics, National Cancer Institute,
National Institutes of Health, Bethesda, MD 20892, USA

SAGE, R.D., Department of Cell and Molecular Biology, Medical College
of Georgia, Augusta, GA 30912, USA

SAMPSELL, B.M., Department of Biology, State University College at
Buffalo, 1300 Elmwood Avenue, Buffalo, NY 14222, USA

SANGSTER, M.Y., Department of Microbiology, University of Western
Australia, Nedlands, 6009, Western Australia

SCHIMENTI, J., Department of Molecular Biology, Princeton University,
Princeton, NJ 08544, USA

SCHÖPFER, R., Max-Planck-Institut für Biologie, Abteilung Immungenetik,
Corrensstrasse 42, D-7400 Tübingen

SCHWARTZ, R.L., Department of Biology, Amherst College, Amherst, MA.
and Laboratory of Genetics, NCI, NIH, Bethesda, MD 20892, USA

SEN, P., Cytogenetics Laboratory, Department of Zoology, Banaras Hindu
University, Varanasi-221005, India.
Present address: Department of Pharmacology, University of Texas
Medical School, Houston, TX 77025, USA

SEN, S., Cytogenetics Laboratory, Department of Zoology, Banaras
Hindu University, Varanasi-221005, India.
Present address: Department of Pathology, M.D. Anderson Hospital
and Tumor Institute, Houston, TX 77030, USA

SHARMA, T., Cytogenetics Laboratory, Department of Zoology,
Banaras Hindu University, Varanasi-221005, India

SHELLAM, G.R., Department of Microbiology, University of Western
Australia, Nedlands, 6009, Western Australia

SHI, L.-I., Department of Biochemistry, Saitama Cancer Center
Research Institute, Kita-Adachi-gun, Saitama, 362, Japan (HY, OG, YT)

SILVER, L.M., Department of Molecular Biology, Princeton University,
Princeton, NJ 08544, USA

SIWARSKI, D.F., Laboratory of Genetics, National Cancer Institute,
National Institutes of Health, Bethesda, MD 20892, USA

STAEHELI, P., Institute for Immunology and Virology, Unversity of
Zürich, Gloriastrasse 30, CH-8028 Zürich.
Present address: Research Institute of Scripps Clinic,
1066 N. Torrey Pines Road, La Jolla, CA 92037, USA

STEINER, L.A., Department of Biology, Massachusetts Institute of
Technology, Cambridge, MA 02139, USA

STEINMETZ, M., Basel Institute for Immunology, Grenzacher Strasse 487,
CH-4058 Basel

SUZUKI, H., Department of Cell Genetics, National Institute of
Genetics, Mishima, Shizuoka-ken, 411, Japan

TAGASHIRA, Y., Department of Biochemistry, Saitama Cancer Center
Research Institute, Kita-Adachi-gun, Saitama, 362, Japan (HY, OG, YT)

THALER, L., Institut des Sciences de l'Evolution, Université de
Montpellier, F-34060 Montpellier

TICHY, H., Max-Planck-Institut für Biologie, Abteilung Immungenetik,
Corrensstrasse 42, D-7400 Tübingen

TUTTER, A., Department of Pathology, Tufts University Medical School,
136 Harrison Avenue, Boston, MA 02111, USA

VARNUM, D., The Jackson Laboratory, Bar Harbor, ME 04609, USA

WAKELAND, E.K., Laboratory of Molecular Biology, Department of Pathology, University of Florida, Gainesville, FL 32610, USA

WALLACE, G.D., Laboratory of Viral Diseases, National Institute of Allergy and Infectious Diseases, National Institutes of Health, Bethesda, MD 20205, USA

WEINSTEIN, D.L., Department of Microbiology, F. Edward Hébert School of Medicine, Uniformed Services University of the Health Sciences, Bethesda, MD 20814-4799, USA

WHITNEY, III, J.B., Department of Cell and Molecular Biology, Medical College of Georgia, Augusta, GA 30912-3331, USA

WILSON, A.C., Department of Biochemistry, University of California, Berkeley, CA 94720, USA

WINKING, H., Institut für Biologie der Medizinischen Universität, Ratzeburger Allee 160, D-2400 Lübeck

YONEKAWA, H., Department of Biochemistry, Saitama Cancer Center Research Institute, Kita-Adachi-gun, Saitama-ken, 362, Japan (HY, OG, YT)

Systematics

Origin and Evolution of Mice:
An Appraisal of Fossil Evidence and Morphological Traits

L. Thaler

MORPHOLOGY AND BIOMETRICS: A LINK BETWEEN GENETICISTS AND PALEONTOLOGY

Systematics of mice has progressed during the last 16 years owing to biochemical genetics (Selander et al. 1969, other references to be found mainly in Marshall and Sage 1981, Thaler et al. 1981a, 1981b, Bonhomme, this symposium). Such studies have brought about the collapse of most older ideas which were based on morphology. However the very progress due to genetics has promoted a revival of morphology. The genus Mus as well as its taxonomic components (species, subspecies, chromosomal races), have recently been redefined. The interactions between these taxa (sympatry, parapatry; syntopy and allopatry; various degrees and modes of introgression; direct and indirect

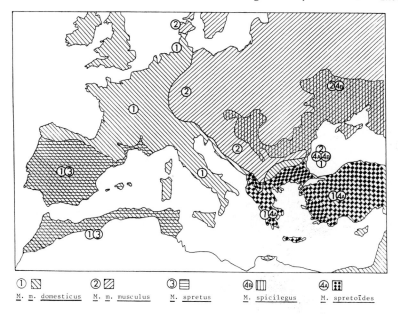

① ▨ M. m. domesticus   ② ▨ M. m. musculus   ③ ☰ M. spretus   ④ᴮ ▥ M. spicilegus   ④ᴬ ▦ M. spretoïdes

Fig. 1 Geographical distribution of the five taxa referable to the genus Mus in Europe (from Bonhomme et al., 1984).

competition) are now better understood. These have revealed complex phylogenetic relationships : diverging and reticulate evolution. It now becomes necessary to place the evolution of mice in real time in history, prehistory and geology. Thus, the fossil and subfossil remains of mice have to be studied, morphologically and biometrically.

The aim of this paper is to evaluate what can be gained from morphology and biometry as the only possible means of linking modern biosystematics, based on genetics, to paleontology dealing only with the remains (i.e. teeth and bones that have been preserved in fossils. The combined paleontological and genetical approach of evolutionary processes is a question of general interest to evolutionary biology and is applicable to the study of certain basic problems.

Rodents play an important role in paleontological as well as in genetical research, and are exceptionally suited for this double approach. The best known fossils (e.g. Apodemus among murids) have not been studied much by geneticists and conversely the rodents best studied by geneticists (e.g. Mus, Rattus) have as yet a very poor fossil record owing to the scarcity of collections from the remote tropical countries where most of their evolutionary history took place.

WHAT KINDS OF MORPHOLOGICAL TRAITS AND HOW TO USE THEM

1. Coat colour and tail length

All mice look alike (and many other species of murids look like mice). Two characters only vary conspicuously: 1) The belly coat colour may be about the same as that of the back or much lighter, 2) The length of the tail varies from longer than the body to much shorter. In addition some systematists of the typological era used the faintest variations of fur shade and of overall size in order to create an absurdly high number of species and subspecies.

The advent of the "new systematics" based on the population concept of species resulted, as far as mice are concerned, in the 1943 revision of Schwarz and Schwarz. It is sad to say that this work was not a step forward. Since that time text-books as recent as Corbet's second edition of "The mammals of the palaearctic region" maintain that there is only one species of mice, Mus musculus in Europe. The lumping of all European mice in one species was based on simplistic univariate or bivariate statistical analyses failing to show any clear-cut differences among them except for tail length which was discarded as insignificant. This was contrary to the long accepted opinion of zoologists like Miller (1912) who proposed that in most Mediterranean countries two sympatric species of mice could be distinguished not only by their tail length but by their habitat preference: short tailed mice are outdoor dwellers, while long tailed mice occur almost always indoors.

When using electrophoretic markers we were able for the first time to demonstrate complete reproductive isolation of two species of mice in a Mediterranean country (Britton & Thaler, 1978). We found as a by-product of the work that tail length was indeed a good character for species identification (fig.2). On the contrary colour of the belly, a character widely used by Schwarz and Schwarz as well as older students to define subspecies of Mus musculus proved to be loosely correlated with electrophoretic groupings. This led us eventually to drop the popular distinction between the grey bellied M. musculus domesticus and the white-bellied M. m. brevirostris (Britton & Thaler, 1978).

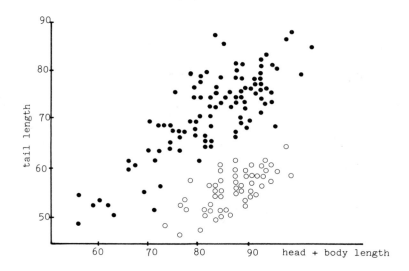

Fig. 2 Relative length of tail among mice from southern France referred
to as <u>Mus</u> <u>musculus</u> <u>domesticus</u> (black dots) and <u>Mus</u> <u>spretus</u> (open dots)
according to electrophoretic markers.

Among the five biochemical groups of mice occurring in Europe (four
species, one of them subdivided into two subspecies) only one, the subspecies
<u>M. musculus</u> <u>domesticus</u>, is clearly distinguishable on live specimens: it is the
long tailed mouse. Pairwise comparisons between the four groups of
shorter-tailed mice may produce statistical differences in tail length but this
is obscured by large overlaps due to individual and geographic variation in
each species.

2. Bones

Accurate identification of specimens by way of electrophoresis has enabled
morphologists to search skulls for meaningfull qualitative features. Characters
have been found for identifying European species and subspecies (Darviche &
Orsini, 1982) and are readily usable for identification of remains such as
those found in owl pellets. Admitedly though, <u>M</u>. <u>spicilegus</u> and <u>M</u>. <u>macedonicus</u>
are very difficult to distinguish on this basis and the two subspecies of <u>M</u>.
<u>musculus</u> are not always easy to recognize.
To get any further with skulls and other bones it seems necessary to
perform multivariate analyses based on morphometric traits. Work in progress
has produced good discriminant functions for distinguishing the skulls of the
two closest species, <u>M</u>. <u>spicilegus</u> and <u>M</u>. <u>macedonicus</u> (Gerassimov, in prep.).
Through a morphometric analysis of the mandible Thorpe <u>et al</u>. (1982) were
able to distinguish between a Robertsonian and a non-Robertsonian population of
<u>M</u>. <u>m</u>. <u>domesticus</u> in Northern Italy. Our team has extended this approach to
several others populations. It appears that in this region the various
Robertsonian populations are well separated from each other on the basis of

morphometry while the non-Robertsonian populations are quite uniform. These results point to an intriguing relation between chromosomal and morphologic differentiation. Besides, lower jaws being the best preserved among bone remains, the prospect of identifying the subfossil ancestors of the chromosomal races can now be carried out.

3. Teeth

3.1. Genus level. Even jaw bones are not preserved in most paleontological localities. The common stuff of fossil rodent material is made of isolated teeth. Fortunately it happens that rodent molars are very complicated and informative structures. Not only paleontologists but also zoologists are relying more and more on teeth morphology for establishing diagnoses of species and genera. Only recently has this morphological systematics been checked out by electrophoretic markers.

At the genus level, it appears that in the family of murid rodents morphology and electrophoretical methods agree fairly well. It is worth noting the results of a survey of the so-called hidden variability by way of sequential electrophoresis (Iskandar & Bonhomme, 1984). This technique revealed no new alleles when comparing species belonging to the same genus. Whereas, a huge hidden variability showed up when the comparison involved distinct genera. However, two outstanding exceptions were found concerning the genera Apodemus and Mus:

Apodemus designates a set of Old World field mice united by systematists because they share the presence of a tooth tubercle t7 which was absent in the extinct genus Progonomys, the common ancestor of all Murids. Electrophoretical analysis shows that species of Apodemus fall into two groups as distantly related from each other as they are from other genera such as Mus, Rattus, etc... Actually, some systematists had already differentiated these two groups due to some external characters and designated them as the subgenera Sylvaemus and Apodemus. We have proposed to give them full generic rank (Bonhomme et al., 1984). Concerning teeth, the tubercle t7 is an apomorphy (new character state), not a synapomorphy (shared by common ancestry), and developed independently in Sylvaemus and Apodemus.

In tooth structure, Mus is even more similar to the extinct ancestor Progonomys than is Apodemus. While paleontologists felt it necessary to create an extinct genus Parapodemus for classifying species intermediate in morphology between Progonomys and Apodemus, they did not create any genus intermediate between Progonomys and Mus. The latter differs from its ancestor by small transformations only: size reduction, elongated shape of first molars, rudimentation of third molars, and a few other characters of even smaller magnitude. The many species referred to as Mus look alike but most of the character states they share are plesiomorphic (already present in the ancestor of all Murids, Progonomys). The morphological departure from Progonomys resulting in Mus is so slight that it has probably occurred more than once. So it is not too surprising to find, according to electrophoretical evidence (see Bonhomme, this symposium), that several subgenera of Mus are no more related to each other than they are to other genera like Rattus, Apodemus, etc... They diverged at the same time but experienced less morphological transformation than the line leading to Apodemus, which is evidence of differences of rates of morphological evolution among Murids. Up to now, the subgenera concerned are Nannomys, Mus, Pyromys and Coelomys, our opinion being to give them full generic rank. A special case is that of the subgenus Leggada which was used until recently for grouping the pigmy mice of Africa and India. The two geographic components of the subgenus behave differently in electrophoresis. The Indian pigmy mice, to which belong the type species of Leggada, are so closely related to Mus proper that we question the usefulness of the subgenus Leggada. As to the African pigmy mice, they are no more related to Mus than they are to Rattus or Apodemus for instance, and are referred to as the already mentioned Nannomys.

When this sorting out of discrete groups of species by electrophoresis or other genetical markers will be finished, the genus Mus, of which Mus musculus is the type species, will probably retain at least a dozen species. To sum up, electrophoretical analysis leads to a splitting of the genus Mus as defined until now into several unrelated genera of Murids exhibiting the same Mus-like character states of tooth structure, most of these states having been retained from the common ancestor of Murids, the others having been acquired through parallel evolution.

3.2. Species level. To the eye of a paleontologist studying only teeth, the four species and two subspecies of European mice are so similar that as fossils they would be referred to as a single species. It is only in localities where two species occur together that sometimes statistical differences in teeth size could be used for identification (fig. 3 and fig. 4).

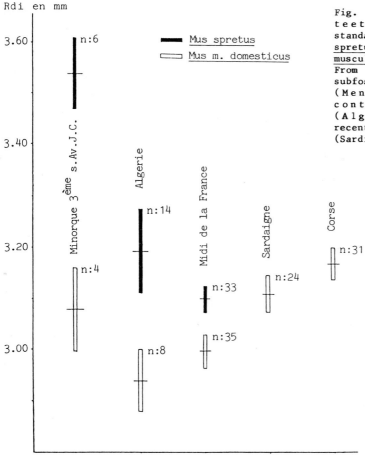

Fig. 3 Length of the lower teeth-row (average and standard deviation) of Mus spretus (black) and Mus musculus domesticus (open). From left to right: a subfossil insular locality (Menorca), two recent continental localities (Algeria, France), two recent insular localities (Sardinia, Corsica).

M. spretus   M. m. domesticus

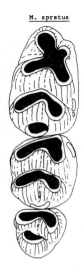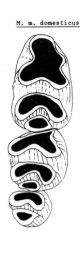

Fig. 4 Lower teeth-rows of subfossil **M. spretus** and **M. m. domesticus** from Menorca (200 - 300 BC).

However the prospect is different when the morphologist deals with specimens previously identified using genetical markers. He is then able to assess the systematic value of characters formerly neglected because it was not possible to decide if they varied between species or within species. This has been done for the sympatric pair of mice Mus musculus domesticus and Mus spretus in Southern France (Darviche & Orsini, 1982). Besides differences in teeth size, very minute qualitative differences have also been found in upper as well as in lower molars.

3.3. Infraspecific level. Geographic variation in a species of mice has not yet been studied except in a few islands (Darviche, 1978). For instance, compared to continental populations, mice from Corsica have tails as long as in Mus m. domesticus and teeth as large as in M. spretus. This puzzling situation was submitted to electrophoretical analysis and resulted in a clear relatedness with M. m. domesticus only. This increase of size, since it is restricted to teeth, is probably not of the same nature as the general trend toward increase of overall size observed in most insular populations of other species of micromammals.

APPLICATIONS AND DISCUSSION

1. Origin of the genus **Mus** and calibration of the molecular evolutionary clocks

Jacobs and Pilbeam (1980) have observed that the time of divergence of 30 MY between Mus and Rattus currently used for calibration of molecular evolutionary clocks is much too old. They rely on fossil evidence from the Sivaliks

(Pakistan) where in beds 8 MY old are found together remains of Mus auctor and of Karnimata an extinct genus more related to Rattus than to Mus. Mus auctor is actually morphologically half-way between Progonomys and Mus. In light of our previous remarks on the high prevalence of parallel evolution of teeth it may be questionned if Mus auctor is really a Mus. Theoretically the line leading to M. musculus could have branched off from Progonomys earlier or later than M. auctor. However this does not matter much if we take into account the whole adaptative radiation of murids. From electrophoretic data it is clear that the lineages leading to recent genera such as Mus, Rattus, Sylvaemus, Apodemus, etc. belong to the earliest radiation of murids and diverged from each other more or less simultaneously. Evidence from European fossils shows that Sylvaemus ancestry can be traced back continuously to Progonomys through Parapodemus (Michaux, 1971). The lineage was well differentiated morphologically 8 to 10 MY ago together with many other lineages most of them now extinct. Considering that morphological differentiation in murid rodents lags usually well behind biological speciations it may be considered that the earliest radiation was well under way 10 MY ago earlier. It could not be earlier than 12 MY when the stem genus Progonomys appeared (Chabbar Ameur et al. 1976). It is difficult to be more precise as long as the lineage leading to Sylvaemus is the only surviving lineage reconstructed. A similar reconstruction is highly desirable for Mus and Rattus but is encountering practical difficulties for the location of the fossil material to look for lies in remote Asiatic countries.

2. Origin of species of mice

There were no mice in Europe during the Last Glacial, so the few findings of fossil mice during an Interglacial in the Pannomic Basin (Janossy, 1961) do not represent direct ancestors of the post-glacial fauna. It is clear that the species and subspecies of mice which have been present in Europe for a few thousand years differentiated elsewhere. Where and when these differentiations occurred are questions paleontologists will not be able to answer as long as they will refer to the European mice as only one morphological species.

Discovery of new morphological characters following genetical identification may help paleontologists to achieve higher systematic resolution. For instance work in progress on pleistocene mice from North Africa has shown that they possess the peculiar teeth character states specific to recent M. spretus but developped to a lower degree. This observation is in favor of the hypothesis according to which M. spretus differentiated as a geographical isolate restricted to North Africa during the Pleistocene before spreading to South Western Europe with the help of Neolithic navigators.

The oldest fossils exhibiting spretus attributes occur in the middle Pleistocene suggesting that the differentiation was under way a few hundred thousand years ago. How much older is the time of divergence, that is to say the geographic isolation which is the initial step in the history of the spretus lineage ? First fossil mice known in North Africa are 3 MY old but the subsequent story of the mammal fauna of the region is characterized by a high rate of extinctions and reappearances by migration. So pending an actual reconstruction of the spretus lineage, a reasonable guess of the time of divergence would be between 1 and 3 MY.

It is by refining this type of approach and extending it to all species, subspecies and chromosomal races that the evolutionary history of mice will be inserted in true time and space.

For the time being we can only attempt to replace the spretus lineage in the phylogenetic tree of the genus Mus sensu stricto as derived from genetical studies and extend our guesses by suggesting that all recent species of Mus sensu stricto diverged during the last very few MY.

3. Insularity

Pleistocene mammal faunas of the Mediterranean islands are composed of endemic extinct species characterized either by "insular dwarfism" (size reduction of large animals) or by "insular gigantism" (size increase of small ones). The dwarf elephants from Sicily are famous. The gigantic mice from Creta are not as popular but their evolution is no less dramatic (Mayhew, 1977). Study of their teeth pattern indicates that despite large transformations they belong to genus Mus. The species is designated as Mus minotaurus. From which continental species lineage did it derive is yet to be found.

Following establishment of man on the islands in post-paleolithic times the highly endemic species became extinct and continental species were introduced, among them mice. In Mallorca (Balearic Islands) the story of these mice is well documented in cave deposits. Using morphological and biometrical criteria it has been possible to ascribe the remains to two species. M. spretus found alone in older deposits and M. musculus coexisting with the former up to the present time. In lower deposits where it is the only species M. spretus exhibits a slight increase in teeth size. After introduction of M. musculus an additional increase is observed in M. spretus. On the contrary there is in M. musculus a decrease of teeth size. This is suggestive of character displacement due to competition between the two species.

CONCLUSION

Progress in systematics due to the use of genetical methods is a challenge to morphologists. The few attempts cited show that in some instances at least it is possible to assess new morphological and biometrical characters allowing the identification of the newly defined species and even of infraspecific units such as chromosomal races. Some of these characters are preserved in fossils, rendering possible the questions of when and where the recent taxa differentiated. This is a very valuable feed-back from paleontology to genetics (think of calibration of molecular evolutionary rates). As yet results of these double-way interaction between paleontology and genetics through morphology are very limited. Limitation is today on the side of morphology and paleontology. Refined morphometrics, especially of teeth and jaws has to be performed in all representatives of the genus Mus. Fossil mice and their ancestors have to be collected in their centers of origin, that is mainly in tropical and central Asia. These laboratory and field investigations will be as money- and time-consuming as genetical programs.

References

Bonhomme F, Iskandar D, Thaler L, Petter F (1984) Electromorphs and phylogeny in muroïd rodents. In : Evolutionary relationships among rodents : A multidisciplinary analysis. WP Luckett & JL Hartenberger, Plenum Pub Corp, New York: 671-684.

Britton J and Thaler L (1978) Evidence for the presence of two sympatric species of mice (Genus Mus L.) in southern France based on biochemical genetics. Biochem genet 16:213-225

Chabbar Ameur R, Jaeger J-J, Michaux J (1976) Radiometric age of early Hipparion fauna in Northwest Africa. Nature 261 (5555): 38-39.

Darviche D (1978) Approche morphologique et biométrique de la biosystématique à la lumière de la génétique biochimique des populations. Application aux genres Mus et Apodemus (Mammalia-Rodentia). Doc. 3ème cycle, Univ. Montpellier 191 p.

Darviche D and Orsini Ph (1982) Critères de différenciation morphologique et biométrique de deux espèces de souris sympatriques: Mus spretus et Mus musculus domesticus. Mammalia 46(2):205-217

Gerassimov S, pers. com.

Iskandar D and Bonhomme F (1984) Variabilité électrophorétique totale à 11 loci structuraux chez les rongeurs muridés (Muridae, Rodentia). Can J Genet Cytol 26 (5):622-627.

Jacobs LL, Pilbeam D (1980) Of Mice and Men : Fossil-based divergence dates and molecular "Clocks". J Human Evol 9 (7):551-555.

Janossy D (1961) Die Entwicklung der kleinsäugerfauna Europas im Pleistozän (Insectivora, Rodentia, Lagomorpha). Z f Säugetierkunde 26:1-11.

Marshall JT and Sage RD (1981) Taxonomy of the House Mouse. Symp Zool Soc Lond 47:15-25.

Mayhew DF (1977) The endemic pleistocene Murids of Crete. I Proc Koninklijke Nederlandse Akademie van Wetenschappen 80:182-201.

Michaux J (1971) Muridae Néogènes d'Europe Sud-Occidentale. Paléobiologie continenetale, Montpellier, II (1):71 p.

Miller GS (1912) Catalogue of the Mammals of Western Europe. British Museum (Natural History), Londres 1019 p.

Schwarz E and Schwarz HK (1943) The wild and commensal stocks of the house mouse, Mus musculus. J Mammal 24:59-72.

Selander RK, Hunt WG and Yang SY (1969) Protein polymorphism and genic heterozygosity in two european subspecies of the house mouse. Evolution 23:379-390.

Thaler L, Bonhomme F, Britton-Davidian J and Hamar M (1981a). The House mouse complex of species : sympatric occurence of biochemical groups Mus 2 and Mus 4 in Rumania. Z f Säugetierkunde 46:169-173.

Thaler L, Bonhomme F and Britton-Davidian J (1981b). Processes of speciation and semi-speciation in the house mouse. Symp Zool Soc Lond 47:27-41.

Thorpe RS, Corti M and Capanna E (1982) Morphometric divergence of Robertsonian populations/species of Mus: A multivariate analysis of size and shape. Experientia 38:920-923.

Systematics of the Genus *Mus*

J. T. Marshall

My purpose is first to show how the geographic color races of Mus
musculus can be identified by coat color and tail length (Fig. 1);
second, to report specimens that appear to link domesticus with musculus
by intergradation around the back way in Asia; and third, to identify
anew specimens in the National Museum of Natural History by means of the
cranial traits discovered by Darviche and Orsini (1982). The resulting
nomenclature of the genus Mus, based on morphology and distribution, is
commensurate in its species-limits with other genera of Muridae that have
not received intensive biochemical study.

A problem with taxonomy of Mus is the occurrence together in the same
meadow of two kinds of mice that are difficult to tell apart. Several
such pairs of species were uncovered before the invention of enzyme
genetics: Matthey and Petter (1968) distinguished Mus booduga from M.
dunni by karyotype and molars, Pantuwatana et al. (1969) separated Mus
caroli from M. cervicolor by differences in feet and tail, and Mishra et
al. (1972) separated sympatric Mus platythrix from M. saxicola by their
unique species of lice.

The genus Mus consists of small Old World rodents possessing a laterally
pointed parietal bone, a first upper molar longer than half the
tooth-row, and upper molars lacking a postero-internal cusp. Most of the
species occupy India and Southeast Asia (Marshall 1977b). There I
discovered a hiatus in the distribution of outdoor Mus musculus; other
species fill the natural and agricultural habitats. They belong to three
subgenera: Coelomys is small-eyed and has broad frontal bones; Mus is
narrow between the orbits; Pyromys has supraorbital ridges like a rat
(Mus saxicola is the one colonized from Mysore by T.H. Yoshida).

Asian species of the subgenus Mus, which prevent the house mouse from
occupying outdoor habitats, exemplify differences among real species.
They are agricultural pests easily dug from paddyfield dikes for
study in a terrarium. They are distinguished from house mice by a long,
shallow rostrum. Below are some of their attributes, more fully described
by Marshall (1977a, 1977b). Copies of the latter reference, with
photographs of living mice taken by Boonsong Lekagul, can be obtained at
the above address. In the following descriptions a "long tail" means as
long as the head plus body length, and "medium size" is the head-and-body
length of the house mouse.

Mus booduga: Small; short-tailed; upper incisors recurved, with a notch;
upper molars broad; the underparts are white. Mus booduga is the type of
Leggada, which name is therefore not available for African pygmy mice.

Mus caroli: Medium size; upper incisors inclined foreward and colored
dark tan, nasals short; the tail is very long.

Fig. 1. Identification of house mice by means of coloration, tail length,
and geography

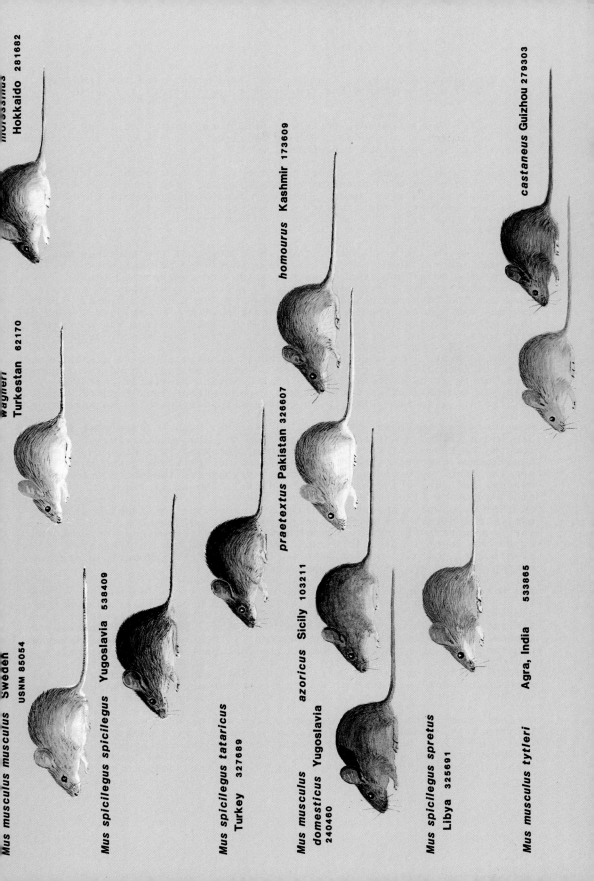

morossinus
Hokkaido 281682

Mus musculus musculus Sweden
USNM 85054

wagneri
Turkestan 62170

Mus spicilegus spicilegus Yugoslavia 538409

Mus spicilegus tataricus
Turkey 327689

praetextus Pakistan 326607

homourus Kashmir 173609

Mus musculus
domesticus Yugoslavia
240460

azoricus Sicily 103211

castaneus Guizhou 279303

Mus spicilegus spretus
Libya 325691

Mus musculus tytleri Agra, India 533865

Mus cervicolor: Pro-odont, nasals long, tail short, and the feet are white. Occurs as medium sized (_annamensis_, _cervicolor_) and large (_popaeus_) races.

Mus cookii: Upper incisors recurved, tail long; teeth are large but the first upper molar is slender. Occurs as large sized (_cookii_) and medium sized (_nagarum_, _palnica_) subspecies.

Mus dunni: Small; upper incisors pro-odont, without notch; upper first molar slender and with anterior accessory cusp; tail long; the white fur of underparts has gray bases. Recently I collected several _M. dunni_ in a ricefield at Medan, Sumatra (now in American Museum of Natural History). They would not enter the cold, wet aluminum traps and had to be taken in snap traps.

Now we come to the house mice. They are members of the subgenus _Mus_ that possess a short, deep rostrum. Figure 1 shows the coloration and tail length of a modal specimen of each species and subspecies. Their arrangement in six tiers corresponds to relative positions on the map of Eurasia. The "zygomatic index," invented by Darviche and Orsini (1982), divides the hillock mouse and its relatives with a broad dorsal root of the zygomatic plate (as in _M. caroli_ and _M. cookii_) from _Mus musculus_ with a narrow root (as in _M. booduga_, _M. cervicolor_, and _M. dunni_).

The house mouse, _Mus musculus_: Most adult specimens can be distinguished from all others in the genus by a broad anterior portion of the zygomatic arch, where it caps the zygomatic plate. Notice in Fig. 1 that _Mus musculus_ consists of an array of geographic subspecies. Each of them intergrades with its neighbor to west and to east within the same tier.

Mus musculus (northern, short-tailed section; Fig. 1, uppermost tier): Specimens traded by Richard D. Sage from the Academia Sinica, Beijing, now in the Museum of Vertebrate Zoology, document intergradation between long-furred _wagneri_ (including the synonymous _gansuensis_ and _mongolius_) and the sleek _molossinus_ (with which I synonymize the short-tailed _manchu_, and pure-white-bellied _yamashinai_). The skull traits distinguishing Linnaean _Mus musculus musculus_ of Uppsala, Sweden, prevail in this sweep of connected populations across the continent: outline of skull in lateral view arched and rounded, tallest at about the level of the fronto-parietal suture; prominent antero-external cusp on both the upper and lower first molars such that the lower one is truncate anteriorly; convexly curved anterior border of the zygomatic plate; and smooth outline of the lateral parietal wing.

Mus musculus (southern, long-tailed section; Fig. 1, fourth tier): The tortuous northern distributional limit of the dark-bellied subspecies _domesticus_, where it comes against _Mus musculus musculus_, runs from the British Isles, across Denmark, along the Elbe, south across Bavaria, and thence toward Yugoslavia, where apparently the two populations diverge. I can find only one specimen from Norway (National Museum of Natural History 84693), along with one of _musculus_ (142602) and one hybrid (199504). The last is the only hybrid I have encountered among several thousand museum specimens of _Mus_; a few other hybrid specimens were mapped by Ursin (1952) and Kraft (1985) from their respective museums.

Because most South American domestic mice are dark, I regard _brevirostris_, named from Uruguay, as synonymous with _domesticus_. The long-tailed, pale-bellied population from the northwestern part of the Mediterranean area can be called _azoricus_. Samples from some French localities contain both dark and light specimens, indicating intergradation with the northern subspecies.

From Morocco to Pakistan Mus musculus praetextus includes all long-tailed
populations that contain pure white-bellied individuals. It is
polychromatic in settlements of the west, including dark individuals and
a silver phase. Dark ones look more like mimics of Mus spretus than
domesticus or azoricus from ships. But at the edge of the desert,
eastward to Pakistan, populations are consistently sandy colored above
and snowy white beneath (= bactrianus, which I synonymize with
praetextus). In northern Pakistan these intergrade uphill with Himalayan
Mus musculus homourus. Nepalese homourus is the easternmost population of
long-tailed domestic mice that can live outside as well as in houses, to
which the high-altitude homourus repairs in winter (as collected by Steve
Frantz). Beyond Sikkim and the Indian desert at Jodhpur is the hiatus
where outdoor habitats are preempted by other species of the
40-chromosome subgenus Mus.

Back in Germany, the skull of Mus musculus domesticus is distinguishable
from that of M. m. musculus. In lateral view, the skull outline of
domesticus is wedge-shaped with the tallest part toward the rear of the
cranium, whence the skull tapers anteriorly in straight lines. The
antero-external cusp of the first molar is insignificant (Darviche and
Orsini 1982), such that the occlusal outline of the lower one is
triangular and pointed anteriorly. Noticeable are the straight, vertical,
anterior border of the zygomatic plate and the squiggly outline of the
lateral parietal wing. These traits prevail in samples of domesticus all
the way to its eastern limit of distribution in Yugoslavia, also in the
the sample of azoricus from Sicily. But east of the Mediterranean, traits
variously become more like musculus.

The overall picture so far shows us two tiers of subspecies: a
transcontinental one in the north with short tail and skull attributes of
the subspecies musculus; a second in the south, abruptly cut off at
Sikkim and eastern India, with long tail and musculus-like skull in the
east, but gradually taking on skull features of domesticus in successive
populations westward. These two tiers are separated by seas amd mountains
except along the secondary contact zone, 20 kilometers wide, in western
Europe. In the east, the width of Southeast Asia and most of India
separates northern molossinus from southern homourus cum praetextus.
Human commerce has injected the strictly indoor Mus musculus castaneus
into the gap.

Mus musculus (Southeast Asian long-tailed section; Fig. 1, bottom tier):
The skull of Mus musculus castaneus is like that of molossinus, its
neighbor to the north, except that the zygomatic plate leans forward.
That one trait makes castaneus the easiest of house mouse taxa to
identify cranially. Coloration resembles domesticus except for chestnut
tints on the upperparts, ochre beneath and on the flanks. M. m. castaneus
is the only completely indoor mouse. (It does occur outdoors in the
Pacific Islands where introduced by man, and occasionally in the
Philippines, because there are no Mus caroli and M. cervicolor to
interfere.) A pale, ochraceous subspecies, tytleri, is found in northern
Indian cities such as Varanasi, New Delhi, and Agra.

Specimens in the National Museum of Natural History and the American
Museum of Natural History collected in Sichuan, labeled Mus musculus
tantillus, are recognizable as molossinus daubed with ochre and sprouting
long tails. These skins are actually intergrades between Yunnan
castaneus and Shaanxi molossinus. The position of the intergrading zone
is probably related to the northern distributional limits of Mus caroli.

The last link of the chain should be between New Delhi (my specimens of Mus musculus tytleri) and Jodhpur to the southwest, where V.C. Agrawal collected M. m. praetextus at the desert research station of the Zoological Survey of India. It should be easy to find the intergrading zone at the edge of the desert. Actually, tytleri is itself the intergrade because its buff underparts are intermediate between dark-bellied castaneus and snow-white-bellied praetextus. This explains the continuation of the musculus-style skull westward into Pakistan from the Orient. Even though tytleri is sequestered indoors it could meet and mate with the indoor contingent of praetextus.

I think that the northern and southern tiers of Mus musculus, having each deployed subspecies adapted to local environments, became separated at the last glacial period. Populations in three far-flung refugia effected genomic reorganisations pointing toward species differentiation of castaneus, domesticus, and musculus. Before they could entirely reach that level, and fail to interbreed, they were thrust back together. Limited interbreeding at the western contact and both sides of castaneus, is just enough to keep the genetic pot boiling and to cut off evolutionary advance.

The short-tailed wild mouse, Mus spicilegus: The mound-building mouse and its close relatives have a short tail, constant color pattern including a white venter with slate bases, plain bevel on the upper incisors or an obtusely angled notch, prominent antero-external cusp on upper and lower first molars, and semicircular line of demarcation between the parietal and frontal bones. The parietal has crept anterolaterally over the frontal, broadening the lateral spine into a crescent. The geographic range of this mouse is superimposed upon that of M. musculus. Aside from western Mediterranean collections of the common form, spretus, specimens are so rare in American collections as to border on the mythical. Three taxa, spicilegus, spretus, and tataricus, apparently are not contiguous geographically. The first builds mounds; the other two do not.

Mus spicilegus spicilegus: Excellent life history studies in Russia refer to the mound-building mouse as Mus hortulanus, the oldest name, with type locality the botanical garden at Odessa. That is an unlikely place for storing grain in mounds. Unless the type specimen can be found and identified as the mound-builder, we should take the advice of Bonhomme et al. (1978) and use spicilegus, meaning "gathering together spikes of grain." The lectotype and former "cotype" of Mus spicilegus from Hungary and six taken by Dr. Sage from mounds in Austria (at Halbturn) and Yugoslavia (two fields near Belgrade) share additional features pictured by Marshall and Sage (1981): skulls are tall dorso-ventrally but short longitudinally. Thus the rostrum is relatively the deepest and shortest in the genus Mus, and the narrow zygomatic plate is tallest, besides being narrowest. In dorsal view the rostrum is narrow and the zygomatic plates seem to have been pinched together; therefore a view from the anterior shows the infraorbital foramen as more of a slit than an open triangle. Paving a store of grain with earth is an inherited skill of this mouse, accomplished to perfection by offspring removed from their parents at an early age (Orsini et al. 1983).

Coloration of the hillock mouse is the same as that of Mus musculus musculus in the same area (although this may not seem obvious from Fig. 1 because the Swedish mice either are paler than those of Yugoslavia or have faded). This tribute to parallel evolution of external characters by related species in the same environment need not detract from the behavioral and internal differences.

Mus spicilegus spretus: The elongated skull is sculptured in graceful curves, teeth are large, the intermolar palatal rugae are reduced to four, and the upper incisors are smoothly beveled. The tail is not only short, but it is slender as well. Luis Thaler told me that spretus can metabolize its own water supply.

Mus spicilegus tataricus: I abandon the name abbotti because the juvenile type specimen (from Turkey) is too small for any member of the house mouse complex. My measurements in millimeters of the type in spirit at the British Museum are 44-50-15.1-9.6, complete upper molar row 3.0. The two Mus species known to occupy Turkey have larger teeth than these and juveniles larger than the type still lack the third molar. The type must be a mislabeled pygmy mouse from Africa or India. Satunin (1908) describes tataricus as a completely wild mouse living in a saline Artemisia steppe near the saltworks at Bank, on the southwest shore of the Caspian Sea; it is grayish brown on the back with some rufous along the flanks; underparts are white with slate gray bases; feet are white and the 69 mm tail is sharply bicolored. Satunin's description could apply to the eastern Mediterranean short-tailed mouse, of which the National Museum of Natural History has specimens from 6 places in Turkey and from 40 km southwest of Asadabad in western Iran. (Some of the latter have pure white underparts.) The teeth and gracile skull of these specimens are exactly like those of spretus except that they are larger and the incisors are usually notched. Thus the Turkish skulls are unlike the few known examples of spicilegus. However, three wild-caught examples that Dr. Sage took at Gradsko in Macedonian Yugoslavia, where they do not build mounds, seem intermediate. They have the tall, narrow zygomatic plate of spicilegus as well as the long skull of tataricus (RDS numbers 10145, 10149, 10150 in the Museum of Vertebrate Zoology, Berkeley, California). The specimens from Egypt (National Museum of Natural History and Field Museum) that I thought were abbotti have a narrow dorsal root of the zygomatic plate and are merely the dark, short-tailed extremes of polychromatic Mus musculus praetextus. I apologize to Lawrence D'Hoostelaere and Harry Hoogstraal for luring them into a search for this non-existent mouse.

Summary: Genus Mus
Subgenus Coelomys, mice of mountain forests.

Mus crociduroides	Sumatra
Mus famulus	Southern India
Mus mayori	Sri Lanka
Mus pahari	SE Asia
Mus vulcani	Java

Subgenus Mus, house mice and their relatives with diploid 40 chromosomes.

Mus booduga	Pakistan, India and Burma (subspecies booduga); Sri Lanka (fulvidiventris)
Mus caroli	Ryukyu Islands, Fujian, and Yunnan (caroli) to Indonesia (ouwensi)
Mus cervicolor	Laos and Vietnam (annamensis), Nepal to Vietnam (cervicolor), Burma and Thailand (popaeus)
Mus cookii	Mountains: Burma and Thailand (cookii); Nepal, northwestern and central India (nagarum), southern India (palnica)
Mus dunni	India and Sumatra
Mus musculus	Eurasia and northern Africa including northern intergrading subspecies from eastern Asia (molossinus) to Europe (musculus) via the midcontinent (wagneri); southern intergrading subspecies in northwestern Mediterranean area (azoricus), western Europe (domesticus), south

slope of Himalayas (homourus), and northern
Africa to Pakistan (praetextus); and
southeastern, indoor subspecies (castaneus,
tytleri)

Mus spicilegus — Separated subspecies on steppes of eastern
Europe (spicilegus); western Mediterranean rim
(spretus); and Macedonia, Turkey, Georgia, and
western Iran (tataricus)

Subgenus Nannomys, African pygmy mice with species minutoides, setulosus
and much, much more!

Subgenus Pyromys, spiny mice.

Mus fernandoni	Sri Lanka
Mus phillipsi	India
Mus platythrix	India
Mus saxicola	Nepal (subspecies gurkha), Pakistan (sadhu), and India (saxicola)
Mus shortridgei	Burma, Thailand, Kampuchea, and Vietnam

References:

Bonhomme F, Britton-Davidian J, Thaler L, Triantaphyllidis C (1978) Sur
l'existence en Europe de quatre groupes de souris (genre Mus L.) du
rang espece et semi-espece, demontree par la genetique biochimique. CR
Acad Sc Paris 287:631-633

Darviche D, Orsini P (1982) Criteres de differenciation mophologique et
biometrique de deux especes de souris sympatrique: Mus spretus et Mus
musculus domesticus. Mammalia 46:205-217

Kraft R (1985) Merkmale und Verbreitung der Hausmause Mus musculus
musculus L., 1758, und Mus musculus domesticus Rutty, 1772 (Rodentia,
Muridae) in Bayern. Saugetierk Mitt 32:1-12

Marshall JT (1977a) Family Muridae: rats and mice. In: Lekagul B, McNeely
J (eds) Mammals of Thailand. Association for Conservation of Wildlife,
Bangkok, p 397

Marshall JT (1977b) A synopsis of Asian species of Mus (Rodentia,
Muridae). Bull Am Museum Nat Hist 158:175-220.

Marshall J, Sage RD (1981) Taxonomy of the house mouse. In: Berry RJ (ed)
Biology of the house mouse. Zool Soc London, London, p 15

Matthey R, Petter F (1968) Existence de deux especes distinctes, l'une
chromosomiquement polymorphe, chez des Mus indiens du groupe booduga.
Rev Suisse Zool 75:461-498

Mishra AC, Bhat HR, Kulkarni SM (1972) Hoplopleura ramgarh sp. nov. and
Hoplopleura sinhgarh sp. nov. (Anopleura: Hoplopleuridae), parasitizing
Mus spp. (Rodentia, Muridae) in India. Parasitology 65:11-21

Orsini P, Bonhomme F, Britton-Davidian J, Croset H, Gerasimov S, Thaler L
(1983) Le complexe d'especes du genre Mus en Europe Centrale et
Orientale. Z Saugetierk 48:86-95

Pantuwatana S, Imlarp S, Marshall J (1969) Vertebrate ecology of Bang
Phra. Nat Hist Bull Siam Soc 23:133-183

Satunin KA (1908) Excursion des Kaukasischen Museums in die Steppen und
Vorberge Ost-Transkaukasiens im Fruhling 1907. Mitt Kaukas Museums
4:41-141

Ursin E (1952) Occurrence of voles, mice, and rats (Muridae) in Denmark.
Vidensk Med Dansk naturh Foren 114:217-244

Evolutionary Relationships in the Genus *Mus*

F. Bonhomme

The Murids, with their many genera, are the most diversified and recent group of Rodents. Mus, along with Rattus and a few others, has been recognized as a separate taxon for a long time. One of its numerous species, the house mouse, has become the most studied vertebrate probably because its habitat is closest to that of man. Because this little brownish animal is well adapted to indoor conditions, it was easy to breed in the laboratory, and has become the universal mammalian model. Although many aspects of its biology have been studied extensively, the biosystematics of its natural populations and the evolutionary relationships between the different members of the genus have only recently begun to be explored.

One of the main reasons for this is that all the taxa referred to currently as Mus seem rather homogeneous in terms of biometry and morphology. Only subtle differences are displayed in dentition, cranial features or tail length (see Thaler, this symposium, for further discussion). Therefore much of what we know has been obtained only recently by such techniques as cytology, protein electrophoresis, mtDNA studies and to a certain extent by RFLP studies of genes and repeated sequences. More is known about the species closely related to the house mouse (M. musculus) than is known about their distant Asian relatives. In this paper, I will recall a few results obtained in the musculus complex of species that may shed some light on phenomena such as reticulate and mosaic evolution which help to understand the evolutionary relationships within the genus as a whole and its position within the Murid phylogeny.

Polytypic species, polymorphic populations.

The study of gene variation within Mus musculus throughout a large geographic area has shown (Selander et al., 1969; Wheeler and Selander, 1972; Minezawa et al., 1976; Bonhomme et al., 1978; Sage. 1981; Bonhomme et al., 1984) that several biochemically differentiated groups ranging from Africa and Western Europe to East Asia can be recognized (see also Moriwaki, this symposium). Our present state of knowledge is based primarily on the variability of mtDNA, rDNA non-transcribed spacer regions, immunoglobulin light and heavy chains, T-cell antigens, t-haplotypes, the major histocompatibility complex, $\beta 2$ microglobulin, maternally-transmitted-antigen, liver gangliosides, hemoglobin and electrophoresis of a variety of soluble proteins. Of course, the geographical coverage is far from complete, and there are still many problems to be solved before we have a complete understanding of the intricate relationships between the different taxonomical units of this differentiated worldwide complex species.

Nevertheless, up to now, four main groups may be recognized, which for the sake of convenience will be referred to by the following widely used latin trinomens : M. m. domesticus (Rutti, 1772- Western Europe and the Mediterranean basin, Africa, Arabia, Middle East and transported by man to the New World and almost anywhere else); M. m. musculus (Linnaeus, 1758 - from Eastern Europe to Japan accross USSR and Northern China), M. m. bactrianus (Blyth, 1846 - from Iran to Pakistan and India), M. m. castaneus (Waterhouse, 1843 - from Ceylon to South East Asia through the Indo-Malayan archipelago).

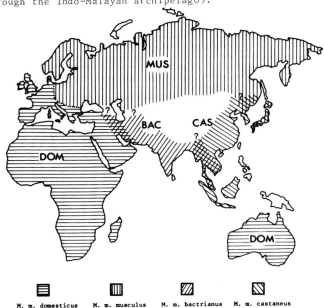

M. m. domesticus   M. m. musculus   M. m. bactrianus   M. m. castaneus

Fig. 1 Geographical distribution of the four main taxonomical
units of the complex species Mus musculus.

Fig. 1 tentatively shows the distribution of these four groups in the Old World. It should be noted that the biochemical definition of these units does not necessarily preclude an internal heterogeneity. For example, M. m. domesticus includes a variety of different morphs which may exhibit variability in characters other than biochemical ones, such as tail length, coat colour and ecological preferenda (e.g. brevirostris from the Mediterranean belt and praetextus from sub-desert biotopes), other morphologic characters (such as changes the ones documented in insular populations) or even chromosomes (there are many populations homogeneous for karyotypes modified by Robertsonian fusions. See Winking, this volume). This differentiation raises questions for the population geneticist concerning the amount of present day gene flow between local populations. Nevertheless, all these phenomena are recent as compared to the intergroup variability. A large number of animals belonging to M. m. domesticus have been screened in our laboratory without revealing much protein variation, whether sampled among Robertsonian races (Britton-Davidian et al., 1980) or otherwise (Britton-Davidian, 1986).

However, the interesting point to deal with here is that these biochemically defined groups, subspecies, semi-species, species or whatever you may call them, exchange genes wherever they come into contact, even though they are already quite differentiated as far as protein variation is concerned. For instance, electrophoresis at 42 loci demonstrates a Nei genetic distance ranging from 0,15 to 0,35 between these four groups (Bonhomme et al., 1984). These exchanges seem to be secondary in the cases studied so far and probably result from range expansion in recent times due to partial commensalism with man.

The best understood cases are those of M. m. musculus/M. m. domesticus in Europe and M. m. musculus/M. m. castaneus in Japan. The latter has been extensively studied by the Japanese authors (see Yonekawa, this symposium). They have shown that the colonization of their archipelago by mice was the result of at least two invasions paralleling those of men. The first one, northward bound from South-eastern Asia, by M. m. castaneus. The second one, eastward bound from China by M. m. musculus. The two taxonomical units have subsequently largely hybridized and given birth to an original population (so called M. m. molossinus) with differentially intermixed nuclear genomes (Minezawa et al., 1981, Miyashita et al., 1985, Suzuki et al., 1985), and mtDNAs of the two types differentiated on a geographical basis. The castaneus mtDNA is restricted to the two extremities of Japan, while musculus mtDNA occupies the center (Yonekawa et al., 1981).

At the other end of Eurasia, M. m. domesticus and M. m. musculus are known to interact along a hybrid zone ranging from Denmark (Selander et al., 1969) to Bulgaria (Bonhomme et al., 1983), where they exchange nuclear genes in a non-random fashion. Extensive mtDNA flow across this line occurs at several points of the zone (Ferris et al., 1983; Boursot et al., 1984), and individuals with nearly 100 % musculus nuclear genome and a domesticus cytoplasm are to be found in Sweden for instance, while the reverse can be found in Greece. However gene flow is asymmetrical and differential depending on which part of the genome is considered. For instance, an entire chromosome such as the Y does not seem to cross the contact zone (Bishop et al., 1985). The blending of the two genomes is thus not complete and there is some occurrence of male sterility in the northern part of the hybrid zone (Denmark N-Germany, H. Winking, pers. comm., S-Germany, R. D. Sage. pers comm.; Czechoslovaky, Forejt and Ivanyi, 1974) whereas a similar phenomenon was not found in Bulgaria (F. Bonhomme, non published). Nevertheless, autosomal alleles characteristic of M. m. domesticus have been found in M. m. musculus populations more than 200 km North of the hybrid zone of East Bulgaria (Vanlerberghe et al., 1986). Thus, it does not appear likely that the process of gene exchange that started some 5000 years ago (Hunt and Selander, 1973) following deforestation of central Europe, is ready to stop. This blending of two different genomes is a reality which concerns more than a narrow hybrid zone, since most classical inbred strains appear to be recombinant between domesticus- and musculus-like genomes (Bishop et al., 1985; Bonhomme and Guénet, 1986).

Much less is known about the interaction of M. m. bactrianus with the remainder of the species. Given its situation south of the Himalayas, it is more likely to come into contact in the west with M. m. domesticus than with M. m. musculus in the north. Although Israëli wild mice are referable to M. m. domesticus, they possess alleles which could have come from M. m. bactrianus (Britton-Davidian, pers. com.) or from a common ancestral stock. Also in a M. m. domesticus individual from Greece, Suzuki et al. (1985) reported the occurrence in moderate frequency of a rDNA-NTS haplotype coming from M. m. bactrianus. To the east, M. m. bactrianus probably interacts with M. m. castaneus. Yonekawa et al. (1981) report having studied two otherwise undistinguishable individuals from Borneo, one with bactrianus type mtDNA, the other with castaneus mtDNA. Suzuki et al. (1985) find a mixture of rDNA-NTS types in all of the M. m. bactrianus or M. m. castaneus they have studied, with their R6 haplotype being found only in castaneus and R8 predominant in bactrianus.

Intraspecific phylogenies.

What are the phylogenetic relationships between taxa within a complex species which shows many primary or secondary genetic exchanges? How have these groups been able to differentiate from a common ancestral stock while still retaining the ability to intercross? A quick look at diverse phylogenies obtained within the M. musculus species complex for different characters shows that there is no simple answer to the first question. In Fig. 2, an "average" phylogeny between the four groups is given, based on electrophoretical data at 42 loci coding for soluble proteins. The divergence is mostly the result of contrasting gene frequencies rather than strict allele specificities.

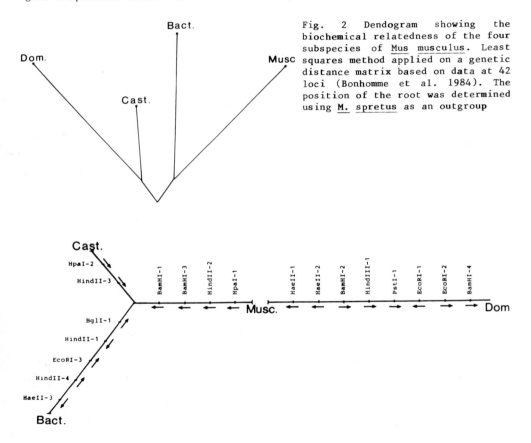

Fig. 2 Dendogram showing the biochemical relatedness of the four subspecies of Mus musculus. Least squares method applied on a genetic distance matrix based on data at 42 loci (Bonhomme et al. 1984). The position of the root was determined using M. spretus as an outgroup

Fig. 3 Mutational pathways between the four main types of mtDNA in Mus musculus. The restriction sites distribution for six enzymes is determined according to Yonekawa et al. (1981). Each site is assigned to a given branch of the tree according to a parsimony criterion. Moving on the tree according to the direction of an arrow indicates gain of a site, and counterwise a loss. No site was found to mutate more than once.

In Fig. 3, we show the mtDNA phylogeny based on endonuclease restriction analyses for the same groups. Four main types of mtDNA have been found so far in wild mice (Yonekawa et al., 1981). This phylogeny is peculiar in at least two respects: firstly, it does not match the previous one very well (Fig. 2) and secondly, it illustrates clearly that the rates of molecular evolution (primarily nucleotide substitutions in mtDNA) may be very different in so far as a given molecule may be evolving much faster in some taxa than in others. Consequently **existing** subspecies possess molecules that are not necessarily at the tips of the branches of the tree, such as is the case here for musculus (Fig. 3).

In Fig. 4, we show a possible reconstitution (based on data from Suzuki et al., 1985) of the evolution of the restriction map of the rDNA non-transcribed spacer which shows the same feature as the mtDNA phylogeny (Fig. 3). Namely, musculus has haplotypes which are "older" than those of domesticus if one takes the root of this net as the middle .

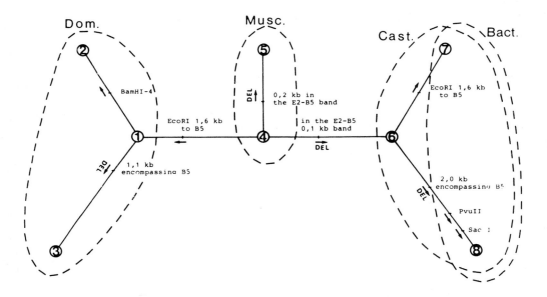

Fig. 4 Possible evolution of the rDNA-non transcribed spacer repeating units in four subspecies of Mus musculus. A parsimony criterion was applied to restriction maps published by Suzuki et al. (1985). Restriction sites are labelled accordingly, and arrows indicate a gain. The polymorphic EcoRI site appears twice.

In Fig. 5, we show the networks obtained with protein electrophoresis allele frequency data (A) and allele frequency data at the H-2 locus (B) between different European populations of musculus and domesticus. The discrepancies obtained clearly show that gene flow may be differential both within and between subspecies depending on which genes are considered.

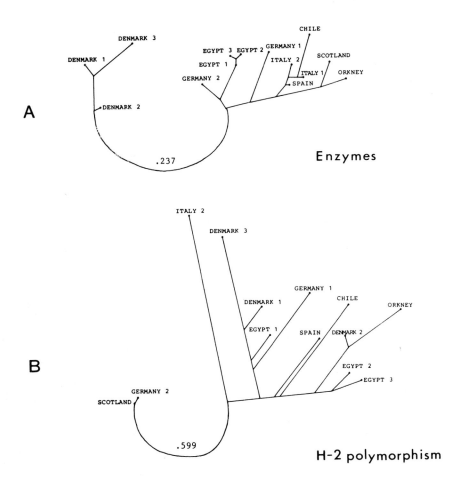

Fig. 5 Dendograms showing the genetic similarities in two data sets, reconstructed by least squares analysis of distance matrices. In A allele frequencies at loci coding for proteins clearly differentiate the M. m. musculus of Denmark from all the other populations referable to M. m. domesticus. In B, the same populations are analyzed for H2 polymorphism and they are clearly not classified according to their taxonomical or geographical affinities (data from Nadeau, Britton-Davidian et al., unpublished).

This type of data implies that the present day taxa of the species Mus musculus will have an unequal share of idiotypic features and commonly shared character states irrespective of whether the traits are ancestral or derived. This is well illustrated in Table 1, which gives the group distribution of haplotypes for some genetic systems. Therefore, phylogenetic relationships cannot be inferred from a single character set (i.e. the study of a single gene or gene family), and reciprocally the knowledge of the phylogenetic proximities of the taxa does not give clues as to the evolutionary history of a given gene, its origin or its divergence time. To a certain extent, the concept of phylogeny itself should be restricted to sets unable to exchange genetic information such as good (sexually isolated) species or non recombinant haploid regions of the genome such as mtDNA or some Y specific sequences. It should be applied only with great caution to genes in diploid organisms or to taxa in a complex species.

	Domesticus	Musculus	Castaneus	Bactrianus	Europ. species	References
Hbb	s d	p d	d	p d	s d	Bonhomme et al., 1984 Miyashita et al., 1985
Y chr.	type 1	type 2	type 2	NK	others	Bishop et al., 1985 Bonhomme et al., (unpul
X chr. C banding	posit.	negat.	posit.	posit.	posit.	Moriwaki et al., 1985
rDNA-NTS haplotype	R1,R2,R3	R4,R5	R6,R7,R8	R7,R8	NK	Suzuki et al., 1985
all. to Thy-1 Lyt-1, Lyt-2	2, 2, 2 2, 2, 1	1, 2, 1	1, 2, 1	1, 2, NK	1, 1, 0 1, 2, 0	Kurihara et al., 1985
Es-3	a b	b c	b c	103	b 70 105	Bonhomme et al.,1984
Es-1	a b	a	a b	98	b 91 92	"
Np-1	a	90 70	a 85	a	a 70	"
Gpd-1	a b	95 90	95	95	a 95	"

Table 1. Group distribution for some genetical systems in Mus Musculus. (NK = unknown)

Students of molecular evolution have to bear in mind that genes are not always found in the genetic background where they originally arose, and this has to be taken into account in order to understand the subtle mechanisms of genomic coevolution. More generally, this implies that different genes may have a different evolutionary fate, and that the phylogeny of a gene is not necessarily concordant with that of the taxa which carries it. The understanding of these mechanisms acting within the complex species Mus musculus may help us to evaluate evolutionary relationships within the other members of the genus.

Interspecific phylogenies.

Other related species may be found in sympatry with representatives of Mus musculus. Three of these species exist in Europe. where their range is rather well known, as illustrated in Fig. 6. These are M. spretus, and two other species, the Eastern mediterranean short-tailed mouse and the mound-building mouse. The latin names of these last two other species are still under debate. because there is a confusion that cannot be resolved concerning the exact nature of the type specimens, since those that have been described come from places where there is sympatry with M. musculus. We wish to recall here that mound-builders and M. m. musculus are often caught and in the same places in the same trap line. We have been able to find subtle morphological characters to discriminate the two species only after first distinguishing them in mixed samples by electrophoretic techniques (Orsini et al., 1983). Marshall and Sage (1981) proposed hortulanus (Nordmann. 1840) for the mound-builder and abotti (for the former), whereas we proposed spicilegus [Mus 4B] (Petenyi, 1882) and spretoides [Mus 4A] (Thaler, in Bonhomme et al.,1984). Earlier, Petrov & Ruzic (1983) have proposed macedonicus (for the latter). However only a careful biometrical analysis of the type specimens. if they still exist in the light of modern knowledge can solve this problem. Controversy of this type explains why we used the numbered biochemical groups, in order not to infringe the rules of systematics. Nevertheless, the following refers provisionally to 4A as macedonicus and to 4B as spicilegus.

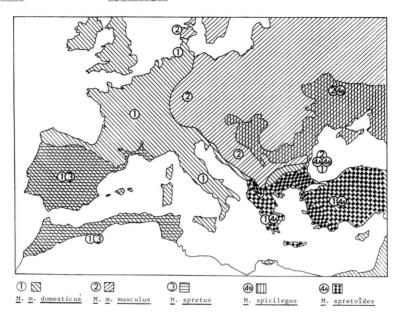

$①\diagdown$ $②\diagup$ $③\equiv$ $④B\;\square$ $④A\;∷$
M. m. domesticus   M. m. musculus   M. spretus   M. spicilegus   M. spretoīdes

Fig. 6 Geographical distribution of the five taxa referable to the genus Mus in Europe (from Bonhomme et al., 1984).

Whatever their names, these two species are interesting since they probably represent the best case of sibling species thus far discovered in mammals. They are very similar morphologically (no obvious character enables us to tell them apart on the basis of the cranium or post-cranium, see also Orsini (1983). Biochemically they display differential alleles at only 4 out of 42 loci studied. The Nei genetic distance is only 0,07. The two mice interact in a narrow part of their range (one coastal plain in Bulgaria) as good sympatric species. Under laboratory conditions, we have never been able to obtain F1 offspring from either of the two reciprocal crosses, although each species will breed with M. musculus laboratory strains.

Mus spretus is the Western mediterranean short-tailed mouse. with the smallest known distribution area being limited to North Africa, Iberia and South France. This species has now been introduced into the laboratory through the construction of one completely inbred and several partially inbred strains. Taking advantage of the possibility of hybridization under laboratory conditions and of the fertility of F1 offspring, many variants of loci so far intractable to genetic analysis have been uncovered and assigned to the chromosome map (Bonhomme et al., 1979 and 1982, Chapman et al., 1983. Robert et al., 1985). This species may represent the most valuable tool offered by wild mice to the mouse geneticists in recent years.

Nevertheless Europe is not really the homeland of the genus. All of the five biochemically differentiated groups that currently inhabit the continent seem to have co-entered with man in the Neolithic times, at least as far as the Western part of the continent is concerned. On the other hand, representatives of this genus have inhabited India and Southeast Asia since their origin. These are M. caroli, M. cervicolor and M. cooki, and in India representatives of the subgenus Leggada such as M. booduga or M. dunni (see Sharma, this symposium, for these two species). There are many other forms described as species belonging to the genus Mus, but for the reasons discussed in the following paragraphs, only biochemical analysis will show whether they have been correctly assigned or really represent anything new.

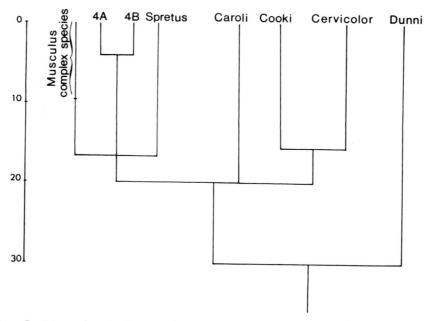

Fig. 7 Schematic dendogram (average clustering) of the biochemical relatedness of several species of the genus Mus, according to distance matrices of the A index of Bonhomme et al. (1984) based on 22-42 protein polymorphism . The ordinate is a measure of the number of differentially fixed loci out of the 42 analyzed.

In Fig. 7, we show a phylogenetic tree obtained for these species based on 22-42 protein electrophoretic polymorphisms. The two trifurcations presented in this tree are points where alternative branching orders are possible. Nevertheless, we have cladistic arguments to favor an early separation of M. spretus. This is detailed in the caption of Fig. 8 which shows a reconstruction of the evolution based on mouse major satellite DNA.

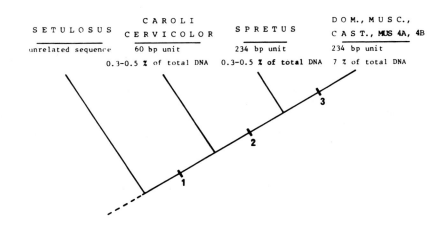

Event n° 1 : generation of the basic 60 bp repeat unit

　　　　n° 2 : generation of the 240 bp unit by amplification
　　　　　　　of the 60 bp unit

　　　　n° 3 : 15 fold increase in amount of satellite DNA

Fig. 8 Evolution of the size and the amount of major satellite DNA in various species of mice. If we exclude the possibility of reversion for event n°3, we have suggestive evidence for an early divergence of M. spretus (from Mottez, Bonhomme & Roizès, unpublished).

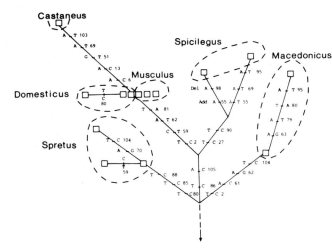

Fig. 9 Cladogram based on differences in the 5'end of 16s mt rDNA in various species and subspecies of the genus Mus according to a parsimony criterion. Point mutations are from left to right. The squares represent different individuals (from Fort et al., 1984).

In Fig. 9, we show a cladogram based on differences in mtDNA by parsimony analysis of a partial sequence of this molecule. The same set of species as in Fig 8 were used. As discussed by Fort et al. (1984), it is interesting to note that this cladogram does not match the one in Fig. 7. 4A and 4B mtDNAs share no branch in the tree whereas they are among the closest groups we know from the stand-point of their nuclear genome. Domesticus, musculus and castaneus also display intriguing relationships in their mitochondrial rDNAs 5' termini that are not shown by their nuclear genomes or by restriction analysis of the whole molecule Within a given species, sequences at different stages in the mutational pathways may occur. These results illustrate well the fact that the gene lineage does not necessarily fit into the species lineage.

Altogether, the phylogeny shown in Fig. 7 gives a reasonable idea of the branching order of the different speciation events. The subgenus Leggada, represented here by the species M. dunni, is in our opinion, the most distantly related group of species still living. The karyotype of M. dunni contains a few submetacentric variations in polymorphic condition (Matthey and Petter, 1968; Sen and Sharma. 1982) but is essentially close to the 40 acrocentric karyotype characteristic of the remainder of the genus, as it is in the closely related Mus booduga. A few embryos have been obtained by artificial insemination of M. m. domesticus with M. dunni sperm (West et al., 1977).

Relationships with other Murids

Many other species have been attributed to the genus Mus in the past, primarily by relying on morphological descriptions of skulls and teeth We have reexamined the taxonomical status of some of those species already used in recent literature and shown that setulosus and minutoïdes, platythrix and pahari are three independant genera (Bonhomme et al., 1984).

In an electrophoretical survey of 21 genera of murids (Bonhomme et al., 1985), we showed that all the 16 African genera studied but one (Acomys), including setulosus and minutoides formerly referred to as the genus Mus (subgenus Nannomys), constituted a monophyletic group independant of the other Eurasian genera. This is evidenced by the existence of clear synapomorphisms at some loci, as underlined in the table of Fig 10. All further attempts to order the dichotomies beyond this point were unsuccessful, regardless of the phenetic or cladistic approach was used. Moreover, the distributions of synapomorphies at different loci appeared to be mutually incompatible, unless reticulate evolution at an early stage within the African murids, or some phenomena occurred as discussed by Bonhomme et al. (1984).

We then reexamined at 28 protein loci the other Asian species platythrix and pahari (trapped and identified as such by J. T. Marshall) and obtained the results given in Table 2 and Fig. 11, which clearly show that platythrix and pahari have to be considered as independent genera of their own (Pyromys and Coelomys respectively), since they are at least as divergent from Mus as the above redefined genus Nannomys. This electrophoretical independence has been confirmed by RFLP studies of a MHC class I gene (Siwarski et al., 1985).

Finally. we are left with the image of many independant Murid genera among which it is difficult to establish a hierarchical order of the different splitting events. Also it is interesting to note that it is not possible to make a cladistic analysis of electromorphic variations in table 2 by taking, let say, Rattus as an out-group. These results match rather well those obtained by E. Viegas-Péquignot et al. (1983) in studying chromosomal rearrangements of ten genera of Murids by various banding techniques. Also they obtained a star-shaped

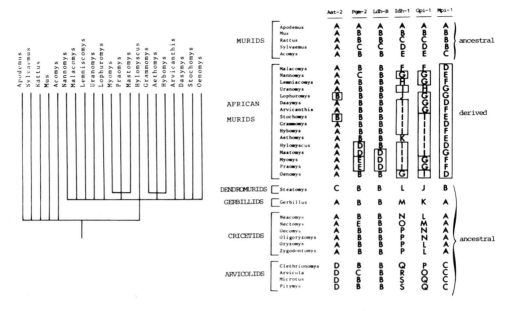

Fig 10 Protein variation and consensus phylogeny in 21 genera of Murids. The protein data were obtained by sequential electrophoresis with 12 buffer conditions. Dendromurids, Gerbillids, Cricetids and Arvicolids are taken as outgroups to define ancestral and derived character states as exemplified for <u>Mpi</u>. From Bonhomme <u>et al</u>. (1985).

	Mor-2	Mor-1	Idh-1	Idh-2	Ldh-1	Ldh-2	Gpi-1	Pgm-2	Gdc-1	Sod-1	Mod-1	Pgd-1	Amy-1	Acp	Ada	Car-2	Glo	Es-14	Mod-2	Sdh	Mpi	Gpd-1	Es-15	Aat-1	Aat-2	Adh-1	Es-10	Alb-1
Europ. Spec.	m	m	mo	m	m	ml	mn	ml	m	lm	mn	m	lmop	m	m	kmn	lm	km	mn	mn	lmo	kmn	mnop	m	m	ijm	lm	lm
M. caroli	m	m	k	m	m	m	m	n	m	m	m	m	p	ij	m	l	j	m	i		p	m	k	m	k	m	m	
M. cervicolor	m	m	k	m	m	m	m	mm	o	o	m		m	o	l	m	m	k	mn	gk	n	mq	mm	l	m	l		
M. cooki	m	m	k	m	m	m	k	m	m	m	m	n	kl	mpq	l	m	l	k	m	n	o	np	mm	l	m	l		
Pyromys	m	lm	l	m	m	m	l	m	m	m	p	q	m	l	m	f	m	l	ij	k	mn	o	st	j	m	lp	m	l
Coelomys	l	n	k	m	m	m	n	m	k	l	q	l	m	m	lm	g	m	l	j	k	f	k	or	k	m	l	m	l
Nannomys	m	m	j	m	l	m	m	l	m	k	n	p	jk	l	m	m	h	m	m	m	m	k	l	pq	jkm	n	m	l
Rattus	m	m	m	m	k	m	l	m	p	p	s	o	p	m	o	mk	n	o	l	l	h	j	s	l	m	o	o	k
Apodemus	m	m	n	m	n	j	n	m	ll	o	r	n	l	n	n	o	m	n	m	k	ij	k	p	m	m	q	n	l
Mastomys	l	m	l	l	m	k	n	n	o	q	n	p	o	n	n	r	n	m	p	o	k	ef	q	o	m	m	m	m	l

Table 2. Variation at 28 loci in several genera of Murids. The <u>domesticus</u> variant is called <u>m</u>, and the others are labeled in the alphabetical order according to increasing electrophoretical mobility.

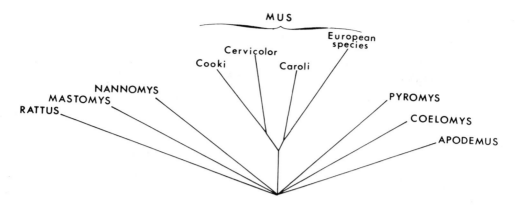

Fig. 11 Consensus phylogeny for seven Murid genera analyzed by standard electrophoresis at 28 protein loci. Data of Table 2 were analyzed by the least squares method. Pyromys and Coelomys were kindly provided by M. Potter, M. cooki by R. Callahan.

cladogram, radiating from a common ancestral karyotype. This is what we expect of rapid and important adaptative radiations, where a family of living creatures arrived to conquer a continent and dispersed to form what we now perceive as genera each time a new ecological opportunity occurred.

This may very well have happened in Asia around -12 MY. since paleontologists link all the Murids to Progonomys cathalai dated 12 MY BP. We see a second radiation in Africa, following the colonization of this continent by this family around -9 MY (first Murids in Ethiopia at this date). All subsequent paleontological data for the genus Mus are doubtful or at least have to be reinterpreted (see Thaler, this symposium). If we want to have provisional estimates of divergence times, we will then have to rely on overall biochemical divergences provided the rates of evolution are constant enough. We think this approach can only give very rough estimates even if one takes into account the reticulation or mosaicism of the evolutionary process we described The significance of the relative lengths of the branches of the dendrograms in terms of evolutionary time therefore has to be interpreted with caution.

Conclusion:

Finally, what about Mus in all this story ? It appears as one of the genera resulting from the great adaptative radiation of Murid rodents with relatively unspecialized forms, at least as far as morphological adaptation is concerned. (This also applies to forms like Nannomys, Pyromys or Coelomys which have been previously described as belonging to Mus on morphological grounds). For other sets of characters, one finds in its species a mixture of ancestral and derived character states, of idiotypic and commonly shared features. This reflects that mosaic and reticulate evolution is what we expect to happen in a fast evolving and exploding taxon, such as the Murid family.

Acknowledgements I am very much indepted to J Catalan. L Thaler. J Britton-Davidian and B Dod for the most invaluable help they gave to me in preparing and discussing this manuscript.

References

Bishop CE, Boursot P, Baron B, Bonhomme F, Hatat D (1985) Most classical Mus musculus domesticus laboratory mouse strains carry a Mus musculus musculus Y chromosome. Nature **325** 6014:70-72

Bonhomme F, Britton-Davidian J, Thaler L, Triantaphyllidis C (1978) Sur l'existence en Europe de quatre groupes de souris (genre Mus L.) du rang espèce et semi-espèce, démontrée par la génétique biochimique. C R Acad Sc Paris D **287** (6):631-633

Bonhomme F, Benmehdi F, Britton-Davidian J, Martin S (1979) Analyse génétique de croisements interspécifiques Mus musculus L. x Mus spretus Lataste : liaison de Adh-1 avec Amy-1 sur le chromosome 3 et de Es-14 avec Mod-1 sur le chromosome 9. C R Acad Sci Paris D **289**:545-548

Bonhomme F, Guénet JL, Catalan J (1982) Présence d'un facteur de sérilité mâle, Hst-2, segrégeant dans les croisements interspécifiques M. musculus x Mus spretus Lataste et lié à Mod-1 et Mpi-1 sur le chromosome 9. C R Acad Sci Paris III **294** (1):691-693

Bonhomme F, Catalan J. Gerasimov S, Orsini Ph, Thaler L (1983) Le complexe d'espèces du genre Mus en Europe centrale et orientale. I. Génétique. Z f Säugetierkunde 1:312-317

Bonhomme F. Catalan J. Britton-Davidian J. Chapman VM, Moriwaki D, Nevo E, Thaler L (1984) Biochemical diversity and evolution in the genus Mus. Biochem Genet 22:275-303

Bonhomme F, Iskandar D, Thaler L. Petter F (1985) Electromorphs and phylogeny in muroîd rodents. In : Evolutionary relationships among rodents : A multidisciplinary analysis. WP Luckett & JL Hartenberger, Plenum Pub Corp, New York:671-684

Bonhomme F and Guénet JL (1985) Do inbred strains of mice really evolve more quickly than expected ? Science (submitted)

Boursot P, Bonhomme F. Britton-Davidian J. Catalan J. Yonekawa H, Orsini Ph, Gerasimov S, Thaler L (1984) Introgression différentielle des génomes nucléaires et mitochondriaux chez deux semi-espèces de Souris. C R Acad Paris III **299** (9):365-370

Britton-Davidian J, Bonhomme F, Croset H, Capanna E , Thaler L (1980) Variabilité génétique chez les populations de souris (genre Mus L.) à nombre chromosomique réduit C.R.Acad.Sci. **290** : 195-198

Britton-Davidian J (1986) Differenciation génique et chromosomique chez les souris M. m. domesticus et M. spretus (in prep.)

Chapman VM, Kratzer PG, Quarantillo BA (1983) Electrophoretic variation for X chromosome linked hypoxanthine phosphoribosyl transferase (HPRT) in wid-derived mice. Genetics 103:785-795.

Ferris SD, Sage RD, Huang CM, Nielsen JT, Ritte U, Wilson AC (1983) Flow of mitochondrial DNA across a species boundary. PNAS USA 80:2290-2294

Forejt J, Ivanyi P (1974) Genetic studies on male sterility of hybrids between laboratory and wild mice (Mus musculus L.). Genet Res 24:189-206

Fort Ph, Bonhomme F, Darlu P, Piechaczyk M, Jeanteur Ph, Thaler L (1984) Clonal divergence of mitochondrial DNA versus populational evolution of nuclear genome. Evol Theo 7 (2):81-90

Hashimoto Y, Suzuki A, Yamakawa T, Wang CH, Bonhomme F, Miyashita N, Moriwaki K (1984) Expression of GM1 and GD1a in liver of wild mice. J Biochem 9 (1):7-12

Hunt WG, Selander RK (1973) Biochemical genetics of hybridisation in European House Mice. Heredity 31:11-33.

Kurihara Y, Miyashita N, Moriwaki K, Wang CH, Petras ML, Bonhomme F, Hoc WI, Kohno SI (1985) Serological survey of T-lymphocyte differentiation antigens in wild mice. Immunogenet. (submitted).

Matthey R, Petter F (1968) Existence de deux espèces distinctes l'une chromosomiquement polymorphe. chez des Mus indiens du groupe booduga. Etude cytogénétique et taxonomique. Rev Suisse Zool 75:471-498

Marshall JT, Sage RD (1981) Taxonomy of the House Mouse. Symp Zool Soc Lond 47:15-25

Minezawa M, Moriwaki K, Kondo K (1976) Studies on protein polymorphism of Japanese wild mouse, Mus musculus molossinus. Ann Rep Natl Inst Genet Japan 26:23-25

Minezawa M, Moriwaki K, Kondo K (1981) Geographical survey of protein variation in wild populations of Japanese house mouse, Mus musculus molossinus. Jap J Genet 56:27-32

Miyashita N, Moriwaki K, Minezawa M, Yu Z, Lu D, Migita S, Yonekawa H, Bonhomme F (1985) Allelic constitution of hemoglobin beta chain in wild populations of the house mouse, Mus musculus. Biochem Genet (in press)

Moriwaki K, Miyashita N, Yonekawa H (1985) Genetic survey of the origin of laboratory mice and its implication in genetic monitoring. ICLAS ?

Orsini Ph, Bonhomme F, Britton-Davidian J, Croset H, Gerasimov S, Thaler L (1983) Le complexe d'espèces du genre Mus en Europe centrale et Orientale. II. Critères d'identification, répartition et caractéristiques écologiques. Z f Säugetierkunde 1:86-95

Petrov B and Ruzic A (1983) Preliminary report of the taxonomical status of the members of the genus Mus in Yougoslavia with description of a new subspecies M. hortulanus macedonicus (sub. nova) Proc. Drugi Simpozyum Osauni pp 175-178 SP Serbie Belgrad.

Robert B, Barton P, Minty A, Daubas Ph, Weydert A, Bonhomme F, Catalan J, Chazottes D, Guénet JL. Buckingham M (1985) Investigation of genetic linkage between myosin and acting genes using an interspecific mouse back-cross. Nature 314:181-183

Sage RD (1981) Wild Mice. Foster Small & Fox, The Mouse in Biomedical Research, Acad Press, New York, 4 (1):39-90

Selander RK, Hunt WG and Yang SY (1969) Protein polymorphism and genic heterozygosity in two european subspecies of the house mouse. Evolution 23:379-390

Sen S, Sharma T (1982) Asynchronous replication of constitutive heterochromatin on X chromosomes in female Mus dunni. Possible influence of facultative heterochromatine on the adjacent constitutive heterochromatin. Chromosoma 85:119-127

Siwarski DF, Barra Y, Jay G, Rogers MJ (1985) Occurence of a unique MHC Class I gene in distantly related members of the genus Mus. Immunogenetics 21: 267-276.

34

Suzuki H, Miyashita N, Moriwaki K, Kominami R, Muramatsu M, Kanehisa T, Bonhomme
    F, Petras ML, Yu Z, Lu D (1985) Evolutionary implication on heterogeneity of
    the Non-transcribed Spacer region of ribosomal DNA repeating units in various
    subspecies of Mus musculus. Mol Genet Evol (in press)
Vanlerberghe F (1986) Genetic interactions between the two semispecies of the
    House Mouse, Mus musculus domesticus and Mus musculus musculus in Bulgaria
Viégas-Péquignot E, Dutrillaux B, Prod'homme M, Petter F (1983) Chromosomal
    phylogeny of Muridae: a study of 10 genera. Cytogenet Cell Genet 35:269-278
West JD, Frels WI, Papaioannou VE, Karr J, Chapman VM (1977) Development on
    interspecific hybrids of Mus. J Emb Exp Morph 41:233-243
Wheeler LL, Selander RK (1972) XIII Genetic variation in populations of the House
    Mouse, Mus musculus, in the Hawaïn Islands. Studies in Genetics VII. Univ
    Texas Publ 7213:269-296
Yonekawa H, Moriwaki K, Gotoh O, Hayashi JI, Watanabe J, Miyashita N, Petras ML,
    Tagashira Y (1981) Evolutionary relationships among five subspecies of Mus
    musculus based on restriction enzyme cleavage patterns of mitochondrial DNA.
    Genetics 98:801-816

Constitutive Heterochromatin and Evolutionary Divergence of *Mus dunni, M. booduga* and *M. musculus*

T. Sharma, N. Cheong, P. Sen, and S. Sen

INTRODUCTION

The Indian pygmy field mice are one of the most interesting groups
of animals from evolutionary point of view and include two
morphologically extremely similar species Mus dunni and Mus booduga
which share widely common natural habitats and until recently were
considered conspecific. They are closely allied to the aboriginal
mice Mus musculus and are distinguished from each other only on the
basis of average characters (Ellerman 1961). The predominant
diploid chromosome number in all the three species is 40 but while
the karyotypes of M. musculus and M. booduga with all acrocentric
chromosomes are identical, that of M. dunni is distinct due to
invariable presence of large submetacentric X and acrocentric Y sex
chromosomes. M. dunni populations from different localities also
exhibit polymorphism in the number of biarmed autosomes (Matthey
and Petter 1968; Sharma and Garg 1975; Markvong et al. 1975;
Manjunatha and Aswathanarayana 1979; Sen and Sharma 1980, 1983).
The close morphometric and cytogenetic alliance of pygmy mice with
a species like M. musculus that has been extensively utilized in
molecular genetic and immunological investigations make these an
attractive choice for detailed phylogenetic considerations. An
attempt toward this direction with the wildly occurring populations
in the Indian subcontinent appears to hold promise, also in view of
the suggestion that these mice would have originated in tropical
Asia (Misonne 1969).

Our study during the last decade on the Indian pygmy field mice
(Sharma and Garg 1975; Sen and Sharma 1980, 1983) has indicated
possible involvement of constitutive heterochromatin in
evolutionary divergence, though hard evidence in support of precise
influence is still lacking.

In this paper we have explored chromosomal, molecular and
ethological approaches in an attempt to understand the possible
roles of constitutive heterochromatin in karyotypic divergence
and speciation and the sequence of events taking place in the
evolution of heterochromatin in these closely related species of
the genus Mus.

MATERIALS AND METHODS

Animals utilized in this study were collected from wild populations of the Indian subcontinent. Chromosome preparations were made from bone marrow of in vivo colchicine-injected individuals and from in vitro spleen cell cultures following the methods routinely done in our laboratory (Sen and Sharma 1983). G- and C-bandings were done according to the methods of Seabright (1971) and Sumner (1972), respectively with slight modifications.

DNA was prepared from freshly excised organs using standard procedure of phenol extraction, ethanol precipitation, treatment with ribonuclease, chloroform extraction and isopropanol precipitation. The DNA samples were digested with each of the restriction enzymes at a ratio of 2 units of the enzyme per microgram of DNA overnight at 37°C. The buffers used for the reactions were according to the specifications of the manufacturers. The enzymes were purchased from Boehringer Mannheim and BRL. The digested DNA samples were run on 1.2% Agarose gel at a constant current of 100 MA. Gels were neutralised according to Southern (1975) and transferred to nitro cellulose paper.

Nick-translation and hybridization: Purified satellite DNA was nick-translated essentially according to the procedure of Rigby et al. (1977). Satellite DNA was labelled with ^{32}PdCTP (2000-3000 Ci/mmol; Amersham) to a specific activity of $1-2 \times 10^7$ cpm/μg. Unincorporated nucleotides were separated from incorporated nucleotides on a Sephadex G-50 column. Labelled satellite DNA was denatured in the presence of 1.7N NaOH. The hybridization was carried out in 5xSSC, 0.1M sodium phosphate, 0.02% of ficoll 400, BSA and polyvinyl pyrolidone at 68°C overnight. Filters were washed extensively at 68°C in phosphate citrate buffer containing 0.5% SDS, dried and autoradiographed at -70°C using Kodak XR-5 film with intensifying screen.

RESULTS AND DISCUSSION

The diploid number of chromosomes in M. musculus, M. booduga and M. dunni is 40 but while the karyotypes of M. musculus and M. booduga are identical that of M. dunni is characterized by invariable presence of a large submetacentric X and a large acrocentric Y; the short arm of the X and entire Y being totally C-band positive. Additionally, M. booduga has a fixed karyotype of 40 acrocentric chromosomes but M. dunni is polymorphic in different localities, exhibiting variation in number and distribution of short arms on the autosomes (Matthey and Petter 1968; Sharma and Garg 1975; Markvong et al. 1975; Manjunatha and Aswathanarayana 1979; Sen and Sharma 1980, 1983). M. dunni populations from peninsular India have 6 to 10 and 4 to 6 biarmed chromosomes, respectively in Madras and Mysore. Of these, pairs 2 and 5 are polymorphic due to pericentric inversions, whereas others (1, 3 and 6) always possess C-band positive prominent short arms in both the homologues.

A study of more than 200 M. dunni individuals from Madras, Tirupati, Madurai and Pondicherry in south India has invariably shown the presence of the autosome pairs 1, 3 and 6 as biarmed with their prominent short arms as C-band positive (Fig. 1a). Only in 4 individuals, one of the homologues of pairs 1 and 6 was with slightly smaller C-band positive short arm. The Mysore and Erode populations (both in south India) are, on the other hand, consistently endowed with only 2 autosomal pairs, 1 and 3, with C-band positive prominent short arms (Fig. 1b). In contrast to this, karyotype of all the 210 M. dunni individuals studied from northern part of India (Varanasi, Jaunpur and Jhansi) is consistent in having all acrocentric autosomes, possessing only minute but perceptible short arms (Fig. 1c) as reported also from populations of Khajuraho (Markvong et al. 1975; Marshall 1977) and of Pune by Dhanda (see Marshall 1977).

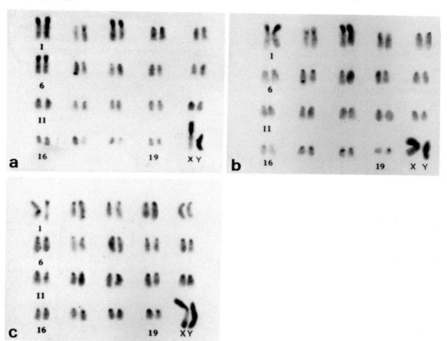

Fig. 1a, b and c. C-band male karyotypes of 3 chromosomal forms of M. dunni: The enlarged X and Y chromosomes with additional heterochromatin are present in all (a) from Madras with 3 pairs (1, 3 and 6) of biarmed autosomes having prominent heterochromatic short arms (b) from Mysore with 2 pairs (1 and 3) of biarmed autosomes having prominent heterochromatic short arms and (c) from Varanasi with all autosomes acrocentric possessing minute heterochromatic short arms

A preliminary study of relative chromosomal DNA contents from 30 metaphases of each species or chromosomal form was done in Leitz MPV-3 cytophotometer after staining with ethidium bromide. The mean values of DNA contents of M. booduga are 0.86±0.01 and of the three chromosomal forms of M. dunni from Varanasi, Mysore and Madras are 0.93±0.01, 1.12±0.011 and 1.28±0.012, respectively relative to 1.0 of M. musculus. Obviously, some change between genomic size of the three species as also of the three chromosomal forms of M. dunni has occurred during their evolutionary divergence. However, the G-band patterns show striking conservation in the euchromatic segments of the genomes of M. musculus, M. booduga and all the 3 chromosomal forms of M. dunni (Fig. 2) which means that

38

no major structural changes involving euchromatin took place during the divergence of these taxa. It, therefore, appears reasonable to believe that the change in genomic size was caused, to a substantial degree, by constitutive heterochromatin. The sporadic occurrence of centric fusions and pericentric inversions in M. dunni are always in polymorphic state only (present study; Sen and Sharma 1983).

The role of constitutive heterochromatin variation in evolutionary divergence of taxa was first suggested in the early 1970s (Duffey 1972; Sharma and Raman 1973; Pathak et al. 1973). This mode of karyotypic change, caused by addition or deletion of constitutive heterochromatin and resulting in alteration of genome size have since been reported in various groups of rodents (see Patton and Sherwood 1982; Gamperl et al. 1982) but the nature of influence of such changes still remains enigmatic. The sequence of events related to mode of evolution of constitutive heterochromatin and in turn of the highly repetitive DNA sequences constituting them is also obscure.

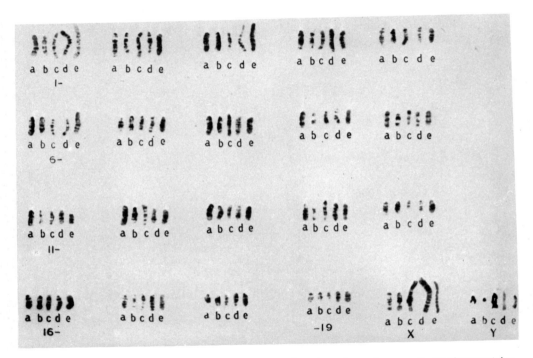

Fig. 2. Composite G-band karyotype showing homology of euchromatic band pattern among the chromosomes of (a) M. musculus (b) M. booduga (c) M. dunni from Varanasi (d) M. dunni from Mysore and (e) M. dunni from Madras; G-band karyotypes are arranged according to the pattern published by Committee on Standardized Genetic Nomenclature of Mice (1972)

Satellite DNA or highly repetitive DNA present in constitutive heterochromatin shows compositional heterogeneity. While the initial studies were suggestive of rigid species specificity, de novo appearance and fast turnover rate of satellite DNA sequences, later investigations revealed that identical repetitive sequences persist in related species, for example, in rodents (Sutton and McCallum 1972; Fry and Salser 1977; Brown and Dover 1980a; Sen and Sharma 1980) and in Drosophila (Gall and Atherton 1974; Peacock et al. 1976; Yamamoto and Miklos 1978). The significance of this is not clear at present. Our earlier in situ hybridization studies using M. musculus satellite DNA as the probe on the chromosomes of M. booduga and M. dunni revealed that musculus satellite-like sequences are present at restricted locations in reduced and varying amounts in these two species (Sen and Sharma 1980). Thus on the basis of this observation and the almost identical situation reported in those species complex where heterogeneous sequence composition of constitutive heterochromatin with relative variation among its constituents exist (Hatch et al. 1976; Peacock et al. 1978), it was postulated that a change in the balance between two or more repetitive sequences in these regions may be more crucial in its evolutionary consequences rather than a mere increase or decrease of a homogeneous repetitive sequence (Sen and Sharma 1980).

Analytical equilibrium sedimentation in neutral CsCl of total DNA of M. dunni and M. booduga did not show a satellite DNA component, unlike M. musculus under identical conditions (Fig. 3).

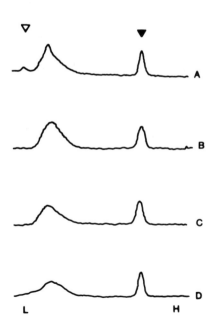

Fig. 3. Analytical UV absorbance profiles in CsCl gradients after sedimentation to equilibrium of DNAs from (A) M. musculus, (B) M. booduga (C) M. dunni from Varanasi and (D) M. dunni from Madras. L and H indicate light and heavy sides of the gradient. (▽) indicates the satellite peak in M. musculus and (▼) indicates the profile of phage 2 C DNA

Despite the apparent absence of a detectable satellite in M. dunni and M. booduga, we wanted to find out if musculus satellite sequences are present in these two species in the two known patterns of organization viz. "type A" and "type B" patterns identifiable following digestion with different restriction enzymes (Hörz and Zachau 1977). The type A pattern is characterized by all satellite

sequences being cut into a regular series of low molecular weight
fragments based on a monomer unit of 234bp by an enzyme like
Eco RII. The type B pattern is produced when only a minor portion
of total satellite sequences is cut into a series of multimers of
234bp by enzymes like Hinf, Alu I, etc. M. musculus, M. booduga and
M. dunni DNAs were restricted with enzymes known to generate either
type A (Eco RII) or type B (Hinf, Alu I) patterns and hybridized
with ^{32}P-labelled M. musculus satellite DNA. It was seen that
hybridization of booduga DNA with mouse satellite resulted in
pattern of bands identical to that seen from the control of mouse
DNA against mouse satellite. In both cases most of the homologous
DNA was digested to monomer of ≈240 bp and lesser amounts of dimer,
trimer, etc., although there was a distinct reduction of type A
segments in booduga genome. In dunni, on the other hand, type A
pattern could not be detected at all (Fig. 4a). The two bands seen
on this autoradiograph are the 1.5kb and 1.7kb Eco RII repeat
family bands also conserved in musculus and booduga genomes.

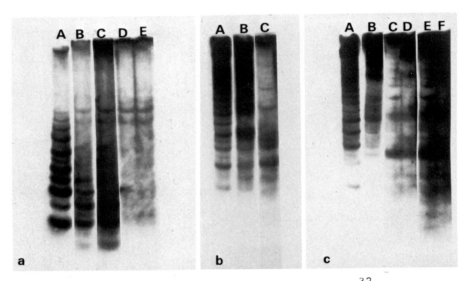

Fig. 4a, b and c. Southern blot hybridization of ^{32}P-labelled
musculus satellite DNA: (a) with Eco RII digested (A) musculus,
(B,C) booduga and (D,E) dunni Varanasi and Madras DNAs: Lane C
is longer exposure of lane B autoradiograph; (b) with Hinf digested
(A) musculus, (B) booduga and (C) dunni DNAs and (c) with Alu I
digested (A) musculus, (B) booduga (C, D, E, F) dunni DNAs:
Lanes E and F are longer exposure of lanes C and D autoradiographs

The band patterns detected in booduga and dunni DNAs digested with
Hinf and Alu I following hybridization with musculus satellite DNA
were similar. It is clear that the proportion of sequences cut by
Hinf in booduga and dunni are quite comparable (Fig. 4b).

The proportion of Alu I sites in booduga and dunni genomes seem to
be distinctly lower than the proportion of Hinf sites. In booduga

while higher multiples of monomers are found to be periodically repeated, in dunni, on the other hand, in addition to a reduction in these segmental variants there is variation in the relative abundance of multimer repeat sizes also (Fig. 4c).

It thus appears that in booduga the basic organization is similar to the bulk mouse satellite DNA, while in dunni the organization looks rather distinctly changed. The small localized segment of musculus satellite-related sequence in dunni perhaps represents a part of the conserved type B segment, while type A segment has been almost totally eliminated. It has earlier been reported that individual chromosomes may have specific distribution and amount of type B segments (Brown and Dover, 1980b). The small segment on dunni X-chromosome heterochromatin may be one such segment conserved during the phylogeny of the species.

The overall similarity in sequence organization of satellite sequences in M. booduga and M. musculus in contrast to that of M. dunni suggests closer phylogenetic relationship between M. musculus and M. booduga compared to M. dunni. It is interesting to note that in 6 individuals of M. dunni collected from Varanasi and Jaunpur in north India, one autosome in 5 of them and two autosomes in 1 of them possessed M. musculus type of centromeric heterochromatin, detected by AT-specific fluorochrome (Hoechst 33258) staining (Sen and Sharma 1983, present study Fig. 5). It appears that the same autosome is not involved in all the individuals. This may represent intermediate steps in the evolution of the centromeric heterochromatin during the process of divergence. This unique situation suggests that the qualitative shift in the composition of constitutive heterochromatin has proceeded in individual chromosome-specific manner and not by wholesale genomic revision.

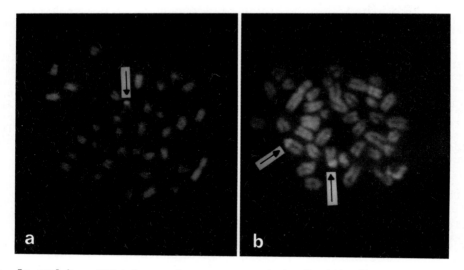

Fig. 5a and b. Metaphase chromosomes stained with fluorochrome Hoechst 33258 showing (a) an autosome (arrow) with bright fluorescence of pericentromeric heterochromatin and (b) two autosomes (arrows) with bright fluorescence of pericentromeric heterochromatin

In a study on mating preference behaviour in individuals of
M. dunni of Varanasi, Madras and Mysore populations with divergent
karyotypes characteristic for each population, a marked preference
by females to males of own chromosomal forms was noticed (Cheong
and Sharma, to be published). The experiment was carried out on
42, 15 and 10 females and 20, 19 and 6 males of Madras, Varanasi
and Mysore populations, respectively. Estrus was induced by
injecting hormone into females. The behaviour of females after
attaining estrus was observed for 35 minutes (5 minutes for
familiarization plus 30 minutes) in each test by placing one female
in an especially designed double-decker cage connected to lower
decks only by detachable tunnels. The design is almost similar to
the one used by Heth and Nevo (1981) in their study of mating
preference behaviour in the mole rats Spalax ehrenbergi complex.
Males of the three chromosomal forms were kept each time along with
a little of their own urine-soaked woodwool and cotton in the upper
decks separately in the 3 terminal cells. The males and the female
do not come in physical contact in the cells separated into upper
and lower decks by wire-mesh. The female is free to move from a
central position through connecting short tunnels to lower decks of
different cells. In the tests, the females of different chromosomal
forms were found predominantly to go and stay in the cells underneath
the males of own chromosomal forms. The preference shown by the
females to own chromosomal forms was statistically highly significant
in each case ($P < 0.001$; Friedmann's test). The striking preference
shown by females to males of own chromosomal forms strongly suggests
that already ethological isolation is in operation between the three
chromosomal forms which are apparently parapatric in distribution.
When the males of different chromosomal forms are brought together
they fight and the male of one chromosomal form goes to the extent
of killing the male of other chromosomal form. It is difficult to
speculate on the factor(s) responsible for the origin and
reinforcement of the isolating mechanism. However, the correlation
found between the three populations showing premating isolation and
divergent karyotypes due to variation of constitutive heterochromatin
is striking.

Although the correlation may be circumstantial, the stable karyotypic
difference achieved between chromosomal forms by establishing
homozygosity for constitutive heterochromatin variation in a group
of fossorial rodents which is in active phase of speciation does
indicate that constitutive heterochromatin might play an important
role in speciation mechanisms in certain groups of organisms. Thus,
a multidirectional approach in a system like the Indian pygmy field
mice might improve our knowledge about the importance of constitutive
heterochromatin.

ACKNOWLEDGEMENTS

This work was supported by a grant from the University Grants
Commission, India and the authors express their thanks to
Dr. Rajiva Raman for going through the manuscript.

REFERENCES

Brown SDM, Dover GA (1980a) Conservation of segmental variants of satellite DNA of Mus musculus in a related species: Mus spretus. Nature (Lond) 285:47-49

Brown SDM, Dover GA (1980b) The specific organization of satellite DNA sequences on the X chromosome of Mus musculus: partial independence of chromosome evolution. Nucleic Acids Res 8:781-792

Committee on standardized genetic nomenclature for mice (1972) Standard karyotype of the mouse, Mus musculus

Duffey PA (1972) Chromosome variation in Peromyscus: a new mechanism. Science 176:1333-1334

Ellerman JR (1961) Fauna of India, Mammalia, Vol III, Rodentia, 2nd edn. Roonwal ML (ed) Zoological Survey of India

Fry K, Salser W (1977) Nucleotide sequences of HS alpha satellite DNA from kangaroo rat Dipodomys ordii and characterization of similar sequences in other rodents. Cell 12:1069-1084

Gall JG, Atherton DD (1974) Satellite DNA sequences in D. virilis. J Mol Biol 85:663-664

Gamperl R, Ehmann C, Bachmann K (1982) Genome size and heterochromatin variation in rodents. Genetica 58:199-212

Hatch FT, Bodner AJ, Mazrimas JA, Moore DH (1976) Satellite DNA and cytogenetic evolution. DNA quantity, satellite DNA and karyotypic variations in kangaroo rats (Genus Dipodomys). Chromosoma (Berl) 58:155-168

Heth G, Nevo E (1981) Origin and evolution of ethological isolation in subterranean mole rats. Evolution 35:259-274

Hörz W, Zachau HG (1977) Characterization of distinct segments in mouse satellite DNA by restriction nucleases. Eur J Biochem 73:383-392

Manjunatha KR, Aswathanarayana NV (1979) Studies on the chromosomes of the genus Mus: Autosomal polymorphism in the Indian pygmy mouse Mus dunni (Wroughton). Curr Sci 48:657-659

Markvong A, Marshall JT, Pathak S, Hsu TC (1975) Chromosomes and DNA of Mus: The karyotype of M. fulvidiventris and M. dunni. Cytogenet Cell Genet 14:116-125

Marshall JT (1977) A synopsis of Asian species of Mus (Rodentia, Muridae). Amer Mus Nat Hist Bull 58:173-220

Matthey R, Petter F (1968) Existence de deux espices distinctes, l'une chromosomiquement polymorphe chez der Mus Indiens de groupe booduga. Etude cytogenetique et taxonomique. Rev Suisse Zool 75:461-498

Misonne X (1969) African and Indo-Australian Muridae, Evolutionary trends. Annls Mus Afr Cent Ser Zool 172:1-219

Pathak S, Hsu TC, Arrighi FE (1973) Chromosomes of Peromyscus (Rodentia, Cricetidae) IV. The role of heterochromatin in karyotypic evolution. Cytogenet Cell Genet 12:315-326

Patton JL, Sherwood SW (1982) Genome evolution in pocket gophers (Genus Thomomys) I. Heterochromatin variation and special potential. Chromosoma (Berl) 85:149-162

Peacock WJ, Appels R, Dunsmuir P, Lohe AR, Gerlach WL (1976) Highly repeated DNA sequences: chromosomal localization and evolutionary conservation in Inter Cell Biol (eds) Brinkley BR, Porter KR. Rockefeller Univ Press 494-506

Peacock WJ, Lohe AR, Gerlach WL, Dunsmuir P, Dennis ES, Appels R (1978) Fine structure and evolution of DNA in heterochromatin. Cold Spring Harb Symp Quant Biol 42:1121-1135

Rigby PWJ, Dieckman M, Rhodes C, Berg P (1977) Labelling
    deoxyribonucleic acid to high specific activity in vitro by
    nick translation with DNA polymerase I. J Mol Biol 113:237-251
Seabright M (1971) A rapid banding technique for human chromosomes.
    Lancet 2:971-972
Sen S, Sharma T (1980) Quantitative variation of "Mus musculus-like"
    constitutive heterochromatin and satellite DNA-sequences in the
    genus Mus. Chromosoma (Berl) 81:393-402
Sen S, Sharma T (1983) Role of constitutive heterochromatin in
    evolutionary divergence: results of chromosome banding and
    condensation inhibition studies in Mus musculus, Mus booduga
    and Mus dunni. Evolution 37:628-636
Sharma T, Raman R (1973) Variation of constitutive heterochromatin
    in the sex chromosomes of the rodent Bandicota b. bengalensis
    (Gray). Chromosoma (Berl) 41:75-84
Sharma T, Garg GS (1975) Constitutive heterochromatin and karyotype
    variation in India pygmy mouse, Mus dunni. Genet Res (Camb)
    25:189-191
Southern EM (1975) Detection of specific sequences among DNA
    fragments separated by gel electrophoresis. J Mol Biol 98:503-517
Sumner AT (1972) A simple technique for demonstrating centromeric
    heterochromatin. Exp Cell Res 75:304-306
Sutton WD, McCallum M (1972) Related satellite DNAs in the genus Mus.
    J Mol Biol 71:633-656
Yamamoto M, Miklos GLG (1978) Genetic studies on heterochromatin in
    Drosophila melanogaster and their implications for the function
    of satellite DNA. Chromosoma (Berl) 66:71-98

The Potential Use of Repetitive Sequences in Phylogenetic Reconstructions

S.C. Hardies

In this paper, I will examine the virtues and problems of using repetitive DNA sequences for molecular systematics in rodents. I will concentrate on a particular family of repetitive sequences called LINES ONE or Ll for short. The prototypes for this family were the KpnI family of primates and the BamHI (also called MIF-1) family of mice (see for review Singer 1982a,b; Singer and Skowronski 1985; Rogers 1985). After the realization that the KpnI and BamHI sequences were homologous (Singer et al. 1983), the entire family was named LINES, which is an acronym for long interspersed repeated sequences (Singer 1982a,b). The family has up to 100,000 copies per genome in rodents (Gebhard and Zachau 1983), with a somewhat lower copy number reported for primates (Grimaldi et al. 1984). Ll is the only mammalian LINES characterized with such a high copy number. It is responsible for many of the ethidium intense restriction bands observed after gel electrophoresis of restricted genomic DNA; hence the tendency to be named after restriction enzymes. Its distinguishing properties are its length and interspersion. Ll sequences are up to 7 kilobases long, although many of the copies consist of only a fragment of the total sequence. Its distribution in the genome is roughly uniform. Therefore, Ll elements have been frequently cloned and characterized because of their chance associations with other genes.

Table 1 contains a survey of other mammals in which Ll has been detected by molecular hybridization. I am aware of no instances in which a mammal was shown not to contain these sequences. Therefore, Ll has the required uniform distribution to make it useful for phylogenetic studies.

Table 1. Mammals known to contain LINES ONE sequences.[a]

Koala	Wallaby	Anteater
Elephant	Goat	Dog
Rabbit	Human	Monkey
Porcupine	Peromyscus	Rat
Chinese Hamster	Apodemus sylvaticus	A. mystacinus
Mus domesticus	M. spretus	M. cervicolor
M. caroli	M. dunni	M. musculus
M. cookii	M. pahari	M. shortridgei
M. castaneus	M. spicilegus (alias	M. hortulanus)
M. platythrix	M. spretoides (alias	M. abboti)
M. nannomys setulosus	M. n. minutiodes	

[a] Compiled from: Cheng and Schildkraut (1980); Heller and Arnheim (1980); Adams et al. (1980); Maio et al. (1981); Brown and Dover (1981); Lueders and Paterson (1982); Martin et al. (1984); Jubier-Maurin et al. (1985); and Burton et al. (1985).

The major advantage of Ll for a systematic study is the ease with which it can be cloned. This is mainly a consequence of the high copy number. Some groups have used the strategy of cutting out one of the ethidium intense bands originating from the repeat and cloning it directly into a vector designed to support dideoxy sequencing (Brown and Piechaczyk 1983; Martin et al. 1985). In this way, a large number of independent isolates can be sequenced in an analogous region very quickly. Unfortunately, the restriction map of the element changes from species to species complicating the problem of getting the analogous sequence from each species. However, with the mapping information derived from the studies tabulated in Table 1 and perhaps the use of synthetic oligonucleotide primers directed at the Ll sequence itself, this problem should be overcome.

On the other hand, there are some problems with using repetitive elements that must be explored before their use can be considered valid. The high copy number of Ll increases the intrinsic risk of making paralogous comparisons. Also, the activity of the element in sequence exchanges may introduce confusion. Finally, since little is known about what constraints may exist on the evolution of these sequences, there is no a priori reason to believe that their rate of evolution will be well behaved.

Although these problems may be exacerbated in Ll, all sequences are subject to such artifacts. Furthermore, all biological traits that might be used in a systematic analysis are encoded by sequences, and therefore subject to these artifacts. Ll provides an opportunity to study them in the context of plentiful sequence information, so that we may know them better.

PARALOGY AND CONCERTED EVOLUTION

Paralogy is a hazard in any multigene family. Consider the two homologous but rather divergent genes: serum albumin, and alpha fetoprotein. If one mistakenly picked serum albumin from one species and compared it to alpha fetoprotein from another in an attempt to gauge when the species diverged, the estimate would be grossly in error. That comparison is paralogous. These two proteins are sufficiently distinct that no one should make such an error, however more subtle cases can, and probably do cause errors in systematic analysis. With the high copy number of Ll, nearly all comparisons are expected to be paralogous. Consequently, without the saving influence of concerted evolution, valid comparisons would be hard to come by in Ll.

Concerted evolution is a process by which related sequences in a species evolve together, somehow acquiring the same mutations. As a result of concerted evolution, as a repetitive sequence evolves in two recently diverged species increased heterogeneity within each species is suppressed, but divergence between the species is not. For a repetitive sequence that has been around as long as Ll has, such a mechanism almost has to exist; otherwise the repetitive nature of the family would have become unrecognizable by now because of intraspecies divergence. Martin et al. (1985) directly measured the concerted evolution of Ll during the descent of Mus domesticus, Mus caroli, and Mus platythrix from their common ancestor. During this interval, heterogeneity within each species has stayed at an average of 4% per base pair. However, the average difference between M. domesticus and M. caroli has increased to 5%, and that between these two species and M. platythrix has increased to about 9%. Thus some homogenizing influence does in fact work within Ll, and the rate is sufficient to homogenize

47

the sequences in about the time it took <u>M</u>. <u>domesticus</u> to diverge from
<u>M</u>. <u>caroli</u>, about 5-7 Myr (Sarich 1985).

 Concerted evolution in L1 is seen in more detail in Fig. 1. This
tree describing the descent of the individual L1 sequences in the above
mentioned studies was taken from Martin et al. (1985). It shows the
individual L1 elements within a species merging with each other, rather
than connecting back to individual ancestral repeats in the common
ancestor. These intraspecies nodes represent individual events in the
concerted evolution process, which might be gene conversions or
duplicative transpositions. The consequence from the standpoint of

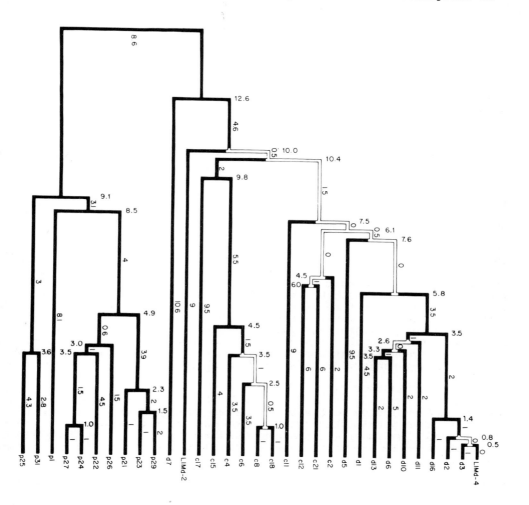

Fig. 1. Phylogenetic tree of LINES ONE sequences constructed by the
method of maximum parsimony. d = <u>Mus domesticus</u>, c = <u>Mus caroli</u>, and p
= <u>Mus platythrix</u>. The figure is taken from Martin et al. (1985) with
permission. Copyright 1985 by The University of Chicago.

species as diverged as M. platythrix and M. domesticus is to limit the influence of paralogous comparisons. One sequence was somehow chosen from the common ancestor to homogenize all of the M. platythrix descendants, and one was chosen to homogenize all of the M. domesticus descendants. Although we can not presume that these two chosen sequences were the same, we can presume that they were about 96% homologous, because all of the Ll sequences in the common ancestor were in that range. Therefore the estimated time of divergence will be off by only a few million years.

Concerted evolution therefore emerges as a favorable influence for the purpose of reconstructing phylogenies from repetitive sequences. The degree to which it suppresses the effects of paralogy is related to the extent of homogenization which is in turn measured by the intraspecies divergence. Of course, there is no assurance that Ll in other species will be homogenized to the same extent as these three, so a number of sequences would have to be taken from each species to guage this property. Species that have diverged within the time that it takes to homogenize their Ll sequences will be more difficult to handle. However, with enough individual Ll sequences sampled, it should be possible to classify the repeats into the subfamilies that appear to develop during incomplete homogenization, and still derive an estimate from the splits in the different subfamilies.

There needs to be some additional consideration of the possibility of very divergent subfamilies of Ll, falling outside of the data discussed above. Both sequencing (Brown and Piechaczyk 1983) and restriction mapping studies (Jubier-Maurin 1985) have pointed to the possible existence of such a divergent subfamily in mice. Members of such a subfamily would not be expected to appear in a sample of sequences such as that described above because the isolation procedure is biased against repeats that are very divergent. If one were consistent about the choice of hybridization probes, the danger of becoming confused by members from a diverged subfamily would be minimized. However, there is always the possibility that a species might be encountered that no longer had representatives of the subfamily most analogous to the probe, and that members of another subfamily would therefore emerge and mislead the analysis. This is Ll's version of the traditional paralogy problem that affects all single gene molecular phylogenies. The only solution is to combine results from independent genes. Therefore, Ll can not be expected to provide a final and independent answer to phylogenetic questions, but it can be one of the sequences used in a combined approach.

RATE OF Ll DIVERGENCE

The rate of evolution of the Ll sequences sets the limits of the range of times within which they may be used to estimate species divergence. The lower limit has been discussed above; the upper limit is constrained by the point at which parallel and back mutations become burdensome. Martin et al. (1985) estimate the divergence rate at 4.1×10^{-9} substitutions per site-year, which is about 1% divergence per million years for two species diverging apart. Therefore, Ll would be ideal for examining species diverging 10 to 20 Myr ago. Species diverging 20 to 40 Myr ago could be examined if sufficient attention were given to correcting for parallel and back mutation. Species diverging more than 40 Myr ago can still be treated, but uncertainty introduced by inadequacies in available corrections for parallel and back mutation will be large.

The finding of a long open reading frame within Ll (Potter 1984;

Martin et al. 1984) has implications with respect to the rate of its evolution. Martin et al. (1984) found that in comparison between mouse and primates there was a suppression of replacement changes amounting to about half of all expected changes. This means that but for the selection to express the protein encoded by this repeat, the divergence rate between species would be closer to 2% than 1%. Also, there is the strong suppression of insertions and deletions that would put translation out of frame. This is an important aid to the comparison of divergent sequences, because the necessity to introduce many gaps to align two sequences can radically increase the uncertainty in measuring their divergence. Consequently, it is probably desirable to avoid the untranslated regions of the Ll repeat when doing quantitative comparisons. For example, the mouse/rat comparison in the 3' untranslated region (Scarpulla 1985) requires a nearly unmanageable alignment even though only about 20 Myr (Sarich 1985) separate these species. Also the selective pressures may vary at different sites in the translated region, thus a common region should be used for all measurements.

RATE CONSTANCY

In considering the potential for fluctuations in the rate of evolution of Ll, I will ignore the debate over rate constancy in ordinary sequences and concentrate on potential sources of extra variation in Ll. There are two separate issues: 1) Within the multiple copies that one might sample, are some evolving faster than others? And 2) should we expect the overall rate of divergence of Ll within a species to vary more than ordinary genes?

I initially thought that there should be variation in rate among individual Ll repeats for the following reason. Some of the repeats are probably experiencing the selective pressure on the reading frame that was discussed earlier. That would be sufficient to eliminate about half of the divergence that would otherwise occur. Others of the repeats are known to be truncated and therefore must be defective for the operation of the reading frame. I presumed that they would be evolving twice as fast.

When I found a way to test this hypothesis, it failed in a surprising way. First I had to find a way to separate the lineages from Fig. 1 into functioning and defective genes. I had guessed that the repeats with active genes would also be those that participated most vigorously in the concerted evolution process. So I divided the lineages from Fig. 1 into those that had participated in many sequence exchanges (lineages with several nodes) and those that did not (lineages with no nodes). When these two classes were examined for the suppression of replacement mutations characteristic of active genes, my

<u>Table 2</u>. Comparison of base changes accumulated during the descent of active and inactive Ll sequences.[a]

	Replacement	Synonymous	Sum
Active	32	32	64
Inactive	48	18	66

[a]Compiled from pairs of lineages descending from selected nodes in Fig. 1.

guess proved correct. Those lineages that were active in sequence exchanges were also showing selective effects of expressing their reading frame, whereas those that were not active in sequence exchanges for long periods were evolving like pseudogenes. The surprising result came when I measured the overall rate of evolution in each of these two classes. Nodes were identified that joined active and inactive sequences, and then all of the changes from active descendants were summed and compared to those of the inactive descendants (Table 2). Although the suppression of replacement mutations is clearly present in the active class and not the other, the overall rate of change is very close.

This result means that there is another influence differentially affecting the rates of change in these two classes. It is a happy coincidence that the suppression of replacement mutations is roughly balanced by this other effect. That means that when picking representative repeats from these species for a phylogenetic reconstruction, it would have made no difference whether active or inactive sequences happened to be picked. However, it is not known if this relationship will hold in all other species, so sampling sufficient numbers of sequences to check on it would be advisable.

The inactive repeats discussed above evolve at a rate close to that traditionally found for pseudogenes (Li et al. 1981), therefore it is the active repeats that are evolving oddly. If one accounts for the suppressed replacement mutations, they would be evolving at twice the speed of nonfunctional sequences. Since the source of this accelerated evolution is not understood, there is cause for concern that it could be a source of rate variability from species to species.

Rodent/rodent divergence can be compared with rodent/primate divergence to get a feeling for variation in rates with time. I'll use only the replacement rates from Martin et al. (1984) because the synonymous sites are saturated in rodent/primate comparisons. The replacement values are also heavily affected by parallel and back mutation, and though corrected should not be considered very accurate. Nonetheless, M. domesticus to M. platythrix was diverged 4.5% at replacement sites while M. domesticus to primates was diverged 34%. Taking 12 Myr as the time of the M. domesticus / M. platythrix split, this extrapolates to 90 Myr for the rodent/primate split, which is roughly correct. Although this calculation is crude, it does suggest that the rate of change in L1 does not undergo excessive shifts.

SUMMARY

Although the potential for a variety of artifacts is indicated by the genetics of L1, its actual behavior seems to be relatively tame with respect to suitability for use in molecular systematics. To be on guard against peculiarities popping up in other species, one should expect to acquire 6 to 10 representative L1 sequences per species and to do a thorough analysis of their properties. The optimal working range is 10-20 Myr. Extension to more closely related species could be accomplished with attention to sorting out the results of partially completed sequence homogenization. Extension to 40 Myr or more could be accomplished with care to properly correct for parallel and back mutation. Given the ease of obtaining L1 sequence, this may be a suitable system for studying the systematics of rodents. As with all such systems, it is best used in combination with other genes to avoid possible artifacts due to paralogy.

REFERENCES

Adams JW, Kaufman RE, Kretschmer PJ, Harrison M (1980) A family of long reiterated DNA sequences, one copy of which is next to the human beta globin gene. Nucl Acids Res 8: 6113-6128

Brown SDM, Dover G (1981) Organization and evolutionary progress of a dispersed repetitive family of sequences in widely separated rodent genomes. J Mol Biol 150:441-466

Brown SDM, Piechaczyk M (1983) Insertion sequences and tandem repetitions as sources of variation in a dispersed repeat family. J Mol Biol 165:249-256

Burton FH, Loeb DD, Voliva CF, Martin SL, Edgell MH, Hutchison CA III (1985) Conservation throughout mammalia and extensive protein encoding capacity of the highly repeated DNA Ll. J Mol Biol, in press.

Cheng SM, Schildkraut CL (1980) A family of moderately repetitive sequences in mouse DNA. Nucl Acids Res 8:4075-4090

Gebhard W, Zachau HG (1983) Organization of the R family and other interspersed repetitive DNA sequences in the mouse genome. J Mol Biol 170:255-270

Grimaldi G, Skowronski J, Singer MF (1983) Defining the beginning and end of KpnI family segments. EMBO 3:1753-1759

Heller R, ArnHeim N (1980) Structure and organization of the highly repeated and interspersed 1.3 kb EcoRI - BglI sequence family in mice. Nucl Acids Res 8:5031-5042

Jubier-Maurin V, Dod BJ, Bellis M, Piechaczyk M, Riozes G (1985) Comparative study of the Ll family in the genus Mus: Possible role of retroposition and conversion events in its concerted evolution. J Mol Biol 184:547-564

Li WH, Gojobori T, Nei M (1981) Pseudogenes as a paradigm of neutral evolution. Nature 292:237-239

Lueders KK, Paterson BM (1982) A short interspersed repetitive element found near some mouse structural genes. Nucl Acids Res 10:7715-7729

Maio JJ, Brown FL, McKenna WG, Musich PR (1981) Toward a molecular paleontology of primate genomes: II The Kpn I families of alphoid DNAs. Chromosoma 83:127-144

Martin SL, Voliva CF, Burton FH, Edgell MH, Hutchison CA III (1984) A large interspersed repeat found in mouse DNA contains a long open reading frame that evolves as if it encodes a protein. Proc Natl Acad Sci USA 81:2308-2312

Martin SL, Voliva CF, Hardies SC, Edgell MG, Hutchison CA III (1985) Tempo and mode of concerted evolution in the Ll repeat family of mice. Mol Biol Evol 2:127-140

Potter SS (1984) Rearranged sequences of a human KpnI element. Proc Natl Acad Sci USA 81:1012-1016

Rogers JH (1985) The origin and evolution of retroposons. Int Rev Cytol 93:187-279

Sarich V (1985) personal communication

Scarpulla RC (1985) Association of a truncated cytochrome c processed pseudogene with a similarly truncated member from a long interspersed repeat family of rat. Nucl Acids Res 13:763-775

Singer MF (1982a) SINEs and LINEs: highly repeated short and long interspersed sequences in mammalian genomes. Cell 28:433-434

Singer MF (1982b) Highly repeated sequences in mammalian genomes. Int Rev Cytol 76:67-112

Singer MF, Thayer RE, Grimaldi G, Lerman MI, Fanning TG (1983) Homology between the Kpn I primate and Bam HI (MIF-1) rodent families of long interspersed repeated sequences. Nucl Acids Res 11:5739-5745

Singer MF, Skowronski J (1985) Making sense out of LINES: long
    interspersed repeat sequences in mammalian genomes. Trends Bioch Sci
    10:119-121
Voliva CF, Jahn CL, Comer MB, Edgell MH, and Hutchison CA III (1983)
    The L1Md long interspersed repeat family in the mouse: almost all
    examples are truncated at one end. Nucl Acids Res 11:8847-8859

Population Genetics

Genetic Features of Major Geographical Isolates of *Mus musculus*

K. Moriwaki, N. Miyashita, H. Suzuki, Y. Kurihara, and H. Yonekawa

INTRODUCTION

Laboratory mice have greatly contributed to the remarkable advances in immunogenetics and mammalian molecular genetics for the last decade. At present many different mouse strains, both classical and newly developed, are available for genetic studies. It is quite reasonable with the extensive development of research in this field, that one would like to know the natural origin of laboratory mice based on their genetic constitution. We have already revealed that the mitochondrial genome and most of the nuclear genomes of the present laboratory mice originated from an European subspecies Mus musculus domesticus (Yonekawa et al 1980, 1982; Moriwaki et al 1982, 1985). From mtDNA sequences, Ferris et al (1982) suggested "Common laboratory strains of inbred mice are descended from a single female". From stand points of either immunogenetics, molecular genetics or evolutionary genetics, it should be desirable to increase further the genetic diversity of the laboratory mice. This could be achieved by utilizing other mouse subspecies. Schwarz and Schwarz (1943) taxonomically discriminated 15 subspecies of mice of Old World origin. In general, taxonomical classification hardly demonstrates how much genetic distance is present among subspecies in a quantitative way. We have attempted to estimate the genetic distance between European domesticus subspecies and Japanese molossinus by Nei's method (1972), which suggested the time of divergence between them around one million years (Moriwaki et al 1979: Minezawa, Moriwaki, Kondo 1981). From mtDNA restriction patterns, Yonekawa et al (1980, 1981) also estimated approximate divergence among domesticus, bactrianus, castaneus and molossinus subspecies to have occurred about one million years ago. A considerable genetic divergence among domesticus, castaneus and molossinus was also demonstrated based on protein similarities (Sage 1981; Bonhomme et al 1984) and on mtDNA (Ferris et al 1983). In this paper, we will present more data on genetic features of those major geographical isolates of Mus musculus and attempt to group them from genetical viewpoints .

Contribution No.1667 from the National Institute of genetics, Japan. Supported in part by Grants-in-Aid from the Ministry of Education, Science and Culture, Japan

GENETIC FEATURES OF MAJOR GEOGRAPHICAL ISOLATES

Chromosome C banding Patterns

Since 1978 we have accumulated the chromosome C banding patterns detected by quinacrine-Hoechst staining in various subspecies of Mus musculus, approximately 300 individuals from 90 localities. Table 1 summarizes the typical patterns of each subspecies. The European, Central Asian and South Asian mice mostly exhibited the even distribution of positive C bands in all the chromosomes (C+ type). On the other hand, the mice from Northern China, Korea and Japan showed clearly different patterns which contained a number of negative C bands and also several larger-sized C bands (C-type). Mus spicilegus which is also considered to be a rather remote species from M. musculus was also C+ type suggesting that this type of C band pattern is evolutionarily older. Some individuals in C+ type subspecies such as bactrianus and castaneus showed a few number of C band negative chromosomes. These were possibly introduced from the surrounding C- type populations. The C band patterns are considered to be a fairly stable genetic traits once established, because the centromeric regions of chromosomes are very rarely involved in the meiotic crossing over. The other Mus species, M. spicilegus, M. spretus and M. caroli, were C+ type, though M. spretus exhibited positive C bands only by Giemsa staining.

Restriction Fragment Length Polymorphism (RFLP) in 28 S Ribosomal RNA Gene and its Non-Transcribed Region

DNA primary structure of 28 S ribosomal RNA region is well conserved among different subspecies, whereas its downstream non-transcribed region (NTR) is quite variable. 0.7 Kb DNA probe encompassing both regions developed by Kominami et al (1982) was used to compare RFLP in various subspecies by Southern blot analysis. Based on the combination of fragment length after EcoRI, BamHI and EcoRI + BamHI digestions, rDNA haplotypes were designated r1-r8 (Suzuki et al, to be published). Subspecies domesticus and brevirostris have r1 and r2 haplotype with 6.6 Kb EcoRI fragment. In musculus-molossinus, r4 and r6 were predominant which exhibited 9.0 Kb EcoRI fragment. r8 haplotype with 7.0 Kb EcoRI fragment was mainly observed in bactrianus and castaneus which also have r7 (6.5 Kb) and r6 (9.0 Kb) as illustrated in Fig. 1 and Fig. 2. Thus, Mus musculus species could be divided into three groups, domesticus-brevirostris, bactrianus-castaneus and musculus-mosossinus, as far as 28 S rDNA and the NTR are concerned.

Allelic Distribution of Lymphocyte Differentiation Antigens in Wild Mice

Allelic distributions of Thy-1 and Ly-2 antigens are character-istic of each Mus musculus subspecies. Eastern mice, molossinus, musculus, castaneus and bactrianus, express Thy-1.1, whereas Western, domesticus and brevirostris, Thy-1.2. Ly-2.1 is distributed in Eastern mice and some Western ones, the remaining of which exhibited Ly-2.2 (Kurihara et al 1985). Polymorphic alleles in beta 2 microglobulin are distributed in the similar pattern as those of Thy-1 and Ly-2 (Bobinson et al 1984). Thy-1.2 and Ly-2.1 alleles were likely differentiated only in domesticus-brevirostris group. Fig. 3 illustrates these findings.

Table 1 Chromosome C-band patterns detected by quinacrine-Hoechst staining in various mouse subspecies (Moriwaki et al 1985)

Subspecies & locality	Chromosome number																			
	1	2	3	4	5	6	7	8	9	10	11	12	13	14	15	16	17	18	19	X
Dom.Lbl	+	+	+	+	+	+	+	+	+	+	+	+	+	+	+	+	+	+	+	+
Dom.Pgn	+	+	+	+	+	+	+	+	+	+	+	+	+	+	+	+	+	+	+	+
Dom.Sey	+	+	+	+	+	+	+	+	+	+	+	+	+	+	+	+	+	+	+	+
Dom.Skm	+	+	+	+	+	+	+	+	+	+	+	+	+	+	+	+	+	+	+	+
Mus.Njl	+	+	+	+	+	+	+	+	+	+	+	+	+	+	+	+	+	+	+	−
Mus.Njl	+	+	+	+	+	+	+	+	+	+	+	+	+	+	+	+	+	+	+	−
Mus.Blg	−	−	+	+	++	+	+	+	+	+	+	+	+	+	+	+	+	+	+	−
Mus.Mbt	−	−	+	+	−	+	+	+	+	+	+	+	+	+	+	+	+	+	+	−
Bac.Lah	+	+	+	+	+	+	+	+	+	+	+	+	+	+	+	+	+	+	+	+
Bac.Lah	−	+	+	+	+	+	+	+	+	+	+/−	+	+	+	+	+	+	+	+	+
Bac.Kab	−	+	+	+	+	+	+/−	+	+	+	+	+	+	+	+	+/−	+/−	+	+	+
Bac.Kab	+	+	+	+	+	+	+	+	+	+	+	+	+	+	+	+	+	+	+	+
Urb.Bdw	+	+	+	+	+/−	+	+	+	+	+	+	+	+	+	+	+	+/−	+	+	+
Urb.Bdw	+	+	+	+	+	+	+	+	+	+	+	+	+	+	+	+	+	+	+	+
Urb.Bdw	+	+	+	+	+/−	+	+	+	+	+	+	+	+	+	+	+	+	+	+	+
Cas.Tch	+	+	+	+	+	+	+	+	+	+	+	+	+	+	+	+	+/−	+	+	+
Cas.Tch	+	+	+	+	+	+/−	+/−	+	+	+	+	+	+	+	+	+	+/−	+/−	+	+
Cas.Tch	+	+	+	+	+	+	+	+	+	+	+	+	+	+	+	+	+	+	+	+
sub.Bjn	+	+	−	+	+	+	+	−	−	+/−	+	−	−	−	−	−	−	+/−	−	−
sub.Chc	+	+/−	−	+/−	+	+	+	+	+	++/−	++/−	+/−	−	−	−	−	+/−	++/−	−	−
sub.Cht	+	+	−	+	+	+	+	+	+/−	+	+/−	+	+	−	−	−	+	−	+	−
sub.Lzh	−	−	−	−	−	−	−	−	−	−	−	−	−	−	−	−	++	++	+	−
sub.Lzh	−	−	−	−	−	−	−	+	−	+/−	−	+/−	+/−	−	+/−	−	++	++	−	−
sub.Urm	−	+	+	−	−	+	+	+	+	+	+/−	+	+	−	+	+	+	+	+	−
Mol.Nsb	+	+	−	+	−	+	−	−	+/−	+	+/−	+	−	−	−	−	−	++	+/−	−
Mol.Ten	−	++	−	+	+	++	−	−	+	+	−	+	−	−	−	−	−	++	−	−
Mol.Msm	−	++	−	+	−	+	+/−	−	+	+	−	−	−	−	−	−	+/−	++	−	−
Mol.Mmy	+	++	−	+	+	+	−	−	+	+	−	+/−	+	−	−	−	−	++	−	−
Mol.Oki	−	++	−	+	+/−	+	+	+/−	+	+	−	+	+	+	−	−	+	++	+	−

Abbreviations of the name of subspecies
Dom:Mus musculus domesticus. Mus:m.m.musculus. Bac:M.m.bactrianus. Urb:M.m.urbanus. Cas:M.m.castaneus. sub:M.m.subspecies collected from China. Mol:M.m.molossinus. Three letters following the name of subspecies represent the localities of collection.

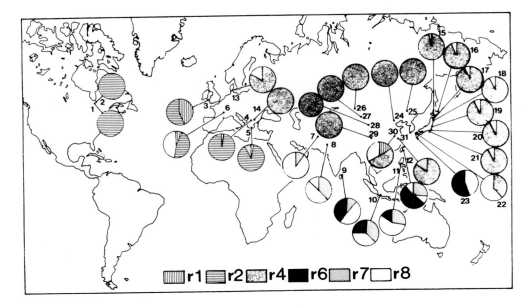

Fig. 1. Geographical distribution of rDNA haplotypes in various mouse subspecies (Suzuki et al To be published).

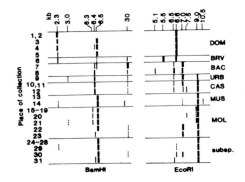

Fig. 2. RFLP of rDNA in the various mouse subspecies demonstrated by BamHI and EcoRI digestion and Southern blotting (Suzuki et al To be published)

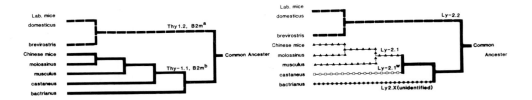

Fig. 3. Allelic distribution of lymphocytic antigens in various mouse subspecies (Kurihara et al 1985; Robinson et al 1984)

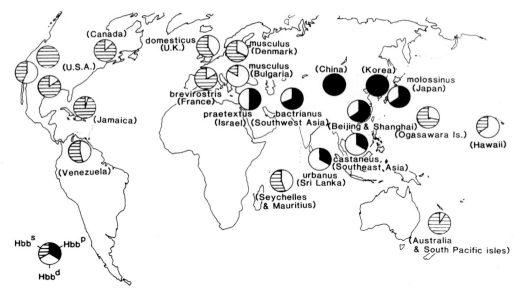

Fig. 4.   Geographical distribution of Hbb alleles in various
mouse subspecies (Miyashita et al 1985)

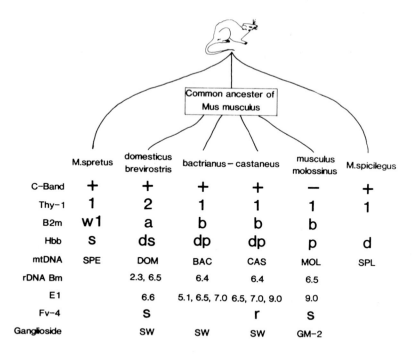

Fig. 5.   Mouse subspecies differentiation and their genetic
features

Polymorphic Alleles and their Geographical Distributions in Hemoglobin Beta Chain Locus

We studied the allelic frequency of the hemoglobin beta chain (Hbb) of wild mice, Mus musculus, collected from 46 localities mostly in Asia and surrounding areas (Fig. 4). The wild populations in the northern part of China, Korea and the central part of Japan exhibited almost monomorphic distribution of Hbb^p. In the southern part of Asia, the frequency of Hbb^p decreased and Hbb^d was predominant. Though Hbb^s and Hbb^d are generally found in Europe, the Hbb^p allele was present in Southeastern Europe (Bulgaria). In the light of these results, the Hbb^p allele might have originated in mice of northern Asia.

How Have Mus musculus Subspecies Been Differentiated ?

Fig. 5 illustrates a presumptive process of Mus musculus species differentiation. A common ancester of Mus musculus had probably been divided into several groups (subspecies) geographically isolated, around one million years ago. After that, mtDNA of each group accumulated a considerable number of mutations which emerged subspecies specific mtDNA types such as DOM, BAC, CAS or MOL. Moreover, in domesticus-brevirostris group Thy-1.1 had been substituted by Thy-1.2, and $B2m^a$ by $B2m^b$. On the other hand, in musculus-molossinus group chromosome C band pattern was changed from C+ type to C- type, hemoglobin beta chain from Hbb^d to Hbb^p and liver ganglioside from SWISS to GM-2. Friend virus resistant gene Fv-4 seems to have been changed from s-allele to r-allele in castaneus group. These findings suggested that domesticus-brevirostris group and musculus-molossinus group had been evolved in fairly independent manner. Evolutionary status of bactrianus and castaneus is rather obscure. They are similar to domesticus-brevirostris group on one hand and to molossinus-musculus group on the other as shown in rDNA RFLP. Genetic characterization of various geographical isolates of Mus musculus seems to be quite helpful to identify each of them. At this moment, it seems to be reasonable from genetical viewpoints to classify Mus musculus species into at least three groups as mentioned above.

REFERENCES

Bonhomme F, Catalan J, Britton-Davidian J, Chapman VM, Moriwaki K, Nevo E, Thaler L (1984) Biochemical diversity and evolution in the genus Mus. Biochem Genet 22:275-303

Ferris SD, Sage RD, Wilson AC (1982) Evidence from mtDNA sequences that common laboratory strains of inbred mice are descended from a single female. Nature 295:163-165

Ferris SD, Sage RD, Prager EM, Ritte U, Wilson AC (1983) Mitochondrial DNA evolution in mice. Genetics 105:681-721

Hashimoto Y, Suzuki A, Yamakawa T, Wang CH, Bonhomme F, Miyashita N, Moriwaki K (1984) Expression of GM1 and GD1a in liver of wild mice. J Biochem 95:7-12

Kominami R, Mishima Y, Urano Y, Sasaki M, Muramatsu M (1982) Cloning and determination of the transcription termination site of ribosomal RNA gene of the mouse. Nucleic Acid Res 10:1963-1979

Kurihara Y, Miyashita N, Moriwaki K, Petras ML, Bonhomme F, Cho WS, Kohno S (1985) Serological survey of T-lymphocyte differentiation antigens in wild mice. Immunogenet 22:211-218

Minezawa M, Moriwaki K, Kondo K (1981) Geographical survey of protein variations in wild populations of Japanese house mouse, Mus musculus molossinus. Jap J Genet 56:27-39

Miyashita N, Moriwaki K, Minezawa M, Yonekawa H, Bonhomme F, Migita S, Yu ZC, Lu DY, Cho WS (1985) Allelic constitution of the hemoglobin beta chain in wild population of the house mouse, Mus musculus. Biochem Genet 23:975-986

Moriwaki K, Miyashita N, Yonekawa H (1985) Genetic survey of the origin of laboratory mice and its implication in genetic monitoring. In:Archibold J, Ditchfield J, Rowsell HC (eds) The contribution of laboratory animal science to the welfare of man and animals, Gustav Fischer Verlag, Stuttgart, p237

Moriwaki K, Shiroishi T, Minezawa M, Aotsuka T, Kondo K (1979) Frequency distribution of histocompatibility-2 antigenic specificities in the Japanese wild mouse genetically remote from the European subspecies. J Immunogenet 6:99-113

Moriwaki K, Shiroishi T, Yonekawa H, Miyashita N, Sagai T (1982) Genetic status of Japanese wild mice and immunological characters of their H-2 antigens. In:Muramatsu T, Cachelin G, Moscona AA, Ikawa Y (eds) Teratocarcinoma and embryonic cell interactions, Japan Scientific Soc Press and Academic Press, Tokyo, p157

Nei M (1972) Genetic distance between population. Am Natur 106:283-292

Odaka T, Ikeda H, Yoshikura H, Moriwaki K, Suzuki S (1981) Fv-4:Gene controlling resistance to NB-tropic Friend murine leukemia virus. Distribution in wild mice, introduction into genetic background of BALB/c mice and mapping of chromosomes. J Nat Cancer Inst 67:1123-1127

Robinson PJ, Steinmetz M, Moriwaki K, Fischer-Lindahl K (1984) Beta-2 microglobulin types in mice of wild origin. Immunogenet 20:655-665

Sage RD (1981) Wild mice. In:Foster HL, Small JD, Fox JG (eds) The mouse in biomedical research, Vol. 1, Academic Press, New York, p39

Schwarz E, Schwarz HK (1943) The wild and commensal stocks of the house mouse. J Mammal 24:59-72

Suzuki H, Miyashita N, Moriwaki K, Kominami R, Muramatsu M, Kanehisa T, Bonhomme F, Petras ML, Yu ZC, Lu DY (to be published) Evolutionary implication of heterogeneity of the non-transcribed spacer region of ribosomal DNA repeating units in various subspecies of Mus musculus. Mol Biol Evol

Yonekawa H, Moriwaki K, Gotoh O, Hayashi JI, Watanabe J, Miyashita N, Petras ML, Tagashira Y (1981) Evolutionary relationship among five subspecies of Mus musculus based on restriction enzyme cleavage patterns of mitochondrial DNA. Genetics 98:801-816

Yonekawa H, Moriwaki K, Gotoh O, Miyashita N, Migita S, Bonhomme F, Hjorth JP, Petras ML, Tagashira Y (1982) Origins of laboratory mice deduced from restriction patterns of mitochondrial DNA. Differentiation 22:222-226

Yonekawa H, Moriwaki K, Gotoh O, Watanabe J, Hayashi JI, Miyashita N, Petras ML, Tagashira Y (1980) Relationship between laboratory mice and the subspecies of Mus musculus domesticus based on restriction endonuclease cleavage patterns of mitochondrial DNA. Jap J Genet 50:289-296

A Hybrid Origin of Japanese Mice
"Mus musculus molossinus"

H. Yonekawa, O. Gotoh, Y. Tagashira, Y. Matsushima, L.-I. Shi, W. S. Cho, N. Miyashita, and K. Moriwaki

INTRODUCTION

Taxonomy of the house mouse, <u>Mus</u> <u>musculus</u> is currently being extensively discussed. Feral and commensal forms of <u>Mus</u> <u>musculus</u> provide an important pool of genes (Morse 1978). In order to unify the taxonomy of the species, it is necessary to accumulate and integrate many lines of experimental evidence. The information on Asiatic mice is still incomplete.

In this regard, we have been studying the genetics of Asiatic mice over the past ten years. Restriction analysis of mtDNA is one of our major subjects. We have analysed mtDNA RFLP of mice in Japan and neighboring countries. The conclusion we thus reached is that Japanese mice, <u>M</u>. <u>m</u>. <u>molossinus</u> were established through the hybridization between <u>M</u>. <u>m</u>. <u>musculus</u> and <u>M</u>. <u>m</u>. <u>castaneus</u>.

MITOCHONDRIAL DNA AS A SUBSPECIES MARKER

After the first attempt to classify <u>Mus</u> <u>musculus</u> by Schwarz and Schwarz (1943), two new schemes have been independently proposed by Thaler et al. (1981) and by Marshall(1981). Marshall identified at least seven morphological groups which he called "species" inside the Genus <u>Mus</u>. His taxonomy was supported by Sage (1983) who analyzed the genus with biochemical markers. On the other hand, Thaler's taxonomy was followed by Bonhomme et al (1984), who reported that there were at least three distinct biochemical groups called "hemi-species" among <u>Mus</u> <u>musculus</u>, and that several other species were identified in the genus <u>Mus</u>. Thus, there are some discordances of terminology between Marshall's and Thaler's taxonomies, although both of them agreed that the taxonomy proposed by Schwarz and Schwarz should be rejected.

Comparing these two new taxonomies, we recognized that at least the following four (sub)species of <u>Mus</u> <u>musculus</u> (complex) could be identi-

Contribution No. 1663 from the National Institute of Genetics Japan

fied as independent ones: <u>M</u>. (<u>m</u>.) <u>domesticus</u> (which contains <u>M</u>. <u>m</u>. <u>brevirostris</u>), <u>M</u>. (<u>m</u>.) <u>musculus</u>, <u>M</u>. (<u>m</u>.) <u>castaneus</u> (which contains <u>M</u>. <u>m</u>. <u>urbanus</u>) and <u>M</u>. (<u>m</u>.) <u>molossinus</u>.

Our first question was whether these subspecies could be distinguished by restriction analysis of their mtDNA. Fig. 1 shows the dendrogram of mtDNA variants among mouse subspecies. If we arbitrarily use an

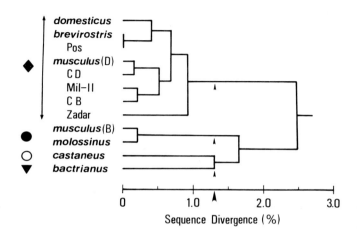

Sequence Divergence (%)

Fig. 1. Dendrogram of mtDNA from representative subspecies of <u>Mus</u> <u>musculus</u> constructed by the UPG method. Letters other than subspecies nomenclatures in this figure are the name of wild <u>domesticus</u> derived strains with Robertsonian translocations (see Moriwaki et al, 1984). Symbols beside the dendrogram represent ◆ <u>domesticus</u>-cluster, ● <u>musculus</u>-cluster, ○ <u>castaneus</u>-cluster and ▼ <u>bactrianus</u>-cluster. These symbols are used in Fig. 2.

mtDNA sequence divergence of 1.3%, four major clusters of variants clearly appeared on the dendrogram: those of <u>M</u>. (<u>m</u>.) <u>domesticus</u>, of <u>M</u>. (<u>m</u>.) <u>musculus</u> and <u>M</u>. (<u>m</u>.) <u>molossinus</u>, of <u>M</u>. (<u>m</u>.) <u>castaneus</u> and of <u>M</u>. (<u>m</u>.) <u>bactrianus</u>. This clustering with mtDNA fits well the clustering with biochemical markers (Sage 1981, Bonhomme et al. 1984) or with morphology (Marshall 1981). Therefore, we conclude that recent mouse taxonomies (Thaler et al. 1981, Marshall 1981) are preferable to the previous one (Schwarz and Schwarz 1943) and that mtDNA is useful as a marker to identify mouse subspecies, even if there are a few exceptions caused by cytoplasmic gene flow (Yonekawa et al. 1982, Ferris et al 1983, Boursot et al 1984).

GEOGRAPHIC DISTRIBUTION OF MTDNA VARIATION IN EURASIAN CONTINENT

Using the four clusters shown in Fig. 1, we constructed a distribution map of mtDNA variants (Fig. 2). We found that the four clusters of mtDNA variants clearly formed geographical clusters. The geographical clusters were superimposed with subspecies distribution, suggesting that mtDNA variation is useful for tracing subspecies distribution.

64

Especially, it should be noticed that the mice with <u>musculus</u>-type mtDNA were found from Eastern Europe to Far East through Central Asia.

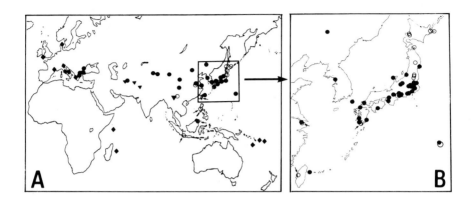

Fig. 2. Geographical distribution of mtDNA variants. ◆ <u>domesticus</u>-cluster, ● <u>musculus</u>-cluster, ○ <u>castaneus</u>-cluster, ▼ <u>bactrianus</u>-cluster, Data on European mice are based on Boursot et al. (1984) and Moriwaki et al. (1984).

JAPANESE MICE CONSIST MAINLY OF TWO MTDNA LINEAGES

We collected mice at 44 localities in Japan. We found that the Japanese mice have no mtDNA variant specific to <u>M</u>. <u>m</u>. <u>molossinus</u> but three clusters of mtDNA variants; <u>musculus</u>-cluster, <u>castaneus</u>-cluster and <u>domesticus</u>-cluster (Yonekawa et al. 1980, 1981, 1982, Ferris et al. 1983, Boursot et al. 1984), although the mice were morphologically identified to be <u>M</u>. <u>m</u>. <u>molossinus</u> (Schwarz and Schwarz 1943, Thaler et al. 1981, Marshall et al. 1981). Since the mice with <u>domesticus</u> mtDNA trapped at two localities were geographical contaminants of European mice (probably from the United States), we exclude them from our further discussion. As for the <u>musculus</u>-cluster, we found a single mtDNA lineage among 31 localities, including our previous data (Yonekawa et al. 1980, 1981, 1982). On the other hand, the <u>castaneus</u>-cluster contained two mtDNA lineages; one of which was found in only one of the ten localities (Yahaba mouse)(Table 1).

A UNIQUE GEOGRAPHICAL DISTRIBUTION OF CASTANEUS-TYPE MTDNA IN JAPAN

The two groups mentioned so far showed a clear geographical distribution in Japan. Namely, the mice with <u>castaneus</u>-type mtDNA are distributed in Hokkaido Island, the Tohoku district of Main Island and the southern distal end of Kyushu Island. Other parts were occupied by the mice with <u>musculus</u>-type mtDNA. There are two points to be emphasized. 1) the northern groups of mice with <u>castaneus</u>-type are sepa-

65

Table 1, The subspecies of <u>Mus musculus</u> used, their sources and the set of restriction enzyme cleavage patterns of mtDNAs obtained from each sample

Subspecies Collection locality	Restriction patterns												
	Bm	Ec	H2	H3	Hp1	He2	Ps	Bg	Hp2	He3	Tq	Hf	Mb*
<u>M. m. castaneus</u>													
Indonesia													
Bogor	C	B	C	B	C	C	B	A	-	-	-**	K	L
Malaysia													
Kota Kinabal	C	B	C	B	C	C	B	A	-	-	-	L	M
Philippines													
Quezon city	C	B	C	B	C	C	B	A	D	-	-	L	J
Taiwan													
Taichun	C	B	C	B	C	C	B	A	E	-	-	L	I
<u>M. m. molossinus</u>													
Japan***													
<u>castaneus</u>-type mtDNA	C	B	C	B	C	C	B	A	D	F	G	J	I
Yahaba	C	B	G	B	-	C	B	A	-	-	-	-	-
<u>musculus</u>-type mtDNA	D	B	A	B	A	C	B	A	A	F	B	B	B
Sasaguri	A	A	A	A	A	A	A	A	A	A	A	A	A
Ogasawara(2)	E	A	A	B	A	A	A	A	-	-	-	-	-
Korea													
Suweon	D	B	A	B	A	C	B	A	-	-	-	C	B
Kojori	D	B	A	B	A	E	B	A	-	-	-	B	B
China													
Changchun	D	B	A	B	A	C	B	A	A	-	B	D	B
Nanking	D	D	A	B	-	-	C	-	-	-	-	-	-
	C	B	C	B	C	C	B	A	-	-	-	-	-
Shanghai	D	B	A	B	A	C	B	A	A	-	C	G	C
	C	B	C	B	C	C	B	A	-	-	-	-	-
Chengtu	D	B	A	B	A	C	B	A	G	-	C	E	C
Lanzhou	D	B	A	B	A	C	B	A	A	-	C	E	C
Jiayuguang	D	B	A	B	A	C	B	A	H	-	C	H	C
Turfan	D	B	A	B	A	C	B	A	I	-	E	E	E
Urumuchi	D	B	A	B	A	C	B	A	J	-	F	I	F
Kunmin	C	B	C	B	C	C	B	A	-	-	-	-	-

* Abbreviation used are Bm: BamHI, Ec: EcoRI, H2: HindII, H3: HindIII, He2: HaeII, Hp1: HpaI, Ps: PstI, Bg: BglI, Hp2: HpaII, He3: HaeIII, Tq: TaqI, Hf: HinfI and Mb: MboI.

** "-" represent "not done".

*** The <u>molossinus</u> mice with <u>castaneus</u>-type mtDNA were collected at 9 different localities, i.e. Nemuro, Nakashibetsu, Sapporo, Teine, Oma, Kurihara, Koriyama, Sukagawa, Izumizaki and Kagoshima. The mice with <u>musculus</u>-type mtDNA were collected at 28 localities, i.e. Ohzuchi, Niigata, Shinanomachi, Iiyama, Wajima, Motegi, Mito, Kuki, Inamachi, Omiya, Ichikawa, Yotsukaido, Koajiro, Mishima, Numazu, Nishio, Anjo, Mizuho, Gobo, Momoyama, Osaka, Kochi, Mine, Hakozaki, Sasaguri, Izumi, Kagoshima, Miyazaki, Tsushima, Ogasawara and Yonaguni.

rated geographically from the native habitat of <u>M</u>. <u>m</u>. <u>castaneus</u> which is Southeastern Asia, Taiwan and Southern China, and 2)there is also a small and probably isolated colony of mice with castaneus mtDNA in Southern Japan (Fig. 2).

A HYBRID ORIGIN OF JAPANESE MICE "<u>M</u>. <u>m</u>. <u>molossinus</u>"

Based on mtDNA data of Japanese mice, we propose the hypothesis that Japanese "<u>M</u>. <u>m</u>. <u>molossinus</u>" was established through the hybridization between Chinese <u>M</u>. <u>m</u>. <u>musculus</u> and <u>M</u>. <u>m</u>. <u>castaneus</u>. This hypothesis is supported by the following facts: Cytogenetical analysis with c-banding showed that Chinese mice had many chromosomes with faintly stained c-bands but <u>M</u>. <u>m</u>. <u>castaneus</u> did not. The frequency of dark c-bands in Japanese mice lay inbetween (Moriwaki et al. 1982). A similar result was obtained by the analysis of Hbb (hemoglobin beta chain) alleles distribution (Miyashita et al. 1985).

Furthermore, we recently found some nuclear markers specific to <u>M</u>. <u>m</u>. <u>castaneus</u>. These genes were found not only in the mice with the <u>castaneus</u>-type mtDNA but also in the mice with <u>musculus</u>-type mtDNA (Kurihara et al. 1985, Suzuki et al. 1985). On the other hand, Japanese "<u>molossinus</u>" mice belong to the same biochemical cluster as that of <u>M</u>. <u>m</u>. <u>musculus</u> (Sage 1981, Bonhomme et al. 1984). These results suggest that there is no gene specific to Japanese mice.

However, the question remains of why only mtDNA has a clear geographical distribution in Japan. One possibility to elucidate this fact is that mtDNA is controlled by some selection mechanism. The other one is that the distribution is a transient state of spatiotemporal processes that are still taking place during the establishment of Japanese mice "<u>M</u>. <u>m</u>. <u>molossinus</u>". The processes can be elucidated as follows: 1) <u>M</u>. <u>m</u>. <u>castaneus</u> first immigrated from Southern China or Southeastern Asia and established their colonies all over Japan; 2) Chinese <u>M</u>. <u>m</u>. <u>musculus</u> then invaded into Japanese <u>castaneus</u> colonies probably from Korea; and 3) these two processes drove the previous occupants to distal area of Japan, Chinese <u>M</u>. <u>m</u>. <u>musculus</u> settled its colonies as the present geographical distribution. It is interesting that this hypothesis meets well one of the major hypotheses on "origins of Japanese human race" based on cultural and physical anthology-pology (Egami et al. 1980).

ACKNOWLEDGMENT

This research was partially supported by a grant of The Naito Foundation. We are grateful to Dr. K. Nakachi and P. Boursot for helpful discussions. We also thank Drs. F. Bonhomme, Y. Furuya, N. Habu, T. Hamada, M. Hozumi, J. P. Hjorth, H. Ikeda, H.T. Imai, K. Kondo, T. H. Ku, Y. Kurihara, T. Kuwahata, D.Y. Lu, Y. Matsuda, J. S. Masanokay, S. Migita, M. Minezawa, F. Nagasawa, M. L. Petras, M. Sakaizumi, T. Sasaba, T. Seno, T. Shiroishi, H. Suzuki, R. Tanaka, M. Tobari, K. Tsuchiya, C.H. Wang, Z.C. Yu, Mr. N. Hanzawa, S. Hiyama, and Ms. T. Sagai, M. Tsuyuki, for providing mice .

REFERENCES

Bonhomme F, Catalan J, Britton-Davidian J, Chapman VM, Moriwaki K,

Nevo E, Thaler L (1984) Biochemical diversity and evolution in the Genus Mus. Biochem Genet 22: 275-303

Boursot P, Bonhomme F, Britton-Davidian J, Catalan J, Yonekawa H, Orisini P, Guerassimov S, Thaler L (1984) Introgression differentielle des Genomes nucleaires et mitochondriaux chez duex semiespeces europeennes de souris. CR Acad Sci Paris 299:365-370

Egami N, Umehara T, Kamiyama S, Nakane C (eds)(1980) Nihonjin towa nanika. (What characters does Japanese human race have in the fields of physical and cultural antholopology?) Proc Amagi Symp, (In Japanese) Kodansha, Tokyo

Ferris SD, Sage RD, Huang CM, Nielsen JT, Ritte U, Wilson AC (1983) Flow of mitochondrial DNA across a species boundary. Proc Natl Acad Sci USA 80: 2290-2294

Kurihara Y, Miyashita N, Wang CH, Petras ML, Bonhomme F, Kono SI, Moriwaki K (1985) Serological survey of T-lymphocyte differentiation antigens in wild mice, Immunogenetics, 22: 211-218

Marshall JT (1981) Taxonomy. In Foster HL, Small JD Fox JG (eds) The mouse in biomedical research, vol 1, Academic Press, New York, p17

Minezawa M, Moriwaki K, Kondo K (1981) Geographical survey of protein variations in wild populations of Japanese house mouse, M. m. molossinus. Jpn J Genet 56: 27-39

Miyashita N, Moriwaki K, Minezawa M, Yonekawa H, Bonhomme F, Migita S, Yu ZC, Lu DY, Cho WS (1985) Allelic constitution of the hemoglobin beta chain in wild populations of the house mouse, Mus musculus. Biochem Genet 23: 975-986

Moriwaki K, Shiroishi T, Yonekawa H, Miyashita N, Sagai T (1982) Genetic status of Japanese wild mice and immunological characters of their H-2 antigens. In Muramatsu T, Gachelin G, Moscona AA, Ikawa Y (eds) Teratocarcinoma and embryonic cell interactions. Japan Scientific Society Press, Tokyo and Academic Press, New York, p157

Moriwaki K, Yonekawa H, Gotoh O, Minezawa M, Winking H, Gropp A (1984) Implications of the genetic divergence between European wild mice with Robertsonian translocations from the view point of mitochondrial DNA. Genet Res Camb 43: 277-287

Morse HC (ed)(1978) Origin of inbred mice, Academic Press, New York

Sage RD (1981) Wild mice. In Foster HL, Small JD, Fox JG (eds) The mouse in biomedical research, vol 1. Academic Press New York p90

Schwarz E, Schwarz HK (1943) The wild and commensal stocks of the house mouse, Mus musculus Linnaeus. J Mammal 24: 59-72

Suzuki H, Miyashita N, Moriwaki K, Kominami R, Muramatsu M, Kanehisa T, Bonhomme F, Wang CH, Lu DY (to be published) Heterogeneity of the non-transcribed spacer region of ribosomal DNA repeating units in various subspecies of Mus musculus. Mol Biol Evol

Thaler L, Bonhomme F, Britton-Davidian J (1981) Processes of speciation and semi-speciation in the house mouse. Symp Zool Soc London 47: 27-41

Yonekawa H, Moriwaki K, Gotoh O, Watanabe J, Hayashi JI, Miyashita N, Petras ML, Tagashira Y (1980) Relationship between laboratory mice and the subspecies Mus musculus domesticus based on restriction endonuclease cleavage patterns of mitochondrial DNA. Jpn J Genet 55: 287-296

Yonekawa H, Moriwaki K, Gotoh O, Hayashi JI, Watanabe J, Miyashita N, Petras ML, Tagashira Y (1981) Evolutionary relationships among five subspecies of Mus musculus based on restriction enzyme cleavage patterns of mitochondrial DNA. Genetics 98: 801-816

Yonekawa H, Moriwaki K, Gotoh O, Miyashita N, Migita S, Bonhomme F, Hjorth JP, Petras ML, Tagashira Y (1982) Origins of Inbred mice deduced from restriction patterns of mitochondrial DNA. Differentiation 22: 222-226

Some Aspects of Robertsonian Karyotype Variation in European Wild Mice

H. Winking

Karyotypically the genus Mus is highly conservative and the most prevalent karyotype consists of 40 acrocentric chromosomes with pericentromeric heterochromatin. In addition, many species of the genus Mus exhibit a homosequential G-band pattern along their chromosomes (Hsu et al. 1978). The 40 all acrocentric karyotype can be considered as the standard karyotype of the house mouse Mus musculus within their world-wide distribution area. In Western Europe, however, several populations with varying chromosome numbers from 2n=39 to 2n=22 are found. The reduction in chromosome number is always associated with a gain of biarmed (metacentric) chromosomes that are equivalent to two acrocentric autosomes. This type of structural rearrangement - the translocation of two acrocentric autosomes on top of each other - is well known as Robertsonian (Rb) translocation, fusion, or exchange. It is generally assumed that prior to whole arm exchange, breaks are simultaneously occurring in both partners. By an analysis of C-banded Rb chromosomes the position of the breakpoints can be ascertained more precisely. Since on both sides of the primary constriction of the rearranged chromosome similar sized blocks of constitutive heterochromatin are present, the breaks must have occurred very close to the centromeric tip of the ancestral acrocentric autosomes (Fig. 1). All Rb chromosomes of the mouse analysed so far show this type of heterochromatin distribution. A substantial loss of constitutive heterochromatin in association with the Rb mutational event therefore seems to be unlikely. The data of Comings and Avelino (1972), who were unable to detect a decrease of satellite DNA in mice with 14 Rb chromosomes by DNA measurements, corroborate the cytogenetic findings.

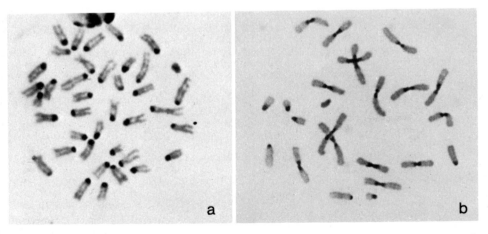

Fig. 1. C-banded metaphases with a)acrocentric chromosomes only and b)with 16 metacentric and eight acrocentric chromosomes

With regard to Rb variation, many aspects are worthwile to discuss, but I will concentrate on two subjects.
1) The rapid evolution of the house mouse karyotype within a limited area of the habitat
2) the consequences of Rb translocations for a heterozygous carrier.

In Europe, the two subspecies M. m. domesticus and M. m. musculus occur. Both subspecies meet along a line running down from the Baltic Sea to the Black Sea and hybridize in a narrow hybrid zone (Fig. 2). Until now Rb chromosomes have been found only in the M. m. domesticus subspecies. About 21 populations with Rb chromosomes have been described in Western Europe (Adolph and Klein 1981; Gropp and Winking 1981; Brooker 1982; Adolph and Klein 1983; Britton-Davidian 1983) plus one in North Africa (Said et al. 1985). Very recently, an additional population has been discovered in Southern Denmark (Winking and Nielsen unpubl. observation). This population is highly remarkable because some of the Rb carrier mice are expected to represent hybrids between musculus and domesticus and some pure domesticus. There is no evidence for the existence of Rb chromosomes north of the hybrid zone within the M. m. musculus habitat. This additionally supports the assumption that the generation of Rb chromosomes is a special trait of the M. m. domesticus subspecies. Within these 23 populations 162 Rb transloca- tions are known to occur. The composition of 76/162 is unique. 86/162 arm combinations have been found in two to 10 karyotypically distinct populations. The most frequent and wide spread combination is 5.15 and is present in mice of Yougoslavia, Central and Northern Italy, Southern Germany and Spain. It is not yet clear whether certain metacentrics shared by different populations are derived from a common ancestor or whether they have been originated independently. Although the chance of creating twice two identical composed metacentrics is low (Sage 1981), both mechanisms seem to be realized in the mouse, whereby spreading of rearranged chromosomes into different areas and populations plays the major role in karyotype diversification of the mouse. With the ex- ception of the sex chromosomes and autosome 19, all other autosomes have been detected as one partner in four to 11 different combinations. It remains obscure why the smallest autosome is not represented within the large sample of biarmed chromosomes, particularly since this chromosome does participate in Rb exchange in laboratory mouse strains. It has been argued that a Rb combination with autosome 19, if hetero- zygous, has a detrimental effect in feral mice, thus leading to elim- ination prior to fixation in a homozygous condition. This hypothesis cannot be ruled out, but it is also conceivable that autosome 19 unlike the other autosomes does not undergo Rb exchanges at all. Are there further indications that individual mouse chromosomes may show a differential proneness to whole arm exchange? Autosome 18 seems to be a good candidate to elucidate this problem. Under the assumption that 76 different Rb chromosomes have been originated in the European and North African mice and autosomes one to 18 (autosome 19 excluded) are randomly involved in Rb combinations, every autosome should be present about 8.4 times among the 152 identified chromosome arms of this sample. In fact, autosome 18 is involved only 5 times in a metacentric chromo- some and is, together with autosome seven, the least represented auto- some. In addition, chromosome 18 as a metacentric arm is present in only one out of nine populations with the submaximal number of six to eight pairs of Rb chromosomes. These observations suggest that the peri- centromeric region of autosome 18, which becomes involved in the process of breakage, exchange, and reunion, is very stable. As a consequence, this chromosome obviously gets fixed in a metacentric late during karyotype evolution. Chromosome seven shows a similar feature and, less pronounced, chromosome one. On the other hand, autosome 12 exhibits a reversed behaviour. In 21/23 populations this chromosome is translocated

on top of several different autosomes. In the Rhine-valley the
Rb(4.12)9Bnr is the only metacentric representative and in populations
of Greece, Scotland, and Spain chromosome 12 is found as a constituent
of metacentrics, although the number of Rb chromosomes is low. In
Scotland the Rb(9.12) is considered of having arisen first within this
country (Brooker 1982). However, chromosome 12 is not necessarily
involved in the Rb chromosome, which appears first in an all acrocentric mouse population. For example, on Ibiza island the only identified metacentric consists of 13.16 and in the Danish population,
despite the presence of three metacentrics, chromosome 12 remained
acrocentric.
At present there is little understanding why the acrocentric chromosomes of the European house mouse are, in general, highly susceptible
to the mutagenic agent that causes so many rearranged chromosomes due
to an exclusive breakage of the pericentromeric region with subsequent
reunion of different acrocentric partners. Whatever the mutagenic
agent might be, it was or is extremely successful in Italy, where it
has created more than 10 highly polymetacentric homozygous mouse populations (Fig. 2). Outside Italy almost all Rb populations are polymorphic with low numbers of Rb chromosomes. If the dynamics of

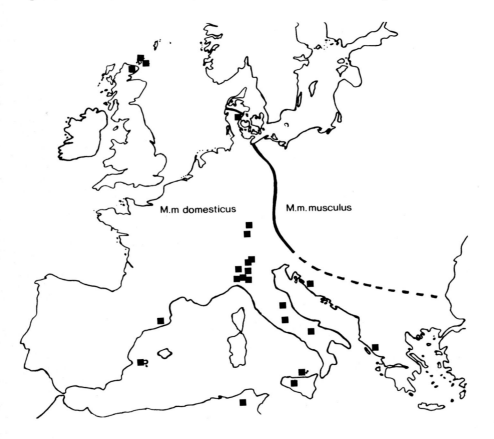

Fig. 2. Geographical map of Europe. Black squares indicate Rb populations. Solid/dashed line represents borderline of M. m. domesticus and
M. m. musculus (see Thaler et al. 1981)

generation and fixation are similar in the European habitat, the karyotypic evolution towards metacentric chromosomes has started much
earlier in Italy than elsewhere. Based on mtDNA analysis, Ferris et al.
(1983) have estimated the rate of Rb fixation to be 1 per 1 000 years
in the CD population of Central Italy. Surprisingly, the mtDNA of mice
from Central Italy is very similar to the mtDNA of Scandinavian animals.
These data suggest common ancestors for both populations that might
have diverged 20 000 to 40 000 years ago (Ferris et al. 1983). Whereas
in the CD population of Central Italy the process of Rb accumulation
has already been finished with the aquired status of Rb homozygosity
for nine pairs of metacentrics, this type of karyotype rearrangement
seems just to start close to and in contact with the hybridization zone
of musculus and domesticus in Southern Denmark. Reasonably the mutagenic
agent became first introduced into populations of Central and Northern
Italy and then has spread from there into regions outside Italy. Since
Rb populations in Western and Northern Europe are geographically
separated, a gradual expansion from Southern Europe to Western and
Northern Europe seems to be unlikely. Considering the geographical map
of Europe it becomes evident that almost all populations with Rb chromosomes outside Italy are located on shores or in coastal regions (Fig. 2).
This distribution pattern favours the assumption of spreading of the
mutagenic agent via ships on human trade routes. Moriwaki et al. (1984)
have claimed that mixing of "foreign" genomes could possibly induce Rb
exchange, since the only identified Rb chromosome of Japanese mice has
been discovered in a population contaminated with European house mice.
If this hypothesis is valid, the transfer of "foreign" mice via ships
into local populations of coastal areas could act as the mutagenic agent
in European wild mice.
I will now again focus on the mode of exchange. First of all, the data
concerning the generation of Rb chromosomes are in favour of an unidirectional process during karyotype evolution, whereby two acrocentric
chromosomes get fused into one metacentric chromosome. However, Crocker
and Cattanach (1981) were first to demonstrate a second type of rearrangement, the exchange between one Rb arm and an acrocentric autosome. This exchange occurred after X-ray exposure of a male homozygous
for three different Rb chromosomes. With this type of exchange the number
of chromosomes and metacentrics remains constant, but the composition
of one Rb chromosome is altered. A third mode of exchange may be an exchange between two arms of two different metacentric chromosomes,
leading to the formation of two differently composed metacentrics by
one mutational event. Evidence for the occurrence of this exchange type
comes from the observation of Rb multivalent rings in males homozygous
for eight pairs of Rb chromosomes of the Mil II type. In an attempt to
evaluate the number of chiasmata in wild mice, multivalent rings were
found in two out of four males tested. Among 100 diakinesis plates of
one male, seven plates showed an Rb ring composed of four metacentrics
and in one plate an Rb ring of six metacentrics was present. In one
further male one among 100 diakinesis plates showed the formation of
an Rb ring of four metacentrics. In the last two males only bivalents
were present. The meiotic multivalent rings in Rb homzygous males are
indistinguishable from those formed by interpopulation hybrids like
Mil I/Mil II (Fig. 3). The latter hybrid karyotype is characterized
by alternating arm homologies of the six following Rb chromosomes:
8.7/7.6/6.3/3.4/4.2/2.8. In prophase of meiosis I the homologous
Rb arms pair and owing to the present alternating arm homologies all
six Rb chromosomes become connected in one pairing unit. In diakinesis
the homologous arms are held together by chiasmata and a ring of six
Rb chromosomes is formed. The striking similarity of rings in meiotic
prophase of Rb homozygous and Rb heterozygous males suggest that in
both cases alternating arm homologies are responsible for this peculiar
phenomenon. Alternating arm homologies leading to a meiotic ring of four

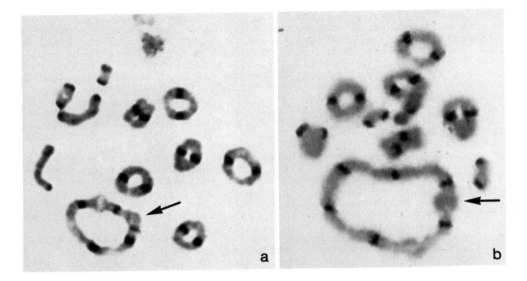

Fig. 3. C-banded dikinesis plates with multivalent rings. a) ring of four in an Rb homozygous male b) ring of six in an interpopulation hybrid. Arrow indicates multivalent

can be generated in an Rb homozygous individual by an intercentric exchange between two arms of two different chromosomes. The formation of a ring of six requires one additional exchange in such a way that both mutations affects the composition of one initial homologous Rb pair.

There is ample evidence that meiotic multivalent rings reduce the fertility of a carrier considerably due to high rates of meiotic non-disjunction leading to gametic and eventually to zygotic aneuploidy (Gropp et al. 1982). In the mouse whole arm aneuploidy is not compatible with postnatal viability. The reduction of fertility is strongly dependent on the rate of meiotic nondisjunction. Nevertheless, animals with meiotic rings, at least with small rings, are able to transmit to a certain extent a balanced haploid genome into viable zygotes. Thus this type of exchange can conserve the newly arisen mutated Rb chromosomes by propagation within a population. It seems likely that different karyotypes can emerge from each other by reorganization of already existing Rb chromosomes. Possibly the karyotypes of Mil I and Mil II have such an origin.
Two further points seem to be of interest. Firstly, the four Mil II males are derived from a stock that has been kept since five years in our laboratory on a wild mouse genomic background. During that time a contamination with mutagens can be excluded. Therefore the observed proneness to exchange whole arms seems to be more likely an inherent trait rather than caused by an environmental mutagen. Secondly, one has to ask, wether Rb generating mutations occur during or prior to meiosis. In order to explain the number of eight multivalents in one animal by meiotic breakage events, nine independent mutations at once have to be postulated. On the other hand, the appearance of eight multivalents can be explained with a minimum of two translocational events, if the mutations have taken place at the spermatogonia level very early during germ cell differentiation. It seems more realistic to favour the premeiotic exchange type.

It is not yet clear to what extent each type of whole arm exchange contributes to the diversification of the house mouse karyotype. There is no doubt about the predominant role of acrocentric-acrocentric fusion, but one should not neglect both other types of exchange, if chromosomal evolution of the house mouse is under discussion.

As stated above Rb heterozygosity may exert a detrimental effect on fertility of a carrier. There are several papers dealing with this type of impairment of fertility, but almost all data have been obtained from laboratory-bred individuals of wild and laboratory mice. It could well be that the results obtained from artificial hybrids bear no or little relation to the situation present in natural hybrids. In order to get the lacking information, the nondisjunction frequencies of six natural hybrids with one to three heterozygous Rb chromosomes without alternating arm homologies were estimated by MII-counts and by karyotypic analysis of 11 days old fetal enbryos in crosses with outbred females. The following Rb chromosomes were present heterozygously: 16.17(2x); 7.18(2x); 8.17; 2.8; 10.12; 3.4; 9.14;. By doubling the hypermodal MII counts the mean nondisjunction frequency per metacentric chromosome was estimated to be 2.2% with a range of 0% to 4% (n = 600 MII plates). Among 398 implants of pregnant females mated with natural Rb hybrids only one trisomic embryo could be identified. This is a yield of 0.25%. Assuming that every disomic sperm has a nullisomic counterpart, the nondisjunction rate can be calculated to be 0.5 %. There is no evidence that Rb heterozygous fathers produce more inviable implants than wild males without structural heterozygosities. The percentage of resorbed implants in crosses with Rb heterozygous males was 6.6± 4.4 (n = 398 implants) compared to 7.2 ± 4.3 (n = 485 implants, nine males tested) in control crosses. This shows that nondisjunction rates caused by Rb heterozygosities are very low in natural hybrids. Some of the Rb chromosomes have been retested again after introduction into a laboratory mouse genome. Interestingly, all Rb chromosomes produce within the laboratory mouse genome high rates of nondisjunction with estimates ranging from 20% to 40%.

The influence of the genetic background on nondisjunction and depression of fertility is apparent. More data are desirable to elucidate the impact of Rb heterozygosity on fertility of natural hybrids within the zone of contact between all acrocentric and polymetacentric mice

REFERENCES

Adolph S, Klein J (1981) Robertsonian variation in Mus musculus from
   Central Europe, Spain, and Scotland. J Hered 72:219-221
Adolph S, Klein J (1983) Genetic variation of wild mouse populations
   in Southern Germany. Genet Res 41:117-134
Britton-Davidian J (1983) Private communication. MNL 69:35
Brooker PC (1982) Robertsonian translocations in Mus musculus from
   N. E. Scotland and Orkney- Heredity 48:305-309
Comings DE, Avelino E (1972) DNA loss during Robertsonian fusion in
   studies of the tobacco mouse. Nature, New Biol 237: 199
Crocker C, Cattanach BM (1981) X-ray induction of translocations in
   mice carrying metacentrics (Robertsonian fusions); detection of
   whole arm chromosome exchanges. Mutation Res 91:353-357
Ferris SD, Sage RD, Prager EM, Ritte U, Wilson AC (1983) Mitochondrial
   DNA evolution in mice. Genetics 105:681-721
Gropp A, Winking H (1981) Robertsonian translocations: cytology meiosis,
   segregation patterns and biological consequences of heterozygosity.
   In: Berry RJ (ed) Biology of the house mouse. Academic Press, London,
   pp 141-181
Gropp A, Winking H, Redi C (1982) Consequences of Robertsonian hetero-

zygosity: Segregational impairment versus male-limited sterility.
In: Crosignani PG, Rubin S (eds) The genetic control of gamete
production and function. Academic Press, Grune & Stratton, pp 115-134
Hsu TC, Markvong A, Marshall JT (1978) G-band patterns of six species
of mice belonging to the subgenus Mus. Cytogenet Cell Genet 20:304-
307
Sage RD (1981) Wild mice.In: Foster HL, Small ID, Fox ID (eds) The
mouse in biomedical research. Academic Press, New York, pp 39-90
Said K, Jacquart T, Montgelard C, Sonjaja H, Helel AN, Britton-
Davidian (1985) Robertsonian house mouse populations in Tunesia:
A karyological and biochemical study. Genetica (in press)

Genetic Analysis of a Hybrid Zone Between Domesticus and Musculus Mice (*Mus musculus* Complex): Hemoglobin Polymorphisms

R.D. Sage, J.B. Whitney, III, and A.C. Wilson

INTRODUCTION

As a result of work by thousands of scientists, the laboratory mouse is the best known vertebrate animal after man. We have a very great understanding of its genetics and physiology. The wild ancestors of this domesticated mouse are also well studied (see reviews by Berry, 1981, and Sage, 1981). Increasing use of stocks of wild house mice indicates the utility of these animals in genetics and immunology (Huang et al., 1982; Arden and Klein, 1982; Dickinson et al., 1984; Nizětić et al., 1984; Robert et al., 1985; Rogers et al., 1985). Thus the mouse holds promise to become the model vertebrate from which a more profound understanding of the interactions of genetics, natural selection, and evolution will emerge.

Domesticus and Musculus in Europe

There is now agreement that the wild mice once lumped as a single species, <u>Mus musculus</u>, belong to two groups. One group of species lives free of mankind, and a second group is strongly commensal in habit. Substantial amounts of divergence at the molecular and morphological levels distinguish these two, ecologically different mouse groups (Britton and Thaler, 1978; Sage, 1978, 1981; Ferris et al., 1983b; Bonhomme et al., 1984). Nevertheless, fertile female hybrids can be made between all of these species. The great range of genetic variation represented in the <u>Mus musculus</u> complex is thus available for genetic analysis.

The commensal mice of Europe, with which this article deals, are further divisible into two closely related species that probably do not exchange genes at a significant rate in nature. One of these species, <u>M. domesticus</u>, lives in western Europe and around the Mediterranean Sea. (The most widely used strains of inbred laboratory mice are of this species.) The other species, <u>M. musculus</u>, lives in most of Scandinavia and eastern Europe (Fig. 1).

Genetic Units and Nomenclature

These two types of commensal mice are sometimes referred to as semi-species, but we regard them provisionally as separate species for both genetic and nomenclatorial reasons. There is strong evidence, from both protein and mitochondrial DNA comparisons, that their gene pools are separate (Sage, 1981; Ferris et al., 1983a, b; Bonhomme et al., 1984; Bishop et al., 1985; Wilson et al., 1985). Indeed, genetic factors cause sterility of male hybrids between these two kinds of

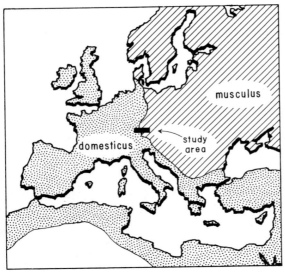

Fig. 1. Map of Europe showing the distribution of two
commensal species of house
mice, M. musculus and M.
domesticus. The limits of
their ranges abut, and hybrid populations form along
the boundary.

mice (Forejt and Iványi, 1975; Forejt, 1981; Sage, unpublished
observations). In addition, the International Code of Zoological
Nomenclature gives no satisfactory way of naming semispecies without
generating confusion as to whether one is referring to subspecies.

The following example epitomizes the problem. The wild populations of
mice living in western Europe and around the Mediterranean Sea have
long been divided taxonomically on the basis of coat color differences
(sometimes caused by genetic variation at only a single locus) into
three "subspecies", formerly known as M. m. domesticus (in the north),
M. m. brevirostris (central), and M. m. praetextus (in the south).
Bonhomme et al. (1984) refer to this group of "subspecies" as the
semispecies M. m. domesticus, which looks like a subspecies name and,
moreover, generates confusion as to whether one is referring to the
northern "subspecies" only or to the whole semispecies. Mayr (1970),
by contrast, uses the binomen, as we prefer, to name semispecies.

Both protein and mitochondrial DNA studies show that, whereas none of
the three "subspecies" appears to be a phylogenetic unit, the group
embracing all three is a well-circumscribed phylogenetic unit (Sage;
1981; Ferris et al., 1983b; Wilson et al., 1985). This domesticus
unit is equivalent in its amount of genetic diversity and phylogenetic
structure to (but entirely distinct genealogically from) the group of
populations of wild commensal mice ranging from eastern Europe across
northern Asia to Japan – the musculus unit (Wilson et al., 1985).

Geneticists have a legitimate and pressing need for a pair of simple
Latin names with which to refer accurately and unambiguously to these
two major genetic units. Mus domesticus and M. musculus are the least
cumbersome and most accurate names for these two genealogically
distinct groups of populations, between which there has been little
genetic exchange during the past million years (Wilson et al., 1985).

We support Ferris et al. (1983b) in preferring that, for now, no subspecies be recognized within M. domesticus. Taxonomic subdivision of
this genetic unit into three "subspecies" on the basis of coat color
receives no support from protein or mitochondrial DNA studies.

Hybrid Zone Between Domesticus and Musculus

This paper reports on the genetic consequences of contact between M. musculus and M. domesticus in southern Germany. These two kinds of mice meet in central and southern Europe (Fig. 1). Where they have been best studied, in Denmark and Germany, the two populations meet and form a narrow band of hybrid populations (Selander et al., 1969; Hunt and Selander, 1973; van Zegeren and van Oortmerssen, 1981; Ferris et al., 1983a).

The fact that domesticus and musculus hybridize where they meet does not necessarily imply that genes flow via hybrids from the gene pool of one species into that of the other. Rather, the hybrid zone may be a genetic sink. Genes certainly flow into the hybrid zone, but it does not follow that they get across the zone from one species into the other. The hybrid zone may be a region in which the mouse populations have a low growth rate, owing to incompatibility between the two gene pools. Male sterility is probably one manifestation of this incompatibility. Each gene pool may be protected against the influx of alien genes by the hybrid zone. By studying the hybrid zone between domesticus and musculus mice we hope to gain insights into the nature of the genetic barriers between species. For reviews of hybrid zones between closely related species, see Barton and Hewitt (1985) and White (1985).

We now present the first report on the genetic structure of the zone of contact between M. domesticus and M. musculus in central Europe, with particular reference to genes encoding the polypeptide chains of adult hemoglobin.

MATERIALS AND METHODS

Mice were collected across a 200 kilometer transect from western Austria into Bavaria, West Germany, where the ranges of M. musculus and M. domesticus are known to meet (Zimmermann, 1949; Kraft, 1985). Animals were collected in June and October, 1984, and June, 1985. To obtain tissue samples, animals were overdosed with sodium pentobarbital. Blood was collected in heparin, and plasma was separated from red cells by centrifugation. The red cells were then washed three times in isotonic saline (0.85 %) to remove residual plasma. The blood fractions and tissues (including kidneys) were frozen in liquid nitrogen. In the laboratory they were maintained at -76°C. Starch gel electrophoresis of plasma, hemolysate, and kidney extract was performed to determine genotypes at the β-globin locus (Hbb), and at four loci that had different alleles in the two species. The electrophoresis methods are described in Table 1 of Sage (1978): Esterase-1, plasma, buffer 3; Esterase-10, kidney, buffer 4; Nucleoside phosphorylase-1 and mannose-phosphate isomerase-1, kidney, buffer 5; and Hbb, hemolysate, buffer 9 (after cystamine treatment as described in Whitney, 1978). Alpha-globin variation was detected using the method of immobilized pH gradient, polyacrylamide gel isoelectric focusing as described by Whitney (1986). The starch-gel work was done in Berkeley by RDS, and the isoelectric focusing was performed in Augusta by JBW. A hybrid index was computed for each animal based on its genotypes at the four diagnostic loci. A -1 value was given for each musculus gene, and a +1 for each domesticus allele. Pure M. musculus and M. domesticus have the maximal values of -8 and +8, respectively.

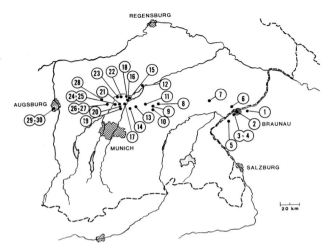

Fig. 2. Collecting localities of house mice in southern Germany and western Austria.

Mice were collected from 30 buildings in 26 different towns across the study area (Fig. 2). Two hundred and eleven mice were killed for tissues and carcasses soon after collection, and 130 animals were sent alive to Berkeley for breeding purposes. This report is based on the study of genotypes of 203 specimens. Complete data at all loci are not available for every mouse.

RESULTS

Analysis of the genotypes at the diagnostic loci shows a sharp transition from the musculus to the domesticus genome in the area just north of Munich. The mean hybrid indices for the 30 populations are listed in Table 1. Figure 3 shows how the index changes along an imaginary line transecting the region. There is an abrupt change from predominantly musculus to domesticus genotypes between localities 12 and 20. Over this distance of a little more than 20 kilometers the average hybrid index changes from about -6 to +6. The central, hybrid

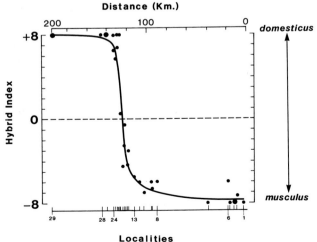

Fig. 3. Mean hybrid indices of 30 mouse populations. The samples are positioned along a line extending between Braunau, Austria, and Augsburg, Germany.

populations contain animals with mixed genotypes, rather than admixtures of pure M. musculus and M. domesticus individuals. This is illustrated in Fig. 4, where the hybrid indices of 26 animals from Neufarhn (locality 19) are portrayed.

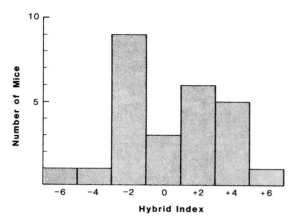

Fig. 4. Hybrid indices of 26 mice collected from one house in Neufahrn, Germany (locality 19). Low values reflect M. musculus genes, and high scores indicate the M. domesticus genome. The maximum possible scores are -8 and +8.

Table 1. The mean hybrid index (HI) and genotypes at the α- and β-globin loci from thirty collections of house mice. Localities 1-5 are in Austria and the others are in Germany

Local-ity[a]	HI	Alpha Locus (and number of mice)	Beta Locus ss	sd	dd
		Eastern Region			
1	-8	nn(1), dn(1), u-1(1)			
2	-7.3	cc[b](1), dn(1)	2	3	
3	-8	nn(1)	2	1	
4	-8	dn(1), u-2(1)	1		1
5	-8[c]	----		1	
6	-6.0	cc(1), nn(1), bn(1), cd(2), cn(1), u-1(1), u-3(1)	1	3	4
7	-8	nn(1)		1	
8	-6	nn(1)		1	
9	-6.6	nn(6), cd(2), cl(1), cn(1), ln(2)	6	4	3
10	-6[b]	----		1	
11	-7.0	cc(1), bn?(1)		2	
12	-6.0	nn(2)			2
		Hybrid Zone			
13	-5.5	nn(2), bn(2)		4	
14	-3.0	nn(1), bc?(1), cl(1), u-1(1)		3	1
15	-4.3	nn(4), cc(2), bc(2), cl(3), cn(5), u-1(1), u-4(1)	10	8	1
16	-0.5	bb(2), nn(1), bn(1)	3	1	
17	-4.5	cc(2), nn(1), bn(1), cd(1), cn(4), dn(1), u-1(3)	8	4	1
18	-2.5	cc(1), nn(1), cd(2)	1	2	1
19	+0.6	cc(13), dd(4), cd(14), cn(1), dn(4)	31	4	

Western Region

20	+6.7	cc(3), cn(2)	6
21	+8	cc(1)	1
22	+8	cc(1)	1
23	+5.7	cc(4), cn(1), u-2(1)	6
24	+6.5	cc(24), nn(1), dn(1)	25 3
25	+7.8	cc(5), cn(4), dn(1)	9 1
26	+8	cc(1), dn(2)	3
27	+8	cc(1)	1
28	+8	cc(1), dn(1)	2
29	+8	cc(3), ff(1), cf(3), ch(1)	8
30	+8	cc(5), cn(1)	6

a Locality names are: 1. Nöfing; 2. Braunau; 3. Ranshofen A; 4. Ranshofen B; 5. Königsaich; 6. Simbach; 7. Mitterskirchen; 8. Tauf-
kirchen; 9. Sonnendorf; 10. Högersdorf; 11. Tittenkofen; 12. Dorn-
haselbach; 13. Schwaig; 14. Gut Wildschwaig; 15. Rudlfing; 16.
Freising; 17. Achering; 18. Tüntenhausen; 19. Neufahrn; 20.
Massenhausen; 21. Giggenhausen; 22. Thalhausen; 23. Eberspoint; 24.
Gesselthausen A; 25. Gesselthausen B; 26. Kammerberg A; 27. Kammerberg B; 28. Ebersbach; 29. Augsburg A; 30. Augsburg B.
b Whitney et al. (1985) note that the c and p haplotypes are indistinguishable by electrophoresis, but differ in their solubility.
Thus, our assignment of the c genotype to all of our electromorphic
patterns is somewhat ambiguous. A more complete analyis of "c"
hapolotypes through breeding studies of wild-caught transect mice is
underway.
c Extrapolated from the three loci examined.

There are also globin differences between the two species of mice.
Table 1 lists the observed genotypes at the alpha and beta loci. Table
2 summarizes the α-locus haplotypes for an eastern, central, and
western grouping of the samples. We found considerable variation at
the α-locus. Seven of the previously described haplotypes (Whitney et
al., 1985) were found in transect mice. The c and n haplotypes were
most frequent. On the eastern side of the contact line n predominates
over c, but in the west there is a reversal in relative frequency of
these two haplotypes. In the eastern region the frequency of the n
haplotype is 0.58 and 0.22 for c. On the western side of the transect
(localities 20-30) the frequency of n declines to only 0.11, and c
increases to 0.81. The central, hybrid populations have more equal

Table 2. Alpha-globin haplotype frequencies for mice from the eastern region (localities 1-12), the hybrid zone (localities 13-19),
and the western region (localities 20-30) of the Bavarian study area.
Cases with unidentified haplotypes were exluded from the calculations

Region	No. of Mice	Frequency of α-globin haplotypes						
		c	n	d	b	l	f	h
Eastern	30	0.22	0.58	0.12	0.03	0.05		
Hybrid Zone	77	0.45	0.25	0.19	0.07	0.03		
Western	68	0.81	0.11	0.04			0.04	0.01

frequencies of these two haplotypes (Table 2). The d haplotype occurs at lower frequencies in populations from all three regions. The remaining four identified haplotypes are present at still lower frequencies. The b and l haplotypes each occur at about five percent frequency in the eastern and central regions. The f and h haplotypes were present only in Augsburg mice (localities 29 and 30).

Some of the observed phenotypes on the gels did not correspond to the known or predicted haplotype patterns found in laboratory mice (Whitney et al., 1985). Seven percent of the 184 samples could not be assigned positive genotypes. These 12 samples had four different phenotypes on the gels, and were arbitrarily identified as u-1 through u-4 in Table 1. They have two or three bands on the gels. One of them, u-1, is three-banded, and presumably represents a heterozygous genotype.

Variation at the β-locus also shows regional differences. In the musculus mice on the east side of the transect, both the s and d chains are present, but in the western, domesticus mice, only the s haplotype occurs (Table 1).

The greatest changes in frequencies of both α- and β-genes occur in the hybrid zone. This is illustrated in Fig. 5, which shows how two of the major alleles have their most abrupt changes in abundance between kilometers 110 and 130. This is the same region where the four diagnostic loci undergo nearly all of their frequency changes (Fig. 3). Thus, these six loci, which are on five separate chromosomes, all show concordant changes in frequency across a short distance of about twenty kilometers.

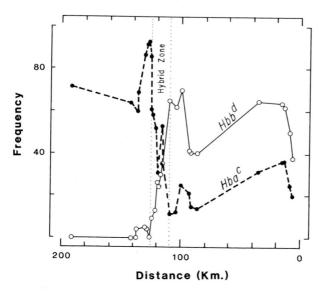

Fig. 5. The average frequencies of the c allele of the α-locus, and the d haplotype of the β-locus across the Bavarian study area.

DISCUSSION

Intensive studies have made the globin gene regions the best known genetic systems of the mouse. The composition of the DNA sequences

(Leder et al., 1980; Leder et al., 1981; Edgell et al., 1983; Erhart et al., 1985), the polypeptide structure (Popp, 1973; Popp and Bailiff, 1973; Popp et al., 1982; Whitney et al., 1985), chromosomal location, in-vitro physiological kinetics (Newton and Peters, 1983), and electrophoretically detectable variability in wild populations (Selander et al., 1969; Berry and Peters, 1977; Britton and Thaler, 1978; Sage, 1978; Minezawa, et al., 1979; Britton-Davidian et al., 1980; Berry et al., 1981; Thaler et al., 1981; Ritte and Neufeld, 1982) are known.

Beta Locus

Two genes, located on chromosome 7, encode the adult β-globin chains (Edgell et al., 1983). Four different haplotypes exist among the commensal house mice, and three of these are readily distinguishable by electrophoresis of the proteins they encode (Whitney, 1978). Surveys of populations of domesticus, musculus, and Japanese molossinus mice show characteristic frequency differences among these three electromorphs. The p-haplotype is common in Japan, and maybe as far west as Israel. But, it is absent from mouse populations to the west and north in Europe. In M. musculus from northern Denmark (Selander et al., 1969), Austria and Yugoslavia (Sage, unpublished observations), and Romania (Thaler et al., 1981), the s and d haplotypes are present in about equal frequencies. The western European, domesticus mice of England (Berry and Peters, 1977), France (Britton and Thaler, 1978), Spain (Sage, 1978), and Italy (Britton-Davidian et al., 1980) have a predominance of the s over the d electromorph.

Across the Bavarian transect the frequencies of the s and d alleles change in a manner consistent with the distributions of these haplotypes in other European populations of musculus and domesticus mice. That is, on the eastern side of the study area both alleles are present (Table 1). But, beginning in the central region the d electromorph declines in abundance, and is absent west of locality 25 (Fig. 5). A reasonable interpretation of this pattern is that the disappearence of the d haplotype on the western side of the study area is due to the absence of the chromosome 7 of M. musculus bearing these genes. Although more samples must be examined to substantiate the hypothesis, these first results suggest that the domesticus mice of southern Germany, which bear metacentric chromomosomes (Adolph and Klein, 1983; Adolph, 1984), lack the d haplotype.

Alpha Locus

The α-globin locus, on chromosome 11, includes two genes in tandem that produce functional polypeptides in adult mice (Leder et al., 1981). Eight haplotypes, detectable by isoelectric focusing, are reported in inbred, laboratory strains, and five others were found in wild-derived stocks of mice identifiable as M. domesticus, M. musculus, and M. molossinus (Whitney et al., 1985). These 13 haplotypes are constructed from combinations of five, distinctive, polypeptide chains. This makes the α-globin complex the most polymorphic "locus" that can be studied by simple laboratory techniques. This is the first large-scale study on α-globin variation in wild mouse populations. Our results suggest that these two mouse species still share haplotypes that were polymorphic in their common ancestor, e.g. the c, n, and d types. Yet, it appears that musculus and domesticus mice differ in the average frequencies of their most common haplotypes, e.g., the n chromosome may be most frequent in M.

musculus, while c is the most frequent form in M. domesticus. Some of the less common alleles may be characteristic of one or the other species. From this first study it appears that the b and l haplotypes occur only in M. musculus, and f and h are unique to the domesticus genome.

This populational survey of α-globin variation also suggests that the maximum chain diversity of this gene complex may not be much greater than what is now reported. No new isoelectric-point classes were observed among our 200 samples. Furthermore, surveys of domesticus mice from Greece, Yugoslavia, Italy, Switzerland, and other parts of Germany revealed no new haplotypes (Whitney, Tichy, and Sage, unpublished observations). These results indicate that for twelve samples, which we could not assign to currently known haplotypes, the patterns are not caused by new substitutions at the DNA level. More likely, they represent products of intergenic recombination. Also, further study is likely to show that these haplotypes are characteristic of the eastern, musculus mice, rather than M. domesticus. This is suggested by their more frequent occurrence on the eastern side of our study area, where the M. musculus genome predominates.

SUMMARY AND CONCLUSIONS

Based on protein and mtDNA divergence patterns, the domesticus gene pool has been diverging from the musculus gene pool for over one million years. These gene pools meet in central Europe, forming a narrow band of hybrid populations. Electrophoretic analysis of diagnostic proteins from over 200 mice trapped in a transect across the hybrid zone in Bavaria shows an abrupt and concordant transition of many genes across a 20 kilometer distance. Other features, such as the mitochondrial DNAs, chromosomes, sterility genes, and morphology also shift in the same place as do the proteins encoded by the nuclear DNA (Sage and Wilson, unpublished observations). Our protein electrophoretic examination of the loci coding for adult hemoglobins shows that they resemble these other genetic systems in their population structure. An allele (d) at the β-locus, present at high frequency in the east, disappears on the western (domesticus) side of the study area. Conversely, an allele (c) at the α-locus that is common in the west becomes relatively rare in the east. The mid-point of these globin transitions occurs at the same place where the alternate, diagnostic proteins change. This first, large survey of alpha locus variability in 200 wild mice suggests that most of the polypeptide chains in the commensal group of species have already been discovered in inbred strains and laboratory stocks of wild mice.

ACKNOWLEDGEMENTS

We thank the many people who allowed RDS to trap mice in their buildings. Without the field support of Mr. F. Seidl, Drs. I. Butler, K. Damme, J. Klein, R. Kraft, H. Tichy, and F. Pirchner this work could not have been accomplished. The National Science Foundation funded this study.

REFERENCES

Adolph S (1984) Robertsonsche Translokationen bei württembergischen
    Hausmäusen (Mus musculus domesticus) -Ein Beispiel zur Chromosomen-
    evolution. Jh Ges Naturkde Wurtt 139:67-92
Adolph S, Klein J (1983) Genetic variation of wild mouse populations
    in southern Germany I. Cytogenetic study. Genet Res Camb 41:117-134
Arden B, Klein J (1982) Biochemical comparison of major histocompat-
    ibility complex molecules from different subspecies of Mus musculus:
    Evidence for trans-specific evolution of alleles. Proc Natl Acad Sci
    USA 79:2342-2346
Barton NH, Hewitt GM (1985) Analysis of hybrid zones. Ann Rev Ecol Syst
    16:113-148
Berry RJ (1981) Town mouse, country mouse: adaptation and adaptability
    in Mus domesticus (M. musculus domesticus). Mamm Rev 11:91-136
Berry RJ, Peters J (1977) Heterogeneous heterozygosities in Mus
    musculus populations. Proc R Soc Lond B 197:485-503
Berry RJ, Sage RD, Lidicker WZ, Jackson WB (1981) Genetical variation
    in three Pacific house mouse (Mus musculus) populations. J Zool,
    Lond 193:391-404
Bishop CE, Boursot P, Baron B, Bonhomme F, Hatat D (1985) Most
    classical Mus musculus domesticus laboratory mouse strains carry a
    Mus musculus musculus Y chromosome. Nature 315:70-72
Bonhomme F, Catalan J, Britton-Davidian J, Chapman VM, Moriwaki K,
    Nevo E, Thaler L (1984) Biochemical diversity and evolution in the
    genus Mus. Biochem Genet 22:275-303
Britton J, Thaler L (1978) Evidence for the presence of two sympatric
    species of mice (genus Mus L.) in southern France based on
    biochemical genetics. Biochem Genet 16:213-225
Britton-Davidian J, Bonhomme F, Croset H, Capanna E, Thaler L (1980)
    Variabilité génétique chez les populations de souris (genre Mus L.)
    à nombre chromosomique réduit. C R Acad Sci, Paris 290:195-198
Dickinson DP, Gross KW, Piccini N, Wilson CM (1984) Evolution and var-
    iation of renin genes in mice. Genetics 108:651-667
Edgell MH, Hardies SC, Brown B, Voliva C, Hill A, Phillips S, Comer M,
    Burton F, Weaver S, Hutchison CA, III (1983) Evolution of the mouse
    ß globin complex locus. In: Nei M, Koehn RK (eds) Evolution of Genes
    and Proteins. Sinauer Assoc., Sunderland, Mass p 1
Erhart MA, Simons KS, Weaver S (1985) Evolution of the mouse ß -Globin
    genes: A recent gene conversion in the Hbb[s] haplotype. Mol Biol Evol
    2:304-320
Ferris, SD, Sage RD, Huang C-M, Nielsen JT, Ritte U, Wilson AC (1983a)
    Flow of mitochondrial DNA across a species boundary. Proc Natl Acad
    Sci USA 80:2290-2294
Ferris SD, Sage RD, Prager EM, Ritte U, Wilson AC (1983b) Mitochon-
    drial DNA evolution in mice. Genetics 105:681-721
Forejt, J (1981) Hybrid sterility gene located in the T/t H-2
    supergene on chromosome 17. In: Reisfeld, RA, Ferrone S (eds)
    Current Trends in Histocompatibility, vol 1. Plenum Press, New York,
    London, p 103
Forejt J, Iványi P (1975) Genetic studies on male sterility of hybrids
    between laboratory and wild mice (Mus musculus L.). Genet Res, Camb
    24:189-206
Huang C-M, Parsons M, Wakeland EK, Moriwaki K, Herzenberg LA (1982)
    New immunoglobulin IgG allotypes and haplotypes found in wild mice
    with monoclonal anti-allotope antibodies. J Immunol 128:661-667
Hunt WG, Selander RK (1973) Biochemical genetics of hybridisation in
    European house mice. Heredity 31:11-33
Kraft R (1985) Merkmale und Verbreitung der Hausmäuse Mus musculus
    musculus L., 1758, und Mus musculus domesticus Rutty, 1772
    (Rodentia, Muridae) in Bayern. Säugetk Mitt 32:1-12
Leder A, Swan D, Ruddle F, D'Eustachio P, Leder P (1981) Dispersion of

α-like globin genes of the mouse to three different chromosomes. Nature 293:196-200

Leder P, Hansen JN, Konkel D, Leder A, Nishioka Y, Talkington C (1980) Mouse globin system: A functional and evolutionary analysis. Science 209:1336-1342

Mayr E (1970) Populations, Species, and Evolutions. Belknap Press, Cambridge

Minezawa M, Moriwaki K, Kondo K (1979) Geographical distribution of HbbP allele in the Japanese wild mouse, Mus musculus molossinus. Jpn J Genet 54:165-173

Newton MF, Peters J (1983) Physiological variation of mouse haemoglobins. Proc R Soc Lond B 218:443-453

Nizetić D, Figueroa F, Klein J (1984) Evolutionary relationships between the t and H-2 haplotypes in the house mouse. Immunogenetics 19:311-320

Popp RA (1973) Sequence of amino acids in the β chain of single hemoglobins from C57BL, SWR, and NB mice. Biochim Biophys Acta 303:52-60

Popp RA, Bailiff EG (1973) Sequence of amino acids in the major and minor β chains of the diffuse hemoglobin from BALB/c mice. Biochim Biophys Acta 303:61-67

Popp RA, Bailiff EG, Skow LC, Whitney JB III (1982) The primary structure of genetic variants of mouse hemoglobin. Biochem Genet 20:199-208

Ritte U, Neufeld E (1982) East Asian hemoglobin type (HbbP) in wild populations of the house mouse in Israel. Biochem Genet 20:475-481

Robert B, Barton P, Minty A, Daubas P, Weydert A, Bonhomme F, Catalan J, Chazottes D, Guénet J-L, Buckingham M (1985) Investigation of genetic linkage between myosin and actin genes using an interspecific mouse back-cross. Nature 314:181-183

Rogers MJ, Germain RN, Hare J, Long E, Singer DS (1985) Comparison of MHC genes among distantly related members of the genus Mus. J Immunol 134: 630-636

Sage RD (1978) Genetic heterogeneity of Spanish house mice (Mus musculus complex). In: Morse HC, III (ed) Origins of Inbred Mice. Academic Press, New York, p 519

Sage RD (1981) Wild mice. In: Foster HL, Small JD, Fox JG (eds) The Mouse in Biomedical Research, vol 1. Academic Press, New York, p 39

Selander RK, Hunt WG, Yang SY (1969) Protein polymorphism and genic heterozygosity in two European subspecies of the house mouse. Evolution 23: 379-390

Thaler L, Bonhomme F, Britton-Davidian J, Hamar M (1981) The house mouse complex of species: Sympatric occurrence of biochemical groups Mus 2 and Mus 4 in Rumania. Z Säugetk 46:169-173

van Zegeren K, van Oortmerssen GA (1981) Frontier disputes between the West- and East-European house mouse in Schleswig-Holstein, West Germany. Z Säugetk 46:363-369

White MJD (1985) Types of hybrid zones. Boll Zool 52:1-20

Whitney JB III (1978) Simplified typing of mouse hemoglobin (Hbb) phenotypes using cystamine. Biochem Genet 16:667-672

Whitney JB III (1986) Immobilized gradient isoelectric focusing: Detection of "silent" biochemical genetic variants. Curr Top Microbiol Immunol, in press

Whitney JB III, Cobb RR, Popp RA, O'Rourke TW (1985) Detection of neutral amino acid substitutions in proteins. Proc Natl Acad Sci USA 82:7646-7650

Wilson, AC, Cann RL, Carr SM, George M, Gyllensten UB, Helm-Bychowski KM, Higuchi RG, Palumbi SR, Prager EM, Sage RD, Stoneking M (1985) Mitochondrial DNA and two perspectives on evolutionary genetics. Biol J Linn Soc 26: 375-400

Zimmermann K (1949) Zur Kenntnis der mitteleuropäischen Hausmäuse. Zool Jahrb Abt Syst (Oekol) Geogr Tiere 78:301-322

Genetical Processes in Wild Mouse Populations. Past Myth and Present Knowledge

R.J. Berry

INTRODUCTION

There is a widely accepted misconception that natural house mouse populations are rigid mosaics of small inbred demes which resist immigration and allow random spread and survival of inherited variation because of their small size and vulnerability to extinction. This myth is understandable, because there is a large amount of data apparently supporting it. Nevertheless it is a misleading perversion of the true situation. This paper is an attempt to provide a more accurate description of the processes that mould mouse populations, and the resulting consequences for the distribution of genetic variants.

The common perception of the population structure of wild mice is well illustrated by the conclusion drawn by Klein (1975) from a review of forty published studies:

"These sources reveal that the mouse population is divided into small subpopulations or demes (breeding units, family units, tribes, colonies), ... occupying not larger than a few square meters .... An average deme consists of 7-12 adult mice."
Ford and Evans (1973) drew a very similar conclusion from their consideration of the origin of mouse chromosomal races characterized by Robertsonian (centric) fusions, which they saw as arising "by chance survival and matings in a very small isolate, despite the infertility of heterozygotes, followed by subsequent expansion with minimal hybridization". De Fries and McClearn (1972) judged likewise: "It is quite conceivable that the effective population size in natural populations of house mice is less than four..... With such a small effective population size, random drift would be an important factor in determining allelic frequencies in local populations" (see also Blair, 1953; Ehrlich and Raven, 1969).

Despite this weight of expert opinion, mouse populations are commonly far less socially rigid and genetically fortuitous than would appear from the above quotations. The house mouse is a weed species, and like all good weeds combines short term inflexibility (and susceptibility to inter-specific competition: Berry and Tricker, 1969; Dueser and Brown, 1980), with longer term adaptability. This adaptability can sometimes be inferred from cross-sectional population surveys but is best investigated in studies lasting several generations. Such studies are necessary to an adequate understanding of the factors which affect the maintenance of polymorphic systems in mouse populations.

SOCIAL CHURNING AND SUCESSFUL IMMIGRATION

There is no doubt that most mouse populations are divided into small, individually defended demes (although high density and resource limitation may interact to disrupt this structure). In stable (usually commensal) populations, a territory holder tends to be replaced by one of his or her own offspring. The extreme of this situation is the hillock mouse (Mus hortulanus) of the Ukraine (Naumov, 1940). In the autumn of each year the adults of a pair gather a supply of weed seeds for the winter. At the beginning of the winter each "hillock" is occupied by a pair of adults and their last litter of the season. There is a high likelihood that the adults will die during the winter, resulting in the territory being taken over by members of the same family.

However, virtually every longitudinal study of mice living in a reasonable stressful environment has shown a degree of population churning. For example, Lidicker (1976) found a small amount of gene flow between established social groups, and more extensive genetic mixing through the formation of new social groups. Similar results have been obtained by Myers (1974a) Stickel (1979), Baker (1981), King (1982), Singleton and Hay (1983), etc. In a seven-year release-recapture experiment on a small Welsh island, Berry and Jakobson (1974) showed that most adult animals were faithful to a locality for extended periods, but more than a quarter of the mice bred at a site other than the one at which they were born. The maximum number of animals in a single group seemed to be about six, but the composition of all groups changed constantly because of the relatively high mortality at all ages (life expectation at birth was c.100 days, compared with over two years in commensal populations: Bellamy, Berry, Jakobson, Lidicker, Morgan and Murphy, 1973; Takada, 1985).

An important experiment was carried out by Anderson, Dunn and Beasley (1964). They released t-heterozygous male mice onto Great Gull Island (7.5 ha) in Long Island Sound, where no t-allele was present. Their expectation was that the introduced t-allele (haplotype) would increase in frequency because of its 95 per cent transmission rate by males (Lewontin and Dunn, 1960). In fact, the t-allele spread very slowly and eventually became extinct (Myers 1974b); Anderson et al (1964) concluded that "social and ecological factors" limited its spread.It is now known that the assumption of no fitness deficit in the heterozygotes was incorrect (Pennycuik, Johnston, Lidicker and Westwood, 1978; Lenington, 1983), but more potently, another island introduction experiment (of mice from Eday in Orkney to the Isle of May in the Firth of Forth, Scotland) led to the rapid spread of introduced allozymes and Robertsonian fusions reaching apparent equilibrium within three years (Berry, Nash and Triggs, unpublished).

A further complication of social dynamics is that there is now clear evidence that female and probably male mice can distinguish between genotypes at both the H-2 and T loci by urinary odour, and choose their mates by discriminating against t/+ heterozygotes and animals of the same H-2 haplotype as themselves (Yamazaki, Boyse, Mike, Thales, Mathieson, Abbott, Boyse, Zayas and Thomas, 1976; Levine, Rockwell and Grassfield, 1980; Boyse, Beauchamp and Yamazaki, 1983; Lenington, 1983; Lenington and Egid, 1983). Pregnancy blockage (i.e. failure of implantation, the "Bruce effect") is increased when pregnant females are exposed to males of a different H-2 type than their mate, indicating that the ability to chemo-recognize H-2 genotypes affects hormonal status (Yamazaki, Beauchamp, Wysocki, Bard, Thomas and Boyse, 1983). Such non-random mating will tend to increas diversity at the H-2 locus (and incidentally reduce inbreeding) and lead to selection against t-alleles.

The unequivocal conclusion from population and breeding studies is that social structure affects gene flow, but that its effect is impermanent, depending on both habitat and genotype; mouse populations behave as completely panmictic units under many conditions and the rigidity of exclusive deme organization is only temporary for any natural mouse line.

NATURAL SELECTION versus NEUTRALITY

Early genetic studies indicated that inherited variants had no effect on fitness in mouse populations: Philip (1938) and Petras (1967) calculated significant heterozygous deficiencies at a number of loci in mice trapped in coal mines and farm buildings; Selander (1970) found that the frequencies of genetic variants were distributed apparently randomly in dense populations living in chicken barns. In contrast, Berry and Murphy (1970) reported that such changes only occurred in seasons when such stress was operating; the important stress seemed to be low temperature (Berry and Jakobson, 1975). Petras and Topping (1983) calculated that the fitnesses of the two heterozygotes at a segregating haemoglobin locus (Hbb) in Berry and Murphy's data were 0.49 and 0.24 (compared to 1.00 for the heterozygote). Newton and Peters (1983) showed that the haemoglobins produced by the alleles involved had different oxygen-binding characteristics.

Confirmation of the link between selection intensity and ecological stress was obtained by Berry, Sage, Lidicker and Jackson (1980), who found no sign of natural selection operating in feral mice trapped in Hawaii or Enewetak Atoll where there was a relatively invariant temperature of c. 25°C, whereas significant allelic differences attributable only to natural selection occurred on the sub-Antarctic Macquarie and Marion Islands (Berry and Peters, 1975; Berry, Peters and Van Aarde, 1978). However, the most intriguing situation was discovered on South Georgia (mean monthly temperature ranging from 4.3°C to -2.5°C), where selection produced genetic changes operating in opposite directions in males and females (Table I) (Berry, Bonner and Peters, 1979).

Table I. Frequencies of $Got-2^a$ in South Georgia mice

	Males	Females
Younger than 3 months	0.159±0.055	0.364±0.073
Older than 3 months	0.350±0.075	0.190±0.061

Most of the change in males took place around the time they would be expected to leave the natal area and establish their own territory; the change in females extended over a longer period.

These results indicate that natural selection may produce rapid and precise adaptive changes in house mouse populations in particular environments (see also Myers, 1974a; Bryant, 1974; Berry and Peters, 1977; Petras and Topping, 1983). Probably most loci have no affect on fitness for most of the time, but clearly high selection intensities may occasionally operate and regulate allele frequencies (Berry, 1978). Such intermittent bouts of selection will have a persisting effect on allele frequencies and levels of polymorphism (Haldane and Jayakar, 1963; Nevo, 1983a, b).

A completely different series of investigations shows also the apparent interaction of chance and adaptation in mouse populations. In 1970, Gropp, Tettenborn and Von Lehmann reported that an isolated Alpine race of house mice ("Mus poschiavinus") had seven pairs of metacentric chromosomes, representing fusions involving fourteen acrocentric elements. Since that time, a large number of chromosome races with different numbers of fusions have been described, mainly in southern Europe (Capanna, 1980; Adolph and Klein, 1981). Any chromosome except the sex chromosomes may be associated with any other. (Fusions involving chromosome 19 have been found only in laboratory stocks). The initial spread of a fresh centric fusion has been claimed to depend on inbreeding within a family unit (Lande, 1979; Sprito, Modesti, Perticone, Cristaldi, Federici and Rizzoni, 1980). However, the finding that pairing behaviour is affected by genotype, and that other behavioural changes may arise from chromosomal alterations (Schroder and Otten, 1985, have reported that an induced 10, 13 reciprocal translocation increased aggressiveness in male heterozygotes) could mean that centric fusions may increase in frequency as a result of preferential mating.

Crosses involving Robertsonian heterozygotes are detrimental, because they involve some gametic or zygotic loss. Consequently, there could be selection for homozygotes. Larson, Prager and Wilson (1984) have argued that the rate of fixation for chromosomal fusions is so rapid that either mutator activity is involved, or that fusions may change social behaviour. The occurrence together of multiple Robertsonian fusions in some populations suggests that a form of mutator may sometimes operate.

The existence of a mechanism facilitating the spread of Robertsonian chromosomes is a necessary inference from the situation in Caithness, Scotland where every mouse examined in the whole of the county (177,400 hectares) has at least two homozygous pairs of fusions (6-13, 9-12); an area in the north-east of the country is also homozygous for 11-17 or both 11-17 and 4-10; a neighbouring area has chromosome 10 fused with chromosome 14. Ten other fusions have been found in single samples, all but two confined to the north-eastern area (Fig. 1) (Brooker, 1982). In the nearby Orkney archipelago eight islands have the usual 2n=40 karyotype; one has two homozygous fusions (6-14, 9-12); one has three (3-14, 4-10, 9-12); one is homozygous for 3-14, 9-12, but is segregating for 4-10 (Nash, Brooks and Davis, 1983, and unpublished). Robertsonian 9-12 is universal in Caithness but 3-14 and 6-14 have not been reported there. No other centric fusions have been found in Britain; Caithness is isolated from mice in the neighbouring county by high moorland where house mice are excluded by Apodemus sylvaticus. The distribution of fused chromosomes in Caithness and Orkney seems inexplicable on the basis of random spread; either natural selection or some "drive" mechanism must be operating.

CONCLUSIONS

Workers who concern themselves mainly with the polymorphism of H-2 haplotypes argue about whether they represent a true polymorphism or whether they are nothing more than a complex of linked loci of similar effect; about stabilizing or frequency-dependent selection, "hitch-hiking", or high mutation rates; and what are the evolutionary rates and relationships between different haplotypes (Klein, 1975, 1979; Nadeau, Collins and Klein, 1982; Miyada, Klofelt, Reyes, McLaughlin-Taylor, 1985; Figueroa, Golubic, Nizetic and Klein, 1985). Some of these questions will be helped by continuing progress in molecular biology and immunology, but a full understanding of the genetical processes operating in mouse populations can only come from a symbiosis of laboratory and population workers (Berry, 1981; Sage, 1981). The unexpected finding of Mus domesticus mitochondrial DNA in M. musculus animals is a good example of the value of such research complementation (Ferris, Sage, Huang, Nielsen, Ritte and Wilson, 1983).

Mouse populations outside the laboratory are far less predictable than their conventional caricature. Migration and adaptation are opportunistic and stochastic processes, and theories based on the analysis of a few animals (or a few legths of DNA) can be grossly misleading. Huxley (1942) believed that the differentiation of mice on the Faroe Islands ("Mus faeroensis") in the 1000 years since the earliest possible date of introduction (by Vikings) gave an upper limit to all rates of evolution. Further study showed that mice colonized one of the islands sometime after 1940, and yet are as distinct from the other Faroe races as the latter are from mainland animals (Berry, Jakobson and Peters, 1978). Comparison of the differences between the island populations suggests that most of the differentiation has been the result of the chance collection of alleles carried by the founding animals. Any subsequent adaptation (or other processes) can only operated on those fortuitous variants. It is

90

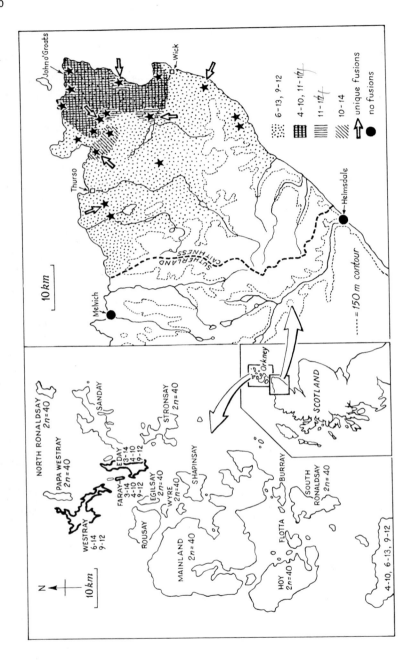

Fig 1. The distribution of Robertsonian chromosomes in Caithness and Orkney

meaningless to calculate evolutionary rates for divergence in such a
situation, because the relative contribution of the founder effect is always
unknown (Berry, 1983). Mice, particularly Mus domesticus, have been
commonly transported enormous distances in association with humans, and
chance differentiation between populations is a normal finding (Moriwaki,
Yonekawa, Gotoh, Minezawa, Winking and Gropp, 1984).

However, it would be wrong to end by over-emphasizing the role of
chance in mouse population dynamics. Natural selection has been shown to
produce genetical changes of a much greater extent than was envisaged before
natural populations were studied genetically. And to this evidence of
adaptation at individual loci (or more accurately, chromosomal segments)
must be added the conservative effect of strong associations between both
linked and unlinked loci in established populations (Berry, Nash and Newton,
in preparation). This strengthens the suggestion repeatedly made from
studies of divergence between inbred strains, that some heterozygositymay
persist despiteintense inbreeding (Deol, Grüneberg, Searle and Truslove,
1960; Wallace, 1965; Whitmore and Whitmore, 1985; Fitch and Atchley, 1985).

The "neutralist" controversy of the 1970s produced a more sensible
recognition of the contributions of chance and selection than existed before
(Berry, 1982). At one time, mouse populations were regarded as almost
paradigmatic of neutral evolution. This interpretation is obviously untrue,
as is the opposite conclusion that all allele frequencies are wholly
controlled by natural selection. The urgent need now is to test the fertile
speculation of many eminent scientists to discover how variation –
especially on chromosome 17- affects fitness under different conditions.

REFERENCES

ADOPLH S. and KLEIN J. (1981) Robertsonian variation in Mus musculus from
    Central Europe, Spain and Scotland. J. Hered. 72 219-221.
ANDERSON P.K., DUNN L.C. and BEASLEY A.B. (1964) Introduction of a lethal
    allele into a feral house mouse population. Am.Nat. 98 57-64
BAKER A.E.M. (1981) Gene flow in house mice: introduction of a new allele
    into free-living populations. Evolution 35 243-58
BELLAMY D., BERRY, R.J., JAKOBSON, M.E., LIDICKER, W.Z., MORGAN, J. and
    MURPHY H.M. (1973) Ageing in an island population of the house mouse.
    Age and Ageing 2 235-50
BERRY R.J. (1978) Genetic variation in wild house mice: where natural
    selection and history meet. Am. Scientist 66 52-60
BERRY R.J. (ed) (1981) The Biology of the House Mouse. London and New
    York: Academic
BERRY R.J. (1982) Neo-Darwinism. London: Edward Arnold
BERRY R.J. (1983) Diversity and differentiation: the importance of island
    biology for general theory. Oikos 41 523-29
BERRY R.J., BONNER W.N. and PETERS, J. (1979) Natural selection in mice
    from South Georgia (South Atlantic Ocean). J. Zool. Lond. 189 385-98
BERRY R.J. and JAKOBSON M.E. (1974) Vagility in an island population of the
    house mouse. J. Zool. Lond. 173 341-54
BERRY R.J. and JAKOBSON M.E. (1975) Ecological genetics of an island
    population of the house mouse. J. Zool. Lond. 175 523-40
BERRY R.J., JAKOBSON M.E. and PETERS J. (1978) The house mouse of the
    Faroe Islands: a study in microdifferentiation. J. Zool. Lond. 185
    73-92
BERRY R.J. and MURPHY H.M. (1970) Biochemical genetics of an island
    population of the house mouse. Proc. R. Soc. B 176 87-103

BERRY R.J. and PETERS J. (1975) Macquarie Island house mice: a genetical isolate on a sub-Antarctic island. J. Zool. Lond. 176 375-89

BERRY R.J. and PETERS J. (1977) Heterogeneous heterozygosities in Mus muculus populations. Proc. R. Soc. Lond. B 197 485-503

BERRY R.J., PETERS J. and VAN AARDE R.J. (1978) Sub-Antarctic house mice: colonization, survival and selection. J. Zool. Lond. 184 127-141

BERRY R.J., SAGE R.D., LIDICKER W.Z. and JACKSON W.B. (1980) Genetical variation in three Pacific house mouse populations. J. Zool. Lond. 193 391-404

BERRY R.J. and TRICKER B.J.K. (1969) Competition and extinction: the mice of Foula, with notes on those of Fair Isle and St Kilda. J. Zool. Lond. 158 247-65

BLAIR W.F. (1953) Population dynamics of rodents and other small mammals. Adv. Genet. 5 1-41.

BOYSE E.A., BEAUCHAMP G.K. and YAMAZAKI K. (1983) Critical review: the sensory perception of genotypic polymorphism of the Major Histocompatibility Complex and other genes: some physiological and phylogenetic implications. Hum. Immunol. 6, 177-84.

BROOKER P. (1982) Robertsonian translocations in Mus musculus from N E Scotland and Orkney. Heredity 48 305-9

BRYANT E.H. (1974) On the adaptive significance of enzyme polymorphisms in relation to environmental variability. Am. Nat. 108 1-19

CAPANNA E. (1980) Chromosomal rearrangement and speciation in progress in Mus musculus. Folia Zool. 29 43-57

DE FRIES J.C and McCLEARN G.E. (1972) Behavioral genetics and the fine structure of mouse populations: a study in microevolution. In Evolutionary Biology 5 279-91. Dobzhansky Th., Hecht M.R. and Steer W.C. (eds) New York: Appleton-Century-Crofts

DEOL M.S., GRÜNEBERG H., SEARLE A.G. and Truslove G.M. (1960) How pure are our inbred strains of mice? Genet. Res. 1 50-8.

DUESER R.D. and BROWN W.C. (1980) Ecological correlates of insular rodent diversity. Ecology 61 50-6

EHRLICH P.R. and RAVEN P.H. (1969) Differentiation of populations. Science, N.Y. 165 1228-32

FERRIS S.D., SAGE R.D., HUANG C-M., NIELSEN J.T., RITTE U. and WILSON A.C. (1983) Flow of mitochondrial DNA across a species boundary. Proc. Natl. Acad. Sci. USA 80 2290-94

FIGUEROA F., GOLUBIC M., NIZETIC D. and KLEIN J. (1985) Evolution of mouse major histocompatibility complex genes borne by t chromosomes. Proc. Natl. Acad. Sci. USA 82 2819-23

FITCH W.M. and ATCHLEY W.R. (1985) Evolution in inbred strains of mice appears rapid. Science N.Y. 228 1169-75

FORD C.E. and EVANS E.P. (1973) Robertsonian translocations in mice: segregational irregularities in male heterozygotes and zygotic unbalance. Chromosomes Today 4 387-97

GROPP A., TETTENBORN U. and LEHMANN E.V. (1970). Chromosomen variation vom Robertson'chen Typus bei der Tabakmaus, M. poschiavinus, und ihren Hybriden mit der Laboratoriumsmaus. Cytogenetics 9 9-23

HALDANE J.B.S. and JAYAKAR S.D. (1963) Polymorphism due to selection of varying direction. J. Genet. 58 237-42

HUXLEY J.S. (1942) Evolution, the Modern Synthesis. London: Allen and Unwin

KING C.M. (1982) Age structure and reproduction in feral New Zealand populations of the house mouse (Mus musculus) in relation to seedfall of southern beech (Nothofagus). New Zealand J. Zool. 9 467-80

KLEIN J. (1975) Biology of the Mouse Histocompatibility-2 Complex. New York: Springer-Verlag

KLEIN J.(1979) Population genetics of the murine chromosome 17. Israel J. med. Sci. 15 859-66

LANDE R. (1979) Effective deme sizes during longterm evolution estimated from rates of chromosomal rearrangement. Evolution 33 234-51

LARSON A., PRAGER E.M. and WILSON A.C. (1984). Chromosomal evolution, speciation and morphological change in vertebrates: the role of social behaviour. Chromosomes Today 8 215-28

LENINGTON S. (1983) Social preferences for partners carrying 'good genes' in wild house mice. Anim. Beh. 31 325-33.

LENINGTON S. and EGID K. (1985) Female discrimination of male odors correlated with male genotype at the T locus: a response to T-locus or H-2-locus variability? Beh. Genet. 15 53-67.

LEWONTIN R.C. and DUNN L.C. (1960) The evolutionary dynamics of a polymorphism in the house mouse. Genetics 45 705-22

LEVINE L., ROCKWELL R.F. and GROSSFIELD J. (1980) Sexual selection in mice. V reproductive competition between +/+ and +/t^5 males. Am. Nat. 116 150-56.

LIDICKER W.Z. (1976) Social behaviour and density regulation in house mice living in large enclosures. J. Anim. Ecol. 45 677-97

MIYADA C.G., KLOFELT, C., REYES, A.A., McLAUGHLIN-TAYLOR E. and WALLACE R.B. (1985). Evidence that polymorphism in the murine major histocompatibility complex may be generated by the assortment of subgene sequences. Proc. Natl. Acad. Sci. USA 82 2890-94

MORIWAKI K., YONEKAWA H., GOTOH O., MINEZAWA M., WINKING H. and GROPP A. (1984) Implications of the genetic divergence between European wild mice with .Robertsonian translocations from the viewpoint of mitochondrial DNA. Genet. Res.43 277-87.

MYERS J. H. (1974a) Genetic and social structure of feral house mouse populations on Grizzly Island, California. Ecology 55 747-59.

MYERS J.H. (1974b) The absence of t alleles in feral populations of house mice. Evolution 27 702-4.

NADEAU J.H., COLLINS R.L. and KLEIN J. (1982). Organization and evolution of the mammalian genome. Genetics 102 583-98

NASH H.R., BROOKER P.C. and DAVIS S.J.M. (1983) The Robertsonian translocation house-mouse populations of north east Scotland: a study of their origin and evolution. Heredity 50 303-10

NAUMOV N.P. (1940) The ecology of the hillock mouse, Mus musculus hortulanus. Nordm. J. Inst. Evolut. Morph. 3 33-77 (In Russian)

NEVO E. (1983a) Population genetics and ecology: the interface. In Evolution from Molecules to Men: 287-321. Bendall D.S. (ed). Cambridge: University Press

NEVO E. (1983b) Adaptive significance of protein variation. In Protein Polymorphism: Adaptive and Taxonomic Significance: 239-82. Oxford, G.S. and Rollinson D. (eds) London and New York: Academic

NEWTON M.F. and PETERS J. (1983) Physiological variation of mouse haemoglobins. Proc. R. Soc. Lond. B 218 443-53

PENNYCUIK P.R., JOHNSTON P.G, LIDICKER W.Z. and WESTWOOD N.H. (1978) Introduction of a male sterile allele (t^{w2}) into a population of house mice housed in a large outdoor enclosure. Aust. J. Zool. 26 69-81

PETRAS M.L. (1967) Studies of natural populations of Mus. I. Biochemical populations and their bearing on breeding structure. Evolution, 21 259-74

PETRAS M.L. and TOPPING J.C. (1983) The maintenance of polymorphisms at two loci in house mouse (Mus musculus) populations. Cand. J. Genet. Cytol. 25 190-201.

PHILIP U. (1938) Mating system in wild populations of Dermestes vulpines and Mus musculus. J. Genet. 36 197-211

SAGE R.D. (1981) Wild mice. In The Mouse in Biomedical Research, vol. 1: 39-90 (Foster H.L., Small, I.D. and Fox I.D., (eds)) New York: Academic.

SCHRÖDER J.H. and OTTEN I-S. (1985) Increase in aggressiveness of male mice carrying a reciprocal translocation T(10,13) in the heterozygous state. Beh. Genet. 15 43-52.

SELANDER R.K. (1970) Behavior and genetic variation in natural populations. Am. Zool. 10 53-66

SINGLETON G.R. and HAY D.A. (1983) The effect of social organization on reproductive success and gene flow in colonies of wild house mice, Mus musculus. Behav. Ecol. Sociobiol. 12 49-56

SPIRITO F., MODESTI A., PERTICONE P., CRISTALDI M., FEDERICI R. and RIZZONI M. (1980) Mechanisms of fixation of accumulation of centric fusions in natural populations of Mus musculus. I. Karyological analysis of a hybrid zone between two populations in the Central Appenines. Evolution 34 453-66

STICKEL L.C. (1979) Population ecology of house mice in unstable habitats. J. Anim. Ecol. 48 871-87

TAKADA Y. (1985) Demography in island and mainland populations of the feral house mouse, Mus musculus molossinus. J. mammal. Soc. Japan feral house mouse, Mus musculus molossinus. J. mammal. Soc. Japan 10 179-91

WALLACE M.E. (1965) The relative homozygosity of inbred lines and closed colonies. J. theoret. Biol. 9 93-116

WHITMORE A.C. and WHITMORE S.P. (1985) Subline divergence within L.C. Strong's C3H and CBA inbred mouse strains. A review. Immunogenetics 21 407-28

YAMAZAKI K., BEAUCHAMP G.K., WYSOCKI C.J., BARD J., THOMAS L. and BOYSE E.A. (1983) Recognition of H-2 types in relation to the blocking of pregnancy in mice. Science N.Y. 221 186-88.

YAMAZAKI K., BOYSE E.A., MIKE V., THAKER H.T., MATHIESON B.J., ABBOTT J., BOYSE J., ZAYAS Z.A. and THOMAS L. (1976) Control of mating preferences in mice by genes in the major histocompatibility complex. J. exp. Med. 144 1324-35.

A Method for Rapid Determination of Male Mouse Genotypes and Transmission Distortion by Breeding with Estrous Females

A. E. Miller Baker

INTRODUCTION

To assess the frequency of haplotypes at the t complex of loci
and their transmission distortion in natural populations of
the house mouse (<u>Mus domesticus</u>) with minimal disruption to
the social organization, it is important to use a technique by
which males can be brought into the laboratory, bred to tester
females (T/+), and then returned to their site of capture. It
would be desirable if males could be returned to the field
within 24 hrs of being captured. Older methods typically
require a period of male retention of several weeks, but this
could compromise conclusions of behavioral ecological
studies. For example, the t complex of loci in house mice is
frequently referred to in marshalling evidence for group
selection (Lewontin 1970; Lacy 1978). Yet the removal of
males from the population for a period of weeks alters the
mating system and territorial structure and could severely
disrupt the spatial and temporal dynamics of alleles at the t
complex. A new method uses DNA from a 1 cm biopsy of the tail
to assess the t haplotype with a specific DNA probe (Silver,
et al. 1984). Whether the tail biopsy influences sexual or
parental behavior is unknown, but seems unlikely. However,
Silver's probe can provide no data on transmission distortion
of undisturbed populations. Transmission distortion of t
haplotypes is known to be influenced by genetic background of
males and females, male age, and time of mating relative to
estrus (reviewed in Lacy 1978; Lyons 1984).

CAN MALES CAGED 12-24 HR WITH FEMALES SIRE LITTERS?

One Litter

The objective of the first experiment was to determine if
newly-caught males could sire pups when caged for only 12 to
24 hrs with an estrous laboratory mouse. Females (CD1, Bagg
Albino, Balb, or random bred) were injected intraperitoneally
at 1600 hrs with a submaximal superovulatory dose of
unextracted serum of pregnant mare (2.5 PMS i.u. in 0.05 ml).
The optimal photoperiod for conception (14L:10D) was used with
the middle of the dark period at 2400 hrs. After 48 h, the
female was injected intraperitoneally with 5 i.u. of human
choriogonadotrophic hormone in 0.10 ml of 0.9 percent NaCl to
induce ovulation. Five males were captured from natural
populations, and each prepared female was put into a male's
cage (29 x 18 x 12 cm) where she remained for 12 to 24 h. Two
of the five males sired litters. Within five days of being
caught, a sixth male was caged with three females and he sired
two litters. Within 21 days of being caught, a seventh male

was caged with five females and an eighth male, with one
female and each sired a litter. Subsequent breeding
demonstrated fertility of the three males that failed to sire
pups and of the females with which they were first caged.

Several Litters

The length and shape of tails from a minimum of seven
T-bearing (T/t and T/+) pups are usually scored to designate a
male with a t haplotype (Petras 1967). A field-caught male
may have to sire several litters to produce this minimum. The
objective of the second experiment was to determine if
field-caught males could fertilize several females within 12
to 24 h. Each of eight males was caged for 12 to 24 hrs with
two to five estrous females. Pups were sired in 14 of the 18
times when males had access to females. In most cases, one
female per cage conceived, though I was not always sure how
many females in a cage produced litters (Fig. 1). The success
rate (number pregnant of total females caged) of males varied
from 26 - 83 percent (Fig. 2). Males that fertilized two
females in the same 12 - 24 hr period had the highest success
rates (67, 83 percent).

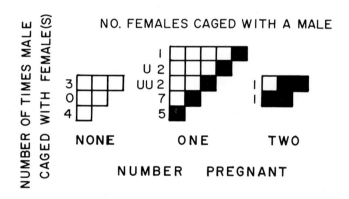

Fig. 1. Pregnancies resulting when 1 - 5 females were caged
with a field-caught male for 12 - 24 h. Nonpregnant and
pregnant females are represented respectively by open and
filled boxes. A row of boxes represents the number of females
caged with a male. Number of times a male was caged with
females is in the column to the left of each row. "U"
designates the three cases where I was unsure if two females
conceived when they were caged simultaneously with the same
male.

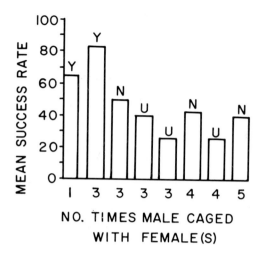

Fig. 2. Rate of successful fertilizations (mean per male of: number of pregnant females out of total available females per cage) by eight males (columns). Above each column is a symbol designating evidence that the male bred two females caged together: Y- certain, U- uncertain, N- none. The number of times each male was caged with females appears below each column.

POSSIBLE INFLUENCES ON CONCEPTION RATE

Four variables may influence conception rate in these experiments. (1) Female age: CD1 females, which were about 2 mos old, had the highest conception rates. Other females were older, but their exact ages were unknown. (2) Female genotype: Genotypes vary in their responsiveness to hormonal treatment and in sexual behavior (e.g., Mosig and Dewsbury 1976). (3) Female dominance order: Dominant females in 1.32 x 0.66 x 0.43 m cages suppressed reproduction by subordinates (Lloyd 1975); whether suppression occurs when females are housed in smaller cages is unknown, but likely. (4) No habituation to the test arena: Studies of sexual behavior usually habituate individuals to the test arena for several days before caging a male and female together.

If a female did not conceive, the hormonal injections were repeated 15 days afer her last HCG injection. During this 15-day period females will not ovulate even if given hormonal injections to bring them into estrus. One female died after her second and another died after her third PMS injection. Repeated injections of the unextracted PMS may have caused anaphylaxis. To prevent anaphylaxis, an antihistamine (0.2 ml pyrilamine) was injected intramuscularly an hour before injecting PMS and no further deaths occurred in 32 injections of PMS. Alternatively, the deaths could be caused by inexperience in giving injections, but no autopsies were done to ascertain this.

GENERAL USES FOR TECHNIQUE

Caging field-caught males with estrous females can be used to assess genotypes other than the t-complex and has advantages over assessing genotypes by biopsy. (1) Though survival in the field is similar for biopsied and nonbiopsied mice (Baker 1983), the mating potential of biopsied mice may be lower. A noninvasive technique, such as caging with estrous females, probably has minimal influence on mating potential (acceptance of males back into the population should be high; e.g. Rowe and Redfern 1969; Myers 1974). (2) Inheritance of alleles at enzyme loci in biopsied tissues (e.g. muscle) must be documented (Fairbairn and Roff (1980). Caging with estrous females allows alleles from tissues to be examined (e.g. heart, brain, testes, spleen, kidney) for which inheritance is already documented. (3) Gene regulation of mice in undisturbed field populations sampled with replacement can be examined by caging field-caught males with laboratory females that have different genetic backgrounds. The use of different genetic backgrounds has played a key role in understanding how transmission distortion is regulated at the t complex. (4) One advantage of biopsy, however, is that genotypes of males, females, and juveniles can be assessed. Only the genotypes of field-caught adult males can be assessed when caging is limited to 12 - 24 hrs after which mice are returned to the field.

CONCLUSION

In conclusion, laboratory females brought into estrous with PMS and HCG conceived when caged 12 to 24 hrs with field-caught males. When males were given simultaneously two to five estrous females, usually only one female conceived.

ACKNOWLEDGEMENTS

Frank Bronson and George Seidel helped formulate this experiment. Kim Pomeroy and Don Nash demonstrated how to give injections. Kim Pomeroy, Tom Gorell, Don Nash, George Seidel, and Mike Baker provided supplies and laboratory space. Don Nash, Bob Behnke, and Charlie Novak allowed mice to be trapped in their barns. Lynn Kesel and Dave Neil provided veterinary advice. Mike Baker, Frank Bronson, Don Dewsbury, Martha McClintock, Kim Pomeroy, and George Seidel helped sharpen the presentation and suggested further experiments. This is dedicated to the memory of Lee Snyder.

REFERENCES

Baker, AEM (1983) Survival of house mice after muscle biopsy. J Mamm 64:704-705
Fairbairn, DJ and Roff, DA (1980) Testing genetic models of isozyme variability without breeding data: can we depend on Chi square? Can J Fish Aquat Sci 37:1149-1159

Lacy, RC (1978) Dynamics of t-alleles in <u>Mus musculus</u> populations: Review and speculation. Biologist 60:41-67

Lewontin, RC (1970) The units of selection. Ann Rev Ecol System 1:1-18

Lloyd, JA (1975) Social structure and reproduction in two freely-growing populations of house mice (<u>Mus musculus</u> L.). Anim Behav 23:413-424

Lyon, MF (1984) Transmission ratio distortion in mouse t-haplotypes is due to multiple distorter genes acting on a responder locus. Cell 37:621-628

Mosig, DW and Dewsbury, DA (1976) Studies of the copulation behavior of house mice (<u>Mus musculus</u>). Behav Biol 16:463-473

Myers, JH (1974) Genetic and social structure of feral house mouse populations on Grizzly Island, California. Ecology 55:747-759

Petras, ML (1967) Studies of natural populations of Mus. II. Polymorphism at the T locus. Evolution. 21:466-478

Rowe, FP and Redfern, R (1969) Aggressive behaviour in related and unrelated wild house mice (<u>Mus musculus</u> L.). Ann Appl Biol 64:425-431

Silver, LM, Garrels, JI, and Lehrach, H (1984) Molecular studies of mouse chromosome 17 and the t complex. In: Setlow, JK and Hollaender, A (eds) Genetic engineering principles and methods Vol 6, Plenum, New York

MHC Polymorphism in Island Populations of Mice

F. Figueroa, H. Tichy, R.J. Berry, and J. Klein

The major histocompatibility complex of the house mouse, Mus domesticus, contains two highly polymorphic class I loci (H-2K and H-2D) and
two or three highly polymorphic class II loci (H-2A$_\beta$, H-2E$_\beta$, and perhaps H-2A$_\alpha$; see Klein et al. 1983, Klein and Figueroa 1981). Any given
small population of wild mice (e.g., mice living in a farm complex) may
contain from 5 to 10 alleles at each of the polymorphic loci, all occurring at appreciable frequencies (Figueroa et al. 1982). The total
number of alleles at a given polymorphic locus probably exceeds 100 and
virtually all wild mice thus far captured in continental Europe or
North America are heterozygous at the polymorphic loci.

The significance of the Mhc polymorphism remains obscure. According to
a popular notion, the polymorphism is necessary to fight invasions of
parasites of all kinds (Klein 1979). It is known that the Mhc molecules
are required for the initiation of any kind of specific immune response, including of course responses to pathogenic viruses, bacteria,
and protozoal or metazoal parasites. The first step in all these responses is the recognition of the foreign antigens expressed by the
parasites. The antigens are first recognized by T lymphocytes on the
surface of antigen-presenting cells (APC) and the recognition normally
does not occur unless the APC also presents its own Mhc molecules to
the T-cell receptor (Klein et al. 1983). The receptor apparently has a
dual specificity, recognizing nonself (foreign antigen) and self (individual's Mhc molecule) simultaneously. However, certain combinations
of foreign antigen and self Mhc molecules fail to be recognized, probably because the individual has inactivated T lymphocytes bearing receptors specific for this particular combination of self and nonself
molecules. The reason for this inactivation is thought to be the necessity of avoiding an attack by these T lymphocytes on the individual's own tissues (because of a degeneracy in the T-cell receptor
repertoire, some combinations of self Mhc and other self components
may resemble certain combinations of self Mhc and foreign antigen).
The Mhc polymorphism is then interpreted as a way of compensating for
this deficiency in the recognition system: individuals heterozygous at
the H-2 loci should have fewer blind spots in the T-lymphocyte repertoire than homozygous individuals.

Two views have been expressed regarding the origin of the Mhc polymorphism. According to one view, held by many immunologists and, in particular, by molecular biologists, Mhc polymorphism arises very quickly
by special mechanisms that can diversify Mhc molecules within a few
generations. We propound the other view, according to which Mhc polymorphism has evolved slowly and over periods of time that are much

longer than the age of the species (Klein 1980). To test how rapidly
the Mhc molecules diversify under natural conditions, we have H-2 typed
wild mice from several island populations. It is reasonable to assume
that these populations grew from very few founders and that, if our
hypothesis is correct, they should remain relatively homogeneous for
some time after their expansion. This prediction is confirmed by our
studies.

The wild mice were typed by 57 monoclonal or polyclonal antibodies
specific for determinants encoded in the class I and class II H-2
genes. The typing was carried out by the microcytotoxic test with complement consisting of a 1:1:4 mixture of rabbit normal serum, guinea
pig normal serum, and Hanks' balanced salt solution. The titrations
were performed in Terasaki microplates, the source of target cells
was the spleen and the lymph nodes of the donor mice, and the test
was evaluated automatically by the propidium iodide method of Bruning
and his colleagues (1982; for details of the cytotoxic test, see
Zaleska-Rutczynska et al. 1983).

The wild mice were obtained from three islands: Helgoland, which lies
just off the coast of Germany in the North Sea, the Isle of May, and
Fara, just off the coast of Scotland. Helgoland was formed in the tri-
assic and tertiary periods as a cliff-girt bastion of red sandstone on
a rocky platform. This large island was gradually reduced in size by
the continuous breaking of waves against the cliffs, the rise in sea
level, and recently also by human activities. Even as late as A.D. 800,
its periphery was about 194 km; it is now less than 13 km (1.5 km²).
There is evidence that the island has been colonized by humans since
the neolithic period. In historical times, its possession was claimed
by Danes, Britons, and finally by Germans. A lighthouse was erected on
the island in 1670 and a spa was discovered in 1826. In both World War
I and World War II, the island was used by Germany as a naval base.
After both wars the military installations were destroyed and with
them part of the island. Its present population is about 2000, but the
island is also a popular tourist attraction. The presence of mice on
the island was first reported in 1829 but the island must have been
colonized by mice much earlier, perhaps at the same time as human colonization. The mice were studied by Zimmermann (1953) and later again by
Reichstein and Vank (1968). The sample analyzed by Zimmermann consisted
of specimens collected in the winter of 1935/1936; Reichstein and Vank
studied mice captured during the years 1956-1965. Zimmermann described
the mice of Helgoland as a separate subspecies, Mus musculus helgolandicus, which shows some characteristics of M. domesticus (large body
size, long tail), others of M. musculus (coat color consisting of grey-
ish-brown back and white-grey belly), and others still specific for the
new subspecies (slender jaw). It therefore seems likely that the founding population consisted of hybrids between M. domesticus and M. musculus (the island lies close to the border between the two species;
other islands in the North Sea are occupied by M. domesticus and those
in the Baltic Sea by M. musculus). However, the colonization must have
occurred a long time ago to have allowed for the development of the
subspecies-specific traits. It may have taken place at the same time as
the colonization by humans some 5000 years ago. The population of M. m.
helgolandicus must have survived many natural catastrophes as well as
severe bombardments and blasting of the military installations in recent times. A factor contributing to the stability of the population is
undoubtedly the relative mild winters on the island: in sheltered parts
of the island even figs and mulberry trees can be grown out-of-doors.

As far as we could determine, there are only two H-2 haplotypes present
among the wild mice of Helgoland (Table 1). One haplotype is character-

Table 1. H-2 antigenic determinants present in wild mice from island populations

Antigenic determinant (controlling locus)

Population	Group	n	m5 (K)	m47 (K)	m48 (K)	m99 (K)	m6 (K)	m25 (K)	m34 (K)	m57 (K)	m84 (K)	m88 (D)	m90 (D)	m93 (K)	m96 (K)	m97 (D)	m98 (D)	m153 (K)	Tu-A (D)	Tu-B (D)	Tu-C (D)	Tu-D (D)	Tu-E	m19 (A)	m27 (A)	m110 (A)	m118 (A)	m25 (A)	m30 (A)	m48 (A)	m52 (A)	m53 (A)	m119 (A)	m120 (A)	m121 (A)	m7 (E)
Helgoland	1	42	-	-	-	-	+	+	+	+	+	+	+	+	+	+	+	+	+	+	+	+	+	-	-	-	-	+	+	+	+	+	+	+	+	+
Helgoland	2	18	+	+	+	+	+	+	+	+	+	+	+	+	+	+	+	+	+	+	+	+	+	+	+	+	+	+	+	+	+	+	+	+	+	+

Antigenic determinant (controlling locus)

Population	Group	n	m7 (K)	m34 (D)	m40 (D)	m88 (D)	Tu-A (D)	Tu-F	Tu-G	Tu-H	Tu-I	m17 (A)	m110 (A)	m116 (A)	m30 (A)	m54 (A)	m15 (A)	m115 (A)	m120 (A)	m53 (A)	m8 (A)	m117 (E)
Isle of May	1	6	-	+	-	-	-	-	+	-	+	+	+	+	(+)	-	+	+	+	+	+	+
Fara Island	2	7	(+)	+	+	-	+	(+)	-	(+)	-	-	-	-	+	+	-	(+)	+	+	-	(+)
Fara Island	3	9	+	+	+	+	+	+	-	+	-	-	-	-	+	+	-	(+)	+	+	-	+
Fara Island	4	5	+	+	+	+	+	+	-	+	-	-	-	-	+	+	-	(+)	+	+	-	+

n, number of mice in a sample. Tu, class I determinants recognized by polyclonal absorbed antisera. +, presence of determinant. -, absence of determinant.

ized by the presence of antigenic determinants H-2K.m5, m47, m48, and m99 as well as H-2A.m19, m27, m110, and m118; the other haplotype is characterized by the absence of these determinants. Both haplotypes share a number of other determinants, particularly those encoded in the H-2D locus so that they may share alleles at this locus. Both haplotypes fail to react with antibodies specific for class I determinants H-2.2, 4, 9, 12, 14, 15, 16, 17, 18, 19, 20, 21, 22, 23, 26, 30, 31, 32, 33, 103, 104, 110, 111, 113, 114, 115, 116, 118, 130, 132, 137, 143, 144, 146, 156, 160, 162, 163, 164, 167, 169, 106, 107, 108, 109, m7, m46, m61, m64, m65, m89, m94, m117, m139 and class II determinants H-2A(E).m2, m15, m17, m20, m26, m44, m111, m112, m114, m115, m116, m117. Most of the mice appear to be homozygous for the particular haplotype, although we have not carried out any progeny tests to prove this contention.

The Isle of May is a small island in the Firth of Forth, not far from Edinburgh. Fara island belongs to the group of Orkney islands which lie off the north coast of Caithness. The Isle of May is formed of igneous rocks; Fara island is formed of massive red sandstones and grey lime-rich flagstones. The climate is windy but relatively mild; the mean temperature in February, the coldest month, is 3.8°C, and in July, the warmest month, 12.8°C. The climate of the Isle of May is warmer in summer and colder in winter than that of Fara Island. The islands have been occupied by humans since prehistoric times, but most of the time very sparsely. Fara Island is 2.4 km long, about 0.8 km wide, and its surface area covers about 0.7 km². At one time, the island had eight crofts and a human population of 70-80 but the last family was evacuated in 1949, and the island is now uninhabited except for a shepherd who spends several weeks there every year. The first record of mice on the Isle of May dates from 1885 (Berry 1964). The Fara mice are homozygous for two Robertsonian fusions, Rb(9.12)10Tu and Rb(3.14)7Tu and are segregating for another metacentric chromosome, Rb(4.10)8Tu (Adolph and Klein 1981, Brooker 1982, Nash et al. 1983). The mice show 3.4% heterozygosity at allozyme-encoding loci which appears to be higher than that on the neighboring islands (Berry and Peters 1977, Berry 1978). No variation was found among the 77 allozyme-encoding loci in 93 mice from the Isle of May population (Berry and Peters 1977).

The mice on the Isle of May all appear to carry one H-2 haplotype characterized by the presence of class I determinants detected by the Tu-G and Tu-I antibodies and H-2A/E determinants m8, m15, m17, m110, and m116. Similarly, all three samples of wild mice from the Fara Island appear to be homozygous for another H-2 haplotype characterized by class I determinants m7, m40, m88, as well as class I determinants detected by the Tu-A, Tu-H, and Tu-F antibodies, and by H-2A determinants m54 and m117. The haplotypes present on these two islands do not appear to be obviously related to each other. Mice from both mouse populations (Isle of May and Fara) failed to react with antibodies specific for class I determinants H-2.2, 4, 9, 12, 14, 15, 16, 17, 19, 20, 21, 22, 23, 26, 30, 31, 32, 33, 103, 110, 111, 113, 114, 115, 116, 130, 132, 137, 143, 144, 146, 149, 160, 164, 167, 169, 106, 107, 108, 109, m2, m5, m6, m25, m46, m47, m57, m61, m64, m65, m84, m89, m90, m93, m94, m95, m117, m139, m153, m96, m97, m98, m99 and class II determinants H-2A/Em2, m8, m19, m20, m25, m26, m27, m44, m48, m52, m111, m112, m116.

We conclude, therefore, that Mhc polymorphism of wild mice on these three islands is very limited. In the Helgoland population, only two alleles could be found at the otherwise highly polymorphic H-2K and H-2A loci and only one allele at the H-2D locus. On the Isle of May and Fara Island, only one allele could be detected in each of the populations at all of the H-2 loci tested. We could not determine how long the Isle of May and Fara Island mice have been isolated from the mainland populations, but the Helgoland mice could have lived in isolation for several thousand years. Yet, apparently during all this time they have thrived in the absence of any extensive polymorphism. This observation must indicate that the one or two H-2 haplotypes in these populations suffice for the mice to be able to cope with the presumably limited spectrum of mouse pathogens and parasites present on these islands. Although one might be tempted to conclude from this observation that the extent of the Mhc polymorphism may correlate with the diversity of pathogens in a given environment, in fact no such conclusion is justified. The mouse populations in some small farms on the continent may be exposed to a similarly restricted spectrum of pathogens as the mice on the islands, yet they are highly polymorphic at their Mhc loci. It seems more likely that the differences in the extent of Mhc polymorphism between the various mouse populations might be established by differences in the size of the founding populations. What our data do suggest, however, is that oligomorphism or even monomorphism at Mhc loci is not a condition incompatible with the survival of a population. We by no means want to imply that Mhc polymorphism provides no selective advantage to a species, but we are inclined to believe that this advantage becomes apparent only over long periods of time.

Our data also argue strongly against the notion that Mhc genes evolve rapidly. If the Helgoland mice have been isolated for the last 5000 years or so, which we believe could be an underestimate, it would mean that in some 10,000 to 15,000 generations their Mhc genes have not diversified to an extent that could be detected by the methods we used. This conclusion is in accordance with the results we obtained by studying other mouse populations (Arden and Klein 1980, 1982). There is thus no evidence to support the notion that Mhc genes diversify rapidly; all the available data are consistent with the hypothesis that Mhc polymorphism has been generated over periods of time that are much longer than the age of a species.

ACKNOWLEDGMENTS

This work has been supported in part by grant A 14736 from the National Institutes of Health, Bethesda, Maryland.

REFERENCES

Adolph S, Klein J (1981) Robertsonian variation in Mus musculus from central Europe, Spain and Scotland. J Hered 72:219-221

Arden B, Klein J (1982) Biochemical comparison of major histocompatibility complex molecules from different subspecies of Mus musculus: Evidence for trans-specific evolution of alleles. Proc Natl Acad Sci USA 79:2342-2346

Arden B, Wakeland EK, Klein J (1980) Structural comparisons of serologically indistinguishable H-2K-encoded antigens from inbred and wild mice. J Immunol 125:2424-2428

Berry RJ (1964) The evolution of an island population of the house mouse. Evolution 18:468-483

Berry RJ (1978) Genetic variations in wild house mice: Where natural selection and history meet. Am Sci 66:52-60

Berry RJ, Peters J (1977) Heterogeneous heterozygosities in Mus musculus populations. Proc R Soc Lond (Biol) 197:485-503

Brooker PC (1982) Robertsonian translocations in Mus musculus from N.E.
    Scotland and Orkney. Heredity 48:305-309
Bruning JW, Claas FHJ, Kardol MJ, Lansberger Q, Naipol AM, Tanke HJ,
    (1982) Automated reading of HLA-A,B,C typing and screening. The
    propidium iodide method. Hum Immunol 5:225-231
Figueroa F, Zaleska-Rutczynska Z, Adolph S, Nadeau JH, Klein J (1982)
    Genetic variation of wild mouse populations in southern Germany. II.
    Serological study. Genet Res Camb 41:135-144
Klein J (1979) The major histocompatibility complex of the mouse.
    Science 203:516-521
Klein J (1980) Generation of diversity at MHC loci: Implications for
    T-cell receptor repertoires. In: Fougereau F, Dausset J (eds)
    Immunology 80. Academic Press, London, pp 239-253
Klein J, Figueroa F (1981) Polymorphism of the mouse H-2 loci. Immunol
    Rev 60:23-57
Klein J, Figueroa F, Nagy ZA (1983) Genetics of the major histocom-
    patibility complex: The final act. Annu Rev Immunol 1:119-142
Nash HR, Brooker PC, Davis JM (1983) The Robertsonian translocation
    house-mouse populations of north-east Scotland: A study of their
    origin and evolution. Heredity 50:303-310
Reichstein H, Vank G (1968) Beitrag zur Kenntnis der Helgoländer
    Hausmaus, Mus musculus helgolandicus. Zimmermann, 1953 Verh D Zool
    Ges Heidelberg 1967:386-394
Zaleska-Rutczynska Z, Figueroa F, Klein J (1983) Sixteen new H-2
    haplotypes derived from wild mice. Immunogenetics 18:189-203
Zimmermann K (1953) Die Hausmaus von Helgoland, M. musculus helgoland-
    icus. sspec nov Z Säugetierkd 17:163-166

Polymorphisms

The Contribution of Wild Derived Mouse Inbred Strains to Gene Mapping Methodology

J.L. Guénet

INTRODUCTION

All geneticists agree that it is essential to obtain highly
accurate gene mapping data for both man and laboratory mammals.
For this reason different techniques have been used, over the
last fifty years, to try and localize, as precisely as possible,
genes on mammalian chromosomes. Several of these techniques,
particularly when applied to the mouse species, where wild
specimens can be used as a source of polymorphism, represent
really important breakthroughs in formal genetics. We will try
and review the most important of these advances.

AMONG LABORATORY MICE THE GENETIC POLYMORPHISM IS LIMITED

It has always been known from historical records (Morse 1978)
that the major laboratory inbred strains are descended from common ancestors. Moreover it has been established recently that in
almost all the major laboratory inbred strains the maternally
inherited mitochondrial DNA (mt DNA) shows a monomorphic restriction pattern of the *Mus musculus domesticus* type (Ferris et
al 1982). Similarly Bishop et al (1985) have shown, looking
for a specific characteristic of the paternally inherited Y,
that most laboratory strains (except SJL which is of the
Mus m. musculus type) are of the *Mus musculus domesticus* type. The
pool of segregating genes in laboratory mice is thus relatively
limited and probably does not reflect the mouse species as it is
in the wild.
This statement has to be qualified by the observation that mice
have been used for years as the mammal of first choice for the
study of induced mutations thus producing some 100-150 polymorphic genes having normal and abnormal alleles.

Mus spretus AS A PROVIDENTIAL SOURCE OF POLYMORPHISM

Although it apparently never occurs in the wild it has been reported by Bonhomme et al (1978) that the West Mediterranean
species of mice : *Mus spretus* Lataste can interbreed under
laboratory conditions (either spontaneously or after hormonal
treatment) with inbred strains of *Mus musculus domesticus*
(the laboratory strains). The libido of the *Mus spretus* male is
generally irregular and rather low but either one can occasionally find reliable studs or artificial insemination can be performed as a routine technique.
Offspring can be obtained in both directions of this inter-

specific cross. It is however much easier to get a progeny when the female belongs to a laboratory strains.

Whatever the situation, it is generally not a serious problem to get several Fl females which in turn can be backcrossed to *Mus m. domesticus* of the same inbred line to produce backcross progeny. Since inbred lines of *Mus spretus* (SPE/Pas F = 30) are now available for use in such crosses it is possible to analyse the segregation of the *spretus* "S" versus *domesticus* "D" alleles. This provides a ready system for linkage analysis which is extremely efficient and possesses very high resolution due to the extensive divergence between the two genomes which can be easily revealed by looking for Restriction Fragment Length Poly- morphism at the level of genomic D.N.A. Almost any probe, even "anonymous", that correspond to a unique (or moderately repea- ted) sequence(s) will produce restriction fragment length poly- morphism with almost any enzyme...even the cheapest ! This polymorphism is proportional to the divergence between the two species and is, at least, 10^5 times larger than that existing between the most divergent "laboratory" strains.The possibility of using *Mus spretus* as a privileged strain to map mouse genes more accurately is not in itself revolutionary ! It simply re- presents one step further, which we will now explain in techni- cal details. It does however open up and facilitate considerably structural mapping.

HOW TO MAP A GENE WITH THE *Mus spretus* SYSTEM ?

There are two possibilities according to whether a molecular probe exists or not for the gene which is to be mapped.

1 - The Gene to be Mapped has Been Cloned and a Molecular Probe of it Exists.

This case has been examplified for the first time by Robert et al (1985) with the myosin light chain and actin genes but seve- ral other genes have been mapped since this publication (Weydert et al 1985, Dandois et al 1985 ...) with this technique. Usually about 50 to 60 backcross progeny are raised from inter- specific *Mus musculus domesticus* X *Mus spretus* Fl females. In general the laboratory strain is chosen to allow as many genetic (or cytogenetic !) markers as possible to segregate.

50/60 of such backcross animals, when adult, are splenectomized and high molecular weight D.N.A. prepared. In parallel the back- cross animals are typed for as many markers as possible : Allo- morphic proteins, alloenzymes, retroviral insertions, coat colour marker genes, alloantigens and so on ...thus a "species distribution pattern" can be established for every single animal and this pattern is unique. Under normal conditions up to 25 polymorphic markers can be analyzed covering about half of the mouse genome if one assumes that with 50 individuals the chromo- some length which is "swept" is in the range of 30 centimorgans (with a 99 % confidence limit). The molecular probe which is to be mapped is then matched with *spretus* and *domesticus* D.N.A. samples restricted with several en-

donucleases. The endonucleases producing the most suitable
polymorphism are used to restrict the invidual backcross DNA's
prior to Southern blotting. Finally the pattern of polymomor-
phism on the blots is matched to the already established S.D.P.
and linkage eventually detected.
Of course, once a given probe has been matched to the D.N.A.
samples it becomes one more element in the S.D.P. and in turn
can be used to map further probes. Thus as with the Recombinant
Inbred Strain the S.D.P. is a permanent document and it is
obvious that the system is "autocatalytic". In other words :
"the more it works the more powerful it becomes".

2 - No Probe is Available for the Gene to be Mapped

In this case there is one necessary prerequisite : the gene has
to be polymorphic between *M. m. domesticus* and *M. spretus*. That
will be the case for any new mutation discovered in an inbred
line of mouse either as a by-product of inbreeding or as an end-
product of a mutagenic treatment. The genes which produce Hybrid
sterility in male *Mus musculus domesticus* X *Mus spretus* interspecific
Fl's are good examples too. Since we have been studying them for
some years we present some details here.

We have already stated in this article that *Mus spretus* and
Mus musculus domesticus species can interbreed in laboratory condition and produce viable progeny. This is true, but the male
progeny are invariably sterile and only the Fl female can breed.
This is a consequence of the so-called Haldane effect which states that when interspecific hybrids are produced the heterogame-
tic sex is frequently sterile and sometimes inviable. We have
shown that this is due to a number of codominant factors segregating in this cross, the number of which may depend upon the
Mus musculus domesticus partner. In DBA/2 X SPE crosses two genes
are segregating. We call them Hst-2 and Hst-3, to recall the
Hst-1 gene reported by Forejt and Ivanvi (1975) and heterozygous
animals for one or both are sterile. It is thus possible to make
D.N.A. from a set of backcross males segregating for these two
genes and to match the pattern of fertility/sterility with the
other segregating allelic markers. This is, by the way, the
quickest way to map a sterility gene !

Attempts at detecting linkage by analysis of interspecific backcross segregations have several advantages over the use of Recombinant Inbred Strains (R.I.S.).

1 - The use of backcrosses extends the analysis over much
longer distances (30 cM) whereas Recombinant Inbred Strains
tend to keep linked only those loci that are very close together
(see Taylor 1978). With 20/25 segregating genetic markers well
"spread" over the genetic map one can "sweep" almost half the
genome of the mouse with only 40/50 backcross D.N.A's.

2 - During the generation of Recombinant Inbred Strains,
certain associations of genes may be favoured (or selected
against ?) resulting in a non random segregation of loci not observed in a backcross (Guénet 1985).

3 - The use of distantly related species increases the probability of finding R.F.L.P. for a given gene, so that any gene
for which a complementary D.N.A. (c D.N.A.) is available can be
be mapped. This is not true when R.I.S. are used.

It is important to note that, in spite of a very large evolutionary distance between the two species there is no apparent
bias in gene segregation in the F1 female. In all the instances
we have looked at, genes known to be linked in laboratory mice
were also cosegregating in our backcrosses, and the order of
these genes on the genetic map remained strictly the same. In
some instances the genetic distances between two linked genes
have been found to be different but these differences, are not
statistically very important and (or) could result from the
fact that the segregation occurs in the female only. This does
not in any case represent a serious inconvenience or limitation
to the technique. In his report on the localization of the
structural genes coding for the myosin light chains Robert et al
(1985), for example, found a perfect correlation between data
from interspecific backcrosses and data from an appropriate set
of Recombinant Inbred Strain D.N.A's.

THE TECHNIQUE CAN BE IMPROVED IN SEVERAL WAYS

The protocol which we have just reported is universal and ap-
liable in all cases whatever the condition under investigation
is.

As we indicated earlier a molecular probe corresponding to a given gene can be localized on the mouse chromosome by matching
its segregation pattern to the Species Distribution Pattern
established with conventional markers. Of course, this also apply to "anonymous" probes with the advantage that these probes
can be selected according to the type of restriction enzyme
used to produce polymorphism. One can decide, for example, that
only the probes giving a clear cut polymorphism with Eco RI will
be kept for further mapping analysis. By doing this the technique is very much improved since it becomes useless to check for
the best enzyme this being done once and forever. One can thus
dream of a series of probes giving a clear cut polymorphism with
the same enzyme (for example the cheapest one) which could allow
several use of the same blot. If in addition, these probes map
to differents points of the mouse genome the yield is further
increased.

An important limitation of the technique is a consequence of the
obviously limited amount of DNA which can be obtained from a given backcross animal. To by-pass this limitation several possibilities exist. For the time being we are trying to induce
transplantable carcinomas in individual backcross animals, using
Ethyl Nitroso-Urea, with the idea that, *domesticus X spretus* F1
being universal acceptors for the transplant the source of DNA
will become indefinite.

REFERENCES

Bonhomme F, Martin S, and Thaler L. (1978) Hybridization between *Mus m. domesticus* L. and *Mus spretus* Lataste under laboratory conditions.
Experientia 1140-1141

Botstein D, White RL, Skolnick M, and Davis RW. (1980) Construction of a genetic linkage map in man using Restriction Fragment Length Polymorphism
Am. J. Hum. Genet. 32 : 314-331

Bishop CE, Boursot P, Baron B, Bonhomme F and Hatat D (1985) Most classical *Mus musculus domesticus* laboratory mouse strains carry a *Mus musculus musculus* Y chromosome.
Nature 315 70-72

Dandoy F, De Maeyer E, Bonhomme F, Guénet J-L and De Maeyer-Guignard J. (1985) In press.
Segregation of Restriction Fragment Length Polymorphism in an interspecies cross of laboratory and wild mice indicates tight linkage of murine IFN- β Gene to the murine IFN- α Genes

Ferris SD, Sage RD, Wilson AC (1982) Evidence from mt DNA sequences that common laboratory strains of inbred mice are descended from a single female.
Nature 295 : 163-165

Forejt J and Ivanyi P. (1985) Genetic studies on male Sterility of Hybrids between Laboratory and Wild mice (*Mus musculus* L.)
Genet. Res. 24 189-206

Guénet J-L (1985) Do non linked genes really reassort at random ?
Ann. Inst. Pasteur/Immunol. 136C 85-90

Morse HC (1978). Origins of Inbred Mice.
Academic Press New-York

Robert B, Barton P, Minty A, Daubas P, Weydert A, Bonhomme F, Catalan J, Simon D, Guénet J-L and Buckingham ME. (1985) Investigation of genetic linkage between myosin and actin genes using an interspecific mouse backcross.
Nature 314 : 181-183

Taylor BA (1978) Recombinant Inbred Strains : use in gene mapping in : Morse HC (ed) Origins of Inbred Mice Academic Press New-York p. 423-440

Weydert A, Daubas P, Lazaridis I, Barton P, Garner I, Leader DP, Bonhomme F, Catalan J, Simon D, Guénet J-L, Gros F and Buckingham ME (1985) Genes for skeletal muscle myosin heavy chains are clustered and do not map on the same mouse chromosome as cardiac myosin heavy chain genes.
Accepted for publication by Proc. Nat. Acad. Sc. U.S.A.

Alleles of β-Glucuronidase Found in Wild Mice

V. M. Chapman, D. R. Miller, E. Novak, and R. W. Elliott

β-Glucuronidase (Gus) has been extensively studied in the mouse as a model of mammalian gene regulation. The structural gene maps to chromosome 5 and variation for the regulation of Gus gene expression cosegregates with the structural locus. The regulatory phenotypes include variation in systemic levels of gene expression (Pfister et al., 1985), variation in testosterone induction of kidney β-glucuronidase (Palmer et al.,1983; Swank et al., 1973) and variation in Gus expression within individual organs. The various structural and regulatory phenotypes which cosegregate at the GUS locus are designated as haplotypes [Gus] and the different regulatory phenotypes have been designated as separate elements of the haplotype complex (Table 1) (Paigen, 1979).

Three haplotypes of structural and regulatory alleles of GUS have been characterized among inbred strains (Pfister et al., 1982). These combinations of alleles of enzyme structure and regulation are present in all laboratory strains and they have not been separated by recombination either in backcrosses of up to 1000 mice (Swank et al., 1978) or in the construction of congenic and recombinant inbred (RI) strains. More recently, the analysis of genomic DNA restriction patterns using a cDNA probe has revealed that these allelic haplotypes differ at at least three positions along the gene as shown by altered fragment sizes in Southern blot analysis (Elliott et al., 1985). In this instance, the [Gus]^H and [Gus]^B haplotypes do not differ from each other but they both differ from [Gus]^A at all three positions (Table 2).

We have sampled diverse house mouse species for variation in 1) gene structure, 2) gene expression at the level of processing and turnover, and 3) gene regulation at the level of systemic synthesis and in the response of the kidney Gus locus to testosterone. We specifically asked whether there was evidence of independent variation for enzyme structure and regulation of synthesis. We have identified six new alleles of enzyme structure, three new variants of GUS regulation and seven new haplotypes. These provide important new insights into the regulation of GUS expression which might not have been readily determined from a molecular analysis of the GUS genomic structures found among inbred strains.

β-GLUCURONIDASE STRUCTURE AND EXPRESSION

β-Glucuronidase is a tetrameric lysosomal acid hydrolase with a subunit size of about 71,000 Daltons. It shows an unusual pattern of localization to both microsomes and lysosomes in liver, kidney and lung which is determined by an unusual protein-protein interaction with a protein called egasyn (Es-22) (Medda et al., 1985; Lusis et al.,1976). Recent evidence suggests that the interaction with egasyn may also alter post-translational processing of this lysosomal fraction as well as the microsomal enzyme (Swank et al., submitted).

Table 1. β-Glucuronidase structural and regulatory properties associated with different [Gus] haplotypes present on C57BL congenic strains.

[Gus] Haplotype	Origin[3]	Allele	pI	Structure[1] Heat Stability	Subunit MW	Regulation[2] Activity	ROS
		Alleles from Laboratory Mice					
B	C57BL (VIS)[4]	B	5.98	1.0	74	70	1.0
A	A/J (VIS)	A	5.86	1.0	75	158	2.8
H	C3H (VIS)	H	5.98	0.12	74	59	0.5
		Alleles from Wild Mice					
N	domesticus	N	6.15	1.0	72	158	3.3
Cs	castaneus	Cs	5.80	2.0	74	37	0.65
Cl	"	Cl	5.80	0.4	74	79	0.56
W12	domesticus ?	A	5.86	1.0	75	75	1.0
W16	domesticus ?	A	5.86	nd	75	142	2.5
W17	domesticus ?	A	5.86	nd	75	nd	nd
W18	domesticus	A	5.86	nd	75	137	2.4
W5	domesticus	A	5.86	1.0	75	145	2.5
W26	musculus	A	5.86	nd	nd	55	nd
S	spretus	S	6.15	1.0	74	95	1.2
Ho	hortulanus	Ho	5.98	0.1	nd	2.5	nd

[1]Enzyme structure
  Heat stability: half life of inactivation at 71°C relative to GUS-SB.
  Charge: pI of major lysosomal activity band in isoelectric focusing gels.
  Subunit MW: Molecular weight of subunits in SDS gels (6% acrylamide).
[2]Regulation of expression in testosterone induction of kidney enzyme synthesis
  Activity: Units of activity/gram after 14 days of testosterone treatment.
  Rate of synthesis: Relative rate of synthesis determined by immunoprecipitation of isotope in β-glucuronidase expressed as a ratio of cpm in TCA precipitate protein. Expressed relative to BL/6 rate of synthesis.
[3]Origin
  GUS-N   N   PAC, trapped in Pennsylvania, sent to us by Dr. John Conner in 1975

116

GUS-A (W^{12})	W12	Male 23-4-76-C, trapped in Southern Jutland
GUS-A (W^{16})	W16	Male 8/19/76-A, trapped in Southern Jutland
GUS-A (W^{18})	W18	M. domesticus, trapped on the Chapman farm in East Aurora, NY
GUS-A (W^{5})	W5	MOR, trapped in Ohio in 1962 by Jon Bruell, Case Western Reserve University
GUS-Cl	Cl	M. castaneus - heat labile
GUS-Cs	Cs	M. castaneus - heat stable
GUS-S	S	M. spretus, from Spain, Dr. Richard Sage
GUS-A (W^{26})	W26	Hungary, sent to RPMI in 1979 by J.T. Nielson, Aarhus University, Aarhus, Denmark

[4]VIS = Various Inbred Strains

β-Glucuronidase synthesis is increased 50 to 100 fold in the kidneys of female mice following testosterone treatment. The kinetics of the induction have been extensively characterized. Following an initial lag period, the kinetics of induction can be defined in terms of two rate constants in the equation for standard turnover kinetics (Pfister et al., 1984). A zero order rate constant, ka, describes the increase in the acquisition of GUS mRNA and a first order rate constant, kb, describes the loss of this expression. Laboratory haplotypes vary in the ka component but we have also determined that [Gus] haplotypes from M. castaneus differ for the kb component. Functionally, these haplotypes also show altered translational efficiency of GUS mRNA (Pfister et al., 1985).

[Gus] HAPLOTYPES FROM THE WILD

We have established 11 congenic strains of C57BL mice which carry [Gus] haployptes from diverse genetic stocks (Table 1). These haplotypes differ from those observed among inbred mice in either structure, posttranslational processing, DNA fragment sizes, or haplotype combinations of structure and regulation. Many of these haplotypes also differ for systemic levels of expression and regulation of kidney expression following testosterone treatment.

ENZYME STRUCTURE AND PROCESSING

Alleles of GUS structure (GUS-S) are determined by charge, thermal stability, and antigenic interaction with anti β-glucuronidase antibody. Subtle differences in subunit size are also detectable in SDS denaturing gel electrophoresis. The inbred GUS-SA and -SB alleles differ in the pI of the major lysosomal form. Two alleles, GUS-SN and -SS from strain PAC (Figure 1) and M. spretus respectively have a pI of 6.15, more basic than GUS-B. A slight difference in pI between the GUS-SCl and -SCs alleles and the GUS-SA has also been observed.

The relative half-life of enzyme activity during heat inactivation is also shown. The allelic form from M. castaneus shows unusual features of heat inactivation which differ from other allelic forms (Table 1). (Pfister et al., 1985).

Differences in enzyme structure also lead to differences in the relative size of GUS subunits in SDS gel electrophoresis. The GUS-SN shares the same pI as the allele from M. spretus GUS-SS but it differs from the S allele by almost 2,000 Daltons in subunit size. These results indicate that the allelic forms probably carry different amino

acid substitutions which produce the same apparent pI. Recent work
from our laboratory indicates that the relative proportions of microsomal and lysosomal β-glucuronidase differ between GUS-SN and GUS-SB
or -SA mice and that this appears to be a function of the structural
differences. Moreover, the data suggest that the altered subcellular
distribution may be the result of increased rates of turnover of the
N allele in the lysosomal compartment (R. Swank, personal communication).

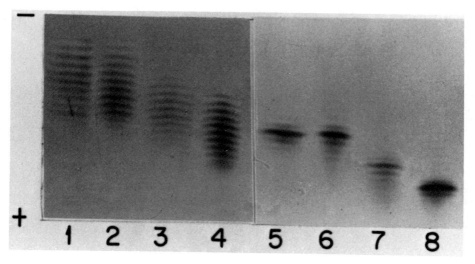

Fig. 1. Isoelectric focusing patterns of β-glucuronidase of microsomal
(lanes 1-4) and lysosomal (lanes 5-8) fractions of kidney homogenates
in 1,5) $[Gus]^N$ in original strain PAC/cv; 2,6)C57BL/6-$[Gus]^N$;
3,7)C57BL/6; 4,8)C57BL/6-$[Gus]^A$.

Finally, we have also identified a GUS-SA like allele in mice trapped
in Hungary which have a marked decrease in liver microsomal GUS
expression. The isoelectric focusing patterns of β-glucuronidase
activity in these mice shows a decrease in the basic microsomal bands
and a high amount of activity in acidic forms of GUS which are highly
sialylated (Figure 2), even in C57BL/6^{W26} mice. These sialylated
forms are found in mutants which lack the egasyn binding protein or
tissues which do not express egasyn (R. Swank et al., in press).
These results suggest that the Hungarian GUS-SA allele may be mutated

118

for the amino acid sequences which are responsible for the β-glucuronidase egasyn interaction.

All of the GUS-S structural alleles have been analyzed as congenic C57BL/6 strains which have undergone 10 or more generations of backcross onto the inbred background. Thus, we would expect that there is a very low probability for genes from the donor strain or mouse unlinked to the GUS locus to remain in these mice and that, on average, there is about 10-20 cMorgans of Gus-linked donor chromosome 5 present. Thus, these congenic strain resources can be used to determine how different GUS-S enzyme structures alter the turnover and/or subcellular processing of the β-glucuronidase molecule.

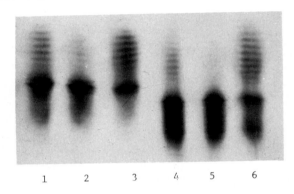

Fig. 2. Isoelectric focusing of liver β-glucuronidase. C57BL/6 in lanes 1-3 and W26 (lanes 4-6). 1,4 whole homogenates; 2,5 lysosomal fractions; 3,6 microsomal fractions.

Table 2. Restriction fragment variants associated with different [Gus] haplotypes

Strain	[Gus] Haplotype	HindIII	BamHI	PstI
C57BL/6	B	3.8	15.5	4.3 ± 0.6
C3H/HeJ	H	3.8	15.5	4.3 ± 0.6
A/J	A	4.0	13.9	5.1
M. domesticus	W15	4.0	15.5	4.9
N. America	W18	4.0	15.5	4.9
M. musculus	W16	3.8	15.5	5.1
Denmark	W17	3.8	15.5	5.1
	W12	3.8	15.5	4.3 ± 0.6

GENOMIC DNA STRUCTURE

The Southern blot analyses of restriction endonuclease fragments using the pGUS-1 cDNA probe have identified three genomic differences among inbred strains (Fig. 3) (Elliott et al., 1985). We have analyzed the restriction fragment patterns of several GUS-SA haplotypes derived from wild mice (Table 3). We observed that the restriction fragment differences between GUS-SA and -SB laboratory mice are not a consistent property of GUS-SA haplotypes recovered from the wild. The North American haplotypes W5 and W18 had the 4.0 kb HindIII fragment similar to the [Gus]^A haplotypes but the 15.5 kb BamHl fragment common to [Gus]^B. By contrast, three GUS-SA haplotypes from Denmark have the same BamHl and HindIII fragments seen in [Gus]^B. One of these haplo-types, W12, has a PstI 4.3 kb fragment similar to GUS-SB while W17 and W18 have GUS-SA-like PstI fragment sizes. Analyses of the enzyme structure shows no differences among these GUS-SA congenic strains in the pI of the lysosomal and microsomal enzyme forms, in heat inactiva-tion, in antigenic sites in the enzyme molecule, and in the charge forms found in cyanogen bromide peptides separated by isoelectric focusing. Moreover, each of these GUS-SA structural alleles shows the peptide charge form previously associated with the GUS-SA allele of inbred strains (Lusis et al., 1980).

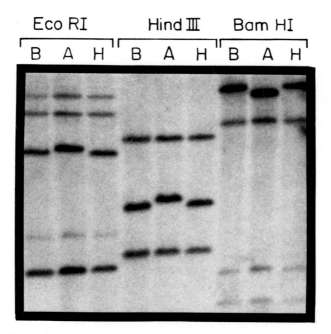

Fig. 3. Southern blot analysis of genomic DNA from C57BL/6 (B), C57BL/6 [Gus]^A (A) and C57BL/6 [Gus]^H (H) digested with the restriction endonucleases EcoRI, HindIII, BamHI.

Taken together, these results indicate that none of the restriction fragment differences observed between laboratory strains is causal of the structural differences between GUS-SA and -SB allelic forms. Moreover, these results indicate that two of these restriction frag-ment differences are not directly concerned with the regulatory differences between GUS-SA and -SB strains in androgen induction of kidney expression.

The most interesting aspect of the results is the difference in restriction fragment pattern for PstI between W12 and W16 and W17. The W12 haplotype expresses a [Gus]^B testosterone induction phenotype while W16 and W17 show [Gus]^A-like induction. Thus, these results suggest that the difference identified by PstI may be related to the induction differences observed between the A and B haplotypes.

VARIATION IN β-GLUCURONIDASE REGULATION

The two M. castaneus haplotypes differ from other strains in tissue levels of synthesis and enzyme activity (Pfister et al., 1985). The Cs and Cl allelic forms differ from each other and from other laboratory haplotypes in systemic levels of expression.

Table 3. Kidney β-glucuronidase activity following 0, 7, and 14 days of subcutaneous implant of testosterone in M. hortulanus (ICR X M. hortulanus)F_1 and Ha/ICR females. Ha/ICR randombred mice are uniformly [Gus]^B. Four females 10-16 weeks of age were used in each group

Genotype	Days of testosterone treatment		
	0	7	14
M. hortulanus	1.83 ± .14	2.78 ± .13	2.49 ± .23
(ICR X M. hortulanus)F_1	2.50 ± .02	23.94 ± 1.33	36.32 ± .83
ICR	4.02 ± .16	40.67 ± 1.10	41.35 ± 1.61

Activity is measured using the substrate 4-methylumbelliferyl-β-D-glucuronic acid and activity is moles/hr/gm tissue weight at 37°C.

One of the more striking differences observed in GUS regulation occurs in the testosterone induction of β-glucuronidase in M. hortulanus. We generally observe a 20 to 50 fold induction in enzyme expression following 7 to 14 days of testosterone treatment of female mice among laboratory strains and most house mouse species, including M. spretus. By contrast, M. hortulanus females show no change in enzyme activity following 14 or more days of testosterone treatment (Table 3). These results could be either a property of the GUS gene in M. hortulanus or the M. hortulanus genetic background. We have derived F_1 hybrids by means of artificial insemination of M. hortulanus sperm into laboratory mouse females (Ha/ICR, randombred) (West et al., 1977). The resulting F_1 hybrid females were testosterone treated and examined for kidney levels of β-glucuronidase expression. We observed levels of activity in F_1 kidneys which were intermediate for β-glucuronidase activity to the levels found in ICR and M. hortulanus. The M. hortulanus GUS-SHo allelic form is less heat stable than the GUS-SB allelic form present in Ha/ICR (Figure 4).

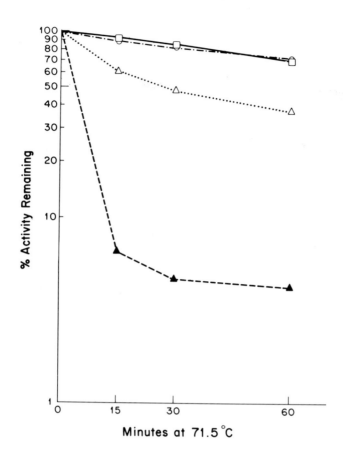

Fig. 4. Heat inactivation of β-glucuronidase in whole kidney homogen-ates expressed as percent activity remaining following 0, 15, 30 or 60 min at 71.5°C. M. hortulanus, (ICR X M. hortulanus)F₁ 0 days testosterone treatment; (ICR X M. hortulanus)F₁ 14 days testos-terone treatment, 0 ICR.

We compared the heat inactivation of β-glucuronidase activity from F_1 kidneys at 0 and 14 days of testosterone treatment. We observed that the heat inactivation kinetics of F_1 β-glucuronidase at 0 days were intermediate between ICR and M. hortulanus. By contrast, the heat inactivation of β-glucuronidase of F_1 and ICR did not differ following 14 days of testosterone treatment. These results indicate that nearly equal levels of M. hortulanus and ICR GUS subunits were present in uninduced female kidneys but that the ICR subunits were the predominant form following testosterone treatment. These findings are consistent with the cis acting regulatory difference between M. hortulanus

122

[Gus]^{Ho} haplotype and [Gus] haplotypes present in house mouse species.

It is of additional interest that other <u>Mus</u> species do not show testosterone induction of kidney β-glucuronidase (Swank et al., 1978) and that these are also probably cis acting differences in regulation. Furthermore, recent work by others suggests that <u>M. hortulanus</u> and <u>M. caroli</u> may lack testosterone induction of other gene sequences (F. Berger, personal communication).

The genetic differences between the house mice and widely diverged <u>Mus</u> species in hormonal and developmental regulation of gene expression in kidney, liver, submandibular gland and other organs have been studied in several laboratories at Roswell Park. In most instances we can only make comparative evaluations of these regulatory phenotypes with little opportunity for a direct genetic analysis. We have been able to produce a small number of F_1 hybrids between <u>M. caroli</u> and laboratory strains (Rossant and Chapman, 1983) and by artificial insemination (West et al., 1977). These hybrids are generally sterile but they provide an experimental test of <u>cis</u> vs. <u>trans</u> regulation for differences in gene regulation (Berger and Baumann, 1985).

The European aboriginal species represented by <u>M. hortulanus</u> provide a similar opportunity to study the genetic basis of regulatory differences but, more importantly, these F_1 hybrid females are fertile in reciprocal matings. This feature provides an opportunity to genetically test specific features of the regulation between species and hopefully we can isolate cis acting differences by molecular cloning and test for trans acting differences by backcrossing known responder alleles into a genetic host which does not normally show hormonal regulation or developmental expression of specific genes.

REFERENCES

Berger FG, Baumann H (1985) An evolutionary switch in tissue-specific gene expression. J Biol Chem 260:1160-1165
Elliott RW, Hohman C, Pazik J, Gallagher PM, Palmer R, Ganschow RE (1985) DNA polymorphisms correlate with glucuronidase haplotypes. J Biol Chem (submitted)
Lusis AJ, Chapman VM, Herbstman C, Paigen K (1980) Quantitation of cis versus trans regulation of mouse β-glucuronidase. J Biol Chem 255: 8959-8962
Lusis AJ, Tomino S, Paigen K (1976) Isolation, characterization and radioimmunoassay of murine egasyn, a protein stabilizing glucuronidase membrane binding. J Biol Chem 251:7753-7760
Medda, S., von Deimling O, Swank RT (1985) Identity of esterase-22 and egasyn, the protein which complexes with microsomal β-glucuronidase. (submitted)
Paigen K (1979) Acid hydrolases as models of genetic control. Ann Rev Genet 13:417-466
Palmer R, Gallagher PM, Boyko WL, Ganschow RE (1983) Genetic control of levels of murine kidney glucuronidase mRNA in response to androgen. Proc Natl Acad Sci USA 80:7596-7600
Pfister K, Chapman V, Watson G, Paigen K (1985) Genetic variation for enzyme structure and systemic regulation in two new haplotypes of the β-glucuronidase gene of <u>Mus musculus castaneus</u>. J Biol Chem (in press)
Pfister K, Paigen K, Watson G, Chapman V (1982) Expression of β-glucuronidase haplotypes in prototype and congenic mouse strains. Biochem Genet 20:519-536

Pfister K, Watson G, Chapman V, Paigen K (1984) Kinetics of β-glucuroni-
  dase induction by androgen. J Biol Chem 259:5816-5820
Rossant J, Chapman VM (1983) Somatic and germline mosaicism in inter-
  specific chimaeras between Mus musculus and Mus caroli. J Embryol exp
  Morph 73:193-205
Swank RT, Paigen K, Davey R, Chapman V, Labarca C, Watson G, Ganschow R,
  Brandt EJ, Novak EK (1978) Genetic regulation of mammalian glucuroni-
  dase. Recent Progress in Hormone Res 34:401-436
Swank RT, Paigen K, Ganschow R (1973) Genetic control of glucuronidase
  induction in mice. J Mol Biol 81:225-243
West JD, Frels WI, Papaioannou VE, Karr J, Chapman VM (1977) Development
  of interspecific hybrids of Mus. J Embryol exp Morph 41:233-243

Genetic Variation in Major Urinary Proteins in Wild Mice

W. A. Held and B. M. Sampsell

INTRODUCTION

The major urinary proteins are a group of closely-related
polypeptides of low molecular weight (17,800) and acidic
isoelectric points. As their name indicates, collectively they
represent the predominant protein fraction of mouse urine, and in
male mice may be excreted at the rate of 20 mg per day (Szoka and
Paigen 1978). These urinary proteins are synthesized in the liver
where MUP mRNA accounts for 5% of the total messenger RNA (Hastie
et al. 1979). Inbred male mice excrete about 20 times more MUP
than females and have about five-fold higher MUP mRNA levels in the
liver. MUP mRNA has also been detected in the submaxillary,
lachrymal, and mammary glands (Shaw et al. 1983). The function of
MUPs and whether they appear in other body secretions besides urine
is not known. The genes coding for the MUPs are members of a
multigene family with approximately 30-35 copies (Hastie et al.
1979; Bishop et al. 1982). The gene cluster has been mapped to
chromosome 4 and is linked to the brown locus (Bennett et al. 1982;
Krauter et al. 1982; Bishop et al. 1982). Recent work (Clark et
al. 1984) indicates that many of the MUP genes on chromosome 4 are
organized pairwise in a divergent fashion with each pair of
consisting of about 45 kb of DNA.

MUP VARIATION IN INBRED STRAINS

Early investigations showed that different inbred strains of mice
had characteristic quantities of at least three different MUPs
which were distinguishable on the basis of electrophoretic mobility
(Finlayson et al. 1963; Szoka and Paigen 1978; Groen and Lagerwerf
1979). Most inbred lines fell into one of two phenotypic classes
on the basis of the relative amounts of each MUP excreted following
testosterone induction. For example, DBA and C57BL/6 belong to
different phenotypic classes. The fact that both classes of mice
could produce all three forms of the protein led Szoka and Paigen
to discard the earlier hypothesis that MUPs 2 and 3 (numbering
system of Knopf et al. 1983) were the products of alternate structural
alleles and to suggest that the two classes differed at a regulatory
locus (denoted Mup-1) which they showed to be linked to the brown
locus.

Because of the apparent complexity of the MUP multigene complex it
now seems more reasonable to interpret the two phenotypes associated
with the Mup-1^a and Mup-1^b genotypes as carrying alternate haplotypes
in which variation may reside in regulatory regions adjacent to each
MUP structural gene as well as within MUP coding regions. (At this
time, the only evidence of the same structural gene in two different

mice is comigration of MUPs. Comigration, however, does not prove
that the amino acid sequences of the proteins are identical, nor
that the proteins are encoded by the same locus.) Inheritance of a
specific MUP multigene complex results in a particular pattern of
gene expression and urinary protein phenotype, as well as in a
characteristic response to testosterone induction.

The use of two-dimensional polyacrylamide electrophoresis has made it
possible to distinguish a number of additional MUPs. Urine from a
C57BL/6 male actually displays at least seven proteins with slightly
different mobilities. We have also used isoelectric focusing alone
(employing a slab gel with a narrow pH range of 4.5 to 5.4) and have
succeeded in resolving more components. For example, in the urine
of a DBA male, MUP 2 is resolved into two bands.

ISOLATION OF MUP GENES

Studies are now in progress in several labs to determine the
organization of individual MUP genes within the complex with respect
to orientation, spacing, and degree of homology. A number of MUP
cDNAs have been isolated for use as probes (Clissold and Bishop
1981; Kuhn et al. 1984). Differential hybridization of various MUP
probes to restriction maps of the genomic clones provide evidence
for several subfamilies of MUP genes with members of each subfamily
showing a greater similarity to one another than to genes of a
different subfamily.

Two MUP cDNA clones (p199 and p499) were derived from C57BL/6
liver RNA. Sequencing has shown that the two genes are divergent
at 20% of their sites in the portion 5' of a common Pvu II site.
These two 5' regions were subcloned and have been used to
discriminate two subsets of MUP genes and their transcripts. There
appear to be a large number of genomic sequences homologous to
p499-5', but only a few (and perhaps only one) copies homologous to
p199-5'. In vitro translation of mRNAs hybridizing to the two
different 5' subclones revealed that the p199-5' sequence represents
about 10% of the liver MUP messenger RNA and codes for MUP-6, a
protein seen in urine at low abundance. Sequences homologous to
p499-5' code for nearly all the abundant urinary proteins namely
MUPs 1, 2, 3, 4, and 5 (Kuhn et al. 1984).

MUP VARIATION IN WILD-DERIVED MICE

We have used the p199 and p499 MUP cDNA clones to survey the level
of activity of MUP genes as well as their genomic organization in
a number of stocks of wild-derived mice maintained by Verne
Chapman at Roswell Park Memorial Institute (Sampsell and Held 1985).
Interesting interspecific variation was observed in both the
quantity of MUP mRNA as well as in the apparent number of genomic
MUP sequences corresponding to the two subfamilies.

Variation in Major Urinary Proteins

Total liver RNA extracts from male mice were hybridized to cloned
cDNA. The selected mRNAs were then translated in vitro and
analyzed by 2-D electrophoresis. Three Mus domesticus stocks (PAC,
MOR, and praetextus) displayed patterns identical to those seen in

126

C57BL/6. M. musculus and M. molossinus each showed acidic proteins
with mobilizes like MUPs 3 and 4, but in addition had one or more
basic proteins unlike any inbred mouse. None of the proteins
synthesized from M. spretus MUP mRNA comigrated with any of the
C57BL/6 proteins being generally more acidic and slightly higher
in molecular weight. Only a few spots were seen on the gels
containing translation products from M. caroli or M. cervicolor
mRNA. This may indicate a lower level of MUP mRNA in these stocks
or may be the consequence of greater divergence between their MUP
coding sequences and the MUP cDNA used for RNA selection. In
general, 2-D gels of urine samples from the stocks were quite similar
to the gels of their translation products.

Table 1. Variation in expression of subfamilies of major urinary
protein genes in wild-derived mice

	p499 Subfamily	p199 Subfamily	Male:Female (Total MUPs)
C57BL/6	90% of liver	10% of liver	5:1
	(wild-derived males compared with C57BL/6 males)		
M. domesticus	1 X	1 X	1:1*
M. musculus	4 X	1/15	10:1
M. molossinus	1 X	1/3	5:1
M. castaneus	2 X	1 X	5:1
M. spretus	2 X	1/20	100:1
M. hortulanus	1/5	1/20	10:1
M. caroli	1/10	2 X	1:1
M. cervicolor	1/40	1 X	5:1

* PAC and MOR; the male:female ratio for M.d. praetextus was
  5:1.

Variation in MUP mRNA Levels

Samples of total liver RNA were used to prepare dot-blots and
Northern blots. Nick-translated p199-5' or p499-5' MUP cDNA was
hybridized to these blots and the intensity of hybridization was
estimated by comparison to a dilution series or by scanning
densitometry (see Table 1). Males of the M. musculus and M.
castaneus stocks had levels of p499 MUP mRNA several-fold higher
than inbred males although the level of p199 sequences in M.
musculus was markedly lower. M. caroli and M. cervicolor seemed
to have few p499-like sequences, but p199-like sequences were as
abundant, or more abundant, than in inbred strains. As previously
observed with the inbred strains, females tended to have lower MUP
mRNA levels than their male conspecifics. An exception was seen
in the wild M. domesticus stocks (PAC and MOR) in which some females

had levels of both p199 and p499 nearly equal to that in males. It
was later observed that while uninduced C57BL/6 females excrete
predominantly MUP 3, PAC and MOR females excrete large amounts of
MUP 3 and 4 and occasionally MUPs 1 and 2 as well.

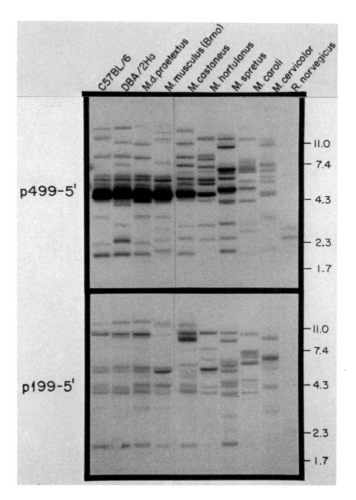

Fig. 1. Southern blots of genomic DNA digested with Pvu II
restriction endonuclease and hybridized to MUP cDNA sequences
indicated on the left. The sizes of lambda restriction fragment
markers are shown on the right. Hybridization and wash
conditions are described in Sampsell and Held 1985.

Variation in Genomic MUP Sequences

Genomic DNAs prepared from males of various stocks were digested
with Pvu II, and the restriction fragments separated by agarose
gel electrophoresis. The Southern blots were probed with the
subcloned MUP cDNAs (Fig. 1). As might be expected, hybridization
intensity and size of hybridizing fragments were most similar to
inbred strains among the closely-related wild-derived stocks. DNA
from distant relatives showed variation in the size of fragments
and a reduced level of hybridization consistent with genetic
divergence of the MUP coding regions as well as with differences
in number of gene copies. Attempts to correlate differences in
MUP mRNA levels with genomic organization produced several
possibilities. As previously noted, males of two different stocks
of M. musculus had relatively low levels of p199 MUP mRNA in their
livers. DNA from both stocks lacked an 11 kb Pvu II fragment to
which p199 cDNA hybridizes strongly in all the M. domesticus
strains examined. Both M. musculus stocks had a strongly hybridizing
5.6 kb fragment instead, suggesting that the p199 gene has undergone
some sort of alteration which may affect its expression.

M. castaneus had a relatively high level of p199 mRNA and an
additional band (approximately 10 kb) to which the p199-5' probe
hybridized suggesting duplication of the p199 gene in this stock.
Very little hybridization was observed between the p499-5' probe
and genomic DNA from M. caroli or M. cervicolor, while the p199-5'
probe hybridized to several fragments at about the same intensity
as in M. domesticus. Neither stock appeared to have the 11 kb
fragment, however. These results suggest that the p199 and p499
subfamilies of MUP genes have had separate evolutionary histories
in this species and that the p199 sequence, in particular, is
widely distributed.

GENETIC BASIS OF MUP VARIATION

Several types of genetic variation may contribute to the
heterogeneity described above. During the evolution of the MUP
multigene family mutations may have accumulated in regions
encoding MUP polypeptides as well as in adjacent control regions.
In addition, the total number of gene copies can vary. Two
proteins with different mobilities (observed in different stocks)
may be the product of alleles at the same locus in which a
nucleotide substitution has led to a detectable amino acid
replacement, or may be the products of genes at different loci -
one of which may be silent or even absent in one of the stocks.
Allelic relationships are especially hard to define in the context
of a clustered multigene system.

The results of genetic crosses performed to date suggest that a
particular MUP phenotype is the product of a specific set of
coding regions and their linked control regions. Thus, F_1 progeny
between stocks with different MUP phenotypes display (in a sex
specific manner) MUP phenotypes which are the combination of the
two parental phenotypes (Hudson et al. 1967; Sampsell and Held
1985).

The MUP phenotypes of M. domesticus PAC males are identical to
those of C57BL/6, but the females excrete a wider range of MUPs.

Crosses between PAC and DBA strains have been carried through two
generations. Urine from F$_2$ animals conformed to one of three
phenotypes: PAC, DBA, or hybrid. These phenotypes were perfectly
correlated with the <u>brown</u> marker on chromosome 4 as determined by
visible coat color or test crosses. One individual appeared to
have inherited a chromosome in which a recombination had occurred
between the MUP genes and <u>brown</u>, and it is being studied in more
detail. These results suggest that the PAC strain has a MUP
haplotype differing from the two carried by the majority of the
lab mice by virtue of a regulatory region affecting expression of
MUPs 1, 2, and especially 4 in females. The levels of MUP mRNA in
the livers of the F$_2$ progeny was examined using dot blots of total
liver RNA probed with p499. The mRNA levels in females of all
three genotypes showed a wide range with some females having levels
equal to or greater than their male sibs, while in others the level
was several fold lower. Thus the high mRNA levels that had been
observed in PAC females did not appear to be the consequence of a
particular MUP complex. Rather the overall level of MUP mRNA is a
polygenic trait influenced by unlinked genes.

SUMMARY AND CONCLUSIONS

Wild-derived stocks of mice clearly represent a source of abundant
genetic variation for the MUP multigene family. Inbred strains of
<u>M. domesticus</u> also contain polymorphisms either for coding regions
or control regions. In one sense the variation may be too profuse
for immediate explanation, since we cannot reliably distinguish
between alleleic variations in coding sequences, mutations in
control regions, and differential gene duplication. Work currently
in progress should lead, however, to the complete cloning, sequencing,
and mapping of the gene cluster for one or more of the inbred
strains within the next few years. At that point, comparative
studies employing the wild-derived stocks may provide answers to
the following sorts of questions: Is there a pattern to the
organization of genes expressed in a particular tissue, at a
particular developmental stage, or in response to a given hormonal
stimulus? Has gene duplication increased the number of copies
belonging to certain subfamilies differentially? What are the
relative roles of gene conversion and natural selection in
maintaining similarities between the different MUP genes and their
products?

REFERENCES

Bennett KL, Lalley PA, Barth RK, Hastie ND (1982) Mapping the
   structural genes coding for the major urinary proteins in the
   mouse: combined use of recombinant inbred strains and somatic
   cell hybrids. Proc Natl Acad Sci 79:1220
Bishop JO, Clark AJ, Clissold PM, Hainey S, Franke U (1982) Two
   main groups of mouse major urinary protein genes, both largely
   located on chromosome 4. EMBO J 1:615-620
Clark AJ, Hickman J, Bishop J (1984) A 45-kb DNA domain with two
   divergently oriented genes is the unit of organization of the
   murine major urinary protein genes. EMBO J 3:2055-2064
Clissold PM, Bishop JO (1981) Molecular cloning of cDNA sequences
   transcribed from mouse liver endoplasmic reticulum poly(A) mRNA.
   Gene 15:225-235
Finlayson JS, Potter M, Runner RC (1963) Electrophoretic variation

and sex dimorphism of the major urinary protein complex in inbred mice: a new genetic marker. J Natl Cancer Inst 31:91-97

Groen A, Lagerwerf AJ (1979) Genetically determined electrophoretic variants of the major urinary protein (Mup) complex in mouse urine. Anim Blood Grps Biochem Genet 10:107-114

Hastie ND, Held WA, Toole JJ (1979) Multiple genes coding for the androgen-regulated major urinary proteins of the mouse. Cell 17:449-457

Hudson DM, Finlayson JS, Potter M (1967) Linkage of one component of the major urinary protein complex of mice to the brown coat color locus. Genet Res 10:195-198

Knopf JL, Gallagher JF, Held WA (1983) Differential, multi-hormonal regulation of the mouse major urinary protein gene family in the liver. Mol Cell Biol 3:2232-2240

Krauter K, Leinwand L, D'Eustachio P, Ruddle F, Darnell JE, Jr (1982) Structural genes of the mouse major urinary protein are on chromosome 4. J Cell Biol 94:414-417

Kuhn NJ, Woodworth M, Gross KW, Held WA (1984) Subfamilies of the mouse major urinary protein (MUP) multi-gene family: sequence analysis of cDNA clones and differential regulation in the liver. Nucleic Acids Res 12:6073-6090

Sampsell B, Held WA (1985) Variation in the major urinary protein multigene family in wild-derived mice. Genetics 109:549-568

Shaw PH, Held WA, Hastie ND (1983) The gene family for major urinary proteins: expression in several secretory tissues of the mouse. Cell 32:755-761

Szoka PR, Paigen K (1978) Regulation of mouse major urinary protein by the Mup-a gene. Genetics 90:597-612

Immobilized-gradient Isoelectric Focusing: Detection of "Silent" Biochemical Genetic Variants

J.B. Whitney III

INTRODUCTION

Electrophoretic methods of various kinds are used to reveal
genetically-encoded variations in enzymes and other proteins. The
variants that are detected provide invaluable genetic markers applicable in a variety of kinds of biological and biomedical research.
It is recognized, however, that many genetically-determined differences in amino acid sequence go undetected in standard electrophoretic
analyses. These "silent" changes involve substitutions of one neutral
amino acid for another neutral amino acid (alanine, glycine, valine,
isoleucine, leucine, serine, threonine, asparagine, glutamine).

A new technique has recently been introduced that promises to make the
detection of neutral amino acid substitutions in proteins as routine
as the current use of regular electrophoretic variants. The new
method -- immobilized gradient isoelectric focusing -- is comparable
in complexity to gradient polyacrylamide gel electrophoresis and comparable in expense to standard isoelectric focusing in 2 mm-thick
polyacrylamide gels. The new method involves the casting of a polyacrylamide gel that polymerizes to incorporate a pH gradient of a
defined span and of a small to medium range. The equipment needed
includes a power supply capable of delivering low milliamperage at
2000 V or more, a cooling platform suitable for electrophoresis at
this high voltage, and a source of cooling liquid at 10°C.

It is calculated that electrophoretically-silent amino acid substitutions are even more common than substitutions that affect protein
size or charge, that generally are electrophoretically detectable.
Many possible changes in codons (particularly at the third base
position) produce no change in the amino acid sequence and therefore
cannot be qualitatively-detectable at the protein level. Other
changes, that have "drastic" effects on protein structure (Modiano
et al., 1981), involve the termination codons. All of the rest of
the codon changes cause substitutions of one amino acid for another.
At pH 8.6, often used for electrophoretic screening studies, only
the amino acids aspartic and glutamic acid and lysine and arginine
are effectively charged (Modiano et al., 1981). Fewer than half of
the possible substitutions in amino acid-encoding codons produce
changes that involve these four charged amino acids (26.7% overall
in the case of human hemoglobin; Modiano et al., 1981). These
changes are generally electrophoretically detectable.

The remainder of the amino acid substitutions, of neutral amino acids
for other neutral amino acids, are usually undetectable or "silent."
This class should include even more variants than does the class of
electrophoretically-detectable substitutions in a particular protein.

Righetti (1983) has estimated that only 40% of all amino acid substitutions are electrophoretically detectable, while 60% are of the heretofore "silent" type.

Substitution of one neutral amino acid for another has a minimal effect on the structure and function of an enzyme or protein, so the variant or mutant gene responsible for such a change would be not unlikely to persist in the population. Unfortunately, because these changes are electrophoretically undectable, there has until now been no easy way to employ this large class of variants as genetic markers for biochemical genetic analyses of wild mice, or for other applications.

MATERIALS AND METHODS

Immobilized Gradient Isoelectric Focusing

The technique for the immobilized gradient isoelectric focusing of hemoglobins from freshly prepared samples of blood from laboratory mice has been described recently (Whitney et al., 1985). Some variations that have often or consistently provein beneficial are described here. Also described below is the storage and re-use of the immobilized gradient polyacrylamide gels. The specific immobilized gradient gel described here was designed to provide information on the mouse hemoglobins, but is suitable for the analyses of some human hemoglobins as well. It should also be suitable for the analyses of enzymes or other proteins that have isoelectric points in the pH 7.2 to 7.55 range. The primary change required to prepare immobilized gradient isoelectric focusing gels suitable for the analyses of other proteins should be the substitution of LKB Immobilines suitable to create the pH span desired (see LKB "Application Notes" 321 and 324).

Using the LKB gradient gel kit, 0.5 mm-thick polyacrylamide gels are cast on Gelbond PAG films approximately 26 cm x 12 cm. Approximately 23 DYMO tape 5 mm squares placed 5 mm apart on the LKB Repelsilane-coated face plate create sample well pockets in the gel. The edges of the casting mold are sealed with autoclave tape, and as many clamps are placed around the edge as are necessary to assure that the volume added to the mold is sufficient to fill it (14.6 to 15.2 ml, generally). The amount of LKB Immobiline pK 3.6 used in the less dense ("pH 7.55") solution can be as much as 170 microliters. The amount of LKB Immobiline pK 3.6 in the more dense ("pH 7.2") solution can be as little as 320 microliters. Each solution receives 863 microliters of pK 7 Immobiline. After polymerization at 50°C for not over one hour, the gel is removed from the mold, weighed, and stored at 4°C in a Tupperware "bacon-keeper" box for one day up to several months in 10 or 20 mM EDTA, pH 7. Storage solutions of 0.05% sodium azide or 0.2 M EDTA, pH 7, have also been used successfully.

Prior to use, free ions are removed by rocking the gel in several changes of deionized water over the course of 1.5 hr or more. An ohmmeter is useful to monitor the deionization: one probe is placed at each end of the gel and the resistance is recorded. At each deionized water change, water is briefly drained from the gel and a new reading is taken. When the resistance reaches a constant maximum, the gel is ready for use. The water is drained off briefly, and two Kimwipes are laid across the surface of the gel to blot away any remaining surface water. The gel is then weighed and allowed to dry at room temperature. The gel is weighed periodically to monitor the evaporation of water. If the gel has not previously been used, grooves are cut to separate each sample lane from the adjacent lanes. Total drying time should be around one hour.

Samples of 5-8 microliters each are applied and the gel is covered with a polyester sheet. If the gel does not quite reach the cathode-edge electrode because the amount of solution added to the gradient maker was inadequate, a two- or four-thickness strip of paper towel wet with deionized water can be used to produce a bridge from the electrode up onto the edge of the gel. Focusing is carried out as previously described (Whitney et al., 1985) at 2000 V overnight or longer, until clear patterns are evident. Focusing can also be carried out overnight at not over 3000 V nor 2.5 W nor 5 mA, with the voltage increased to 5000 V to sharpen the bands for the final hour(s). If there is a tendency for the gel to accumulate water, the polyester cover is removed and Kimwipes are laid atop the gel to absorb it. The gel is then re-covered and the current is reapplied. If there is a tendency for the gel to become too dry, the interior of the apparatus can be humidified by filling the (unused) electrophoresis-reservoirs with water and passing a slow stream of air through the water.

If the gel is to be re-used, the hemoglobin patterns are recorded by photographing or Xerox copying, or the proteins are transferred to filter paper or nitrocellulose membranes that can be stained directly with Ponceau S solution (Helena). Otherwise, fixation and staining can be carried out by standard methods and the gel dried at room temperature.

Re-use of Immobilized Gradient Polyacrylamide Isoelectric Focusing Gels

If a gel is to be re-used, after recording of the patterns it is placed into fresh storage solution and kept at 4°C until the hemoglobins have eluted, then handled in the same manner as a previously unused gel, except, of course, that it does not have to be grooved again. Special care should be taken to remove dislocated bits of gels from previously-used gels after the final water wash step. Gels have been used successfully as many as seven times.

Wild Mouse Samples

For the analyses of the alpha globin genotypes of wild European mice (Sage, Whitney, and Wilson, this volume), red blood cells were washed three times by centrifugation from saline, packed in 0.4 ml poly-propylene tubes, and frozen in liquid nitrogen for long-term storage at -70°C. For isoelectric focusing, hemolysates were prepared by scraping from the partially-defrosted surface an amount of packed cells ranging up to approximately 10 microliters. The cells were expelled into 12 x 75 mm polystyrene tubes, and an amount of deionized water up to approximately 50 microliters was added to produce a hemo-lysate matching or slightly exceeding the depth of color characteristic of the freshly prepared samples described previously (Whitney et al., 1985). When very small samples are available, 2 microliters of erythrocytes is more than adequate if a correspondingly smaller amount of water is used.

134

RESULTS

Mouse Alpha Globin Genetics

The figure shows the variety of hemoglobin alpha chain genotypes that
have been discovered in inbred strains (haplotypes a through h), in
exotic laboratory-maintained stocks, or in wild or feral mice
(Whitney et al., 1979, 1985). Some hemoglobin patterns are observed
in samples from wild mice that cannot be interpreted as products of
any heterozygous combination of the haplotypes already characterized.
Thus, one or more additional haplotypes may exist in these mice,
probably in heterozygous condition. All of the genotypes found in
laboratory-maintained exotic mice probably have been seen again in
wild mice; likewise, almost all of the haplotypes evident in wild mice
were also seen in Dr. M. Potter's laboratory-maintained exotic mice
(Potter, 1981).

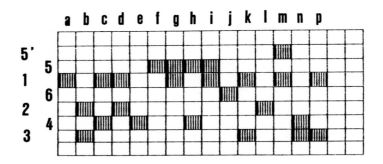

Fig. 1. Alpha globin chains specified by various Hba haplotypes. The
various alpha globin haplotypes ("alleles") characterized thus far are
listed across the top of the chart. Along the left edge are listed
numbers of the individual globin chains encoded by the various haplotypes, in the order of their hemoglobins' pI values (5' (cathodal),
5, 1, 6, 2, 4, 3 (anodal)). A filled box indicates that the chain of
the number listed at the left of its row is specified by the haplotype
of the letter listed at the top of its column. Some haplotypes specify
only one alpha globin chain, while others specify two. Some haplotypes
differ only in the amounts of certain chains produced. The globins
specified by the Hba^j through Hba^p haplotypes have not been sequenced,
so their chain number assignments are tentative. Haplotypes Hba^a
through Hba^h are known in standard inbred strains. At least two
additional uncharacterized Hba haplotypes probably exist in wild mice.

Only five different natural alpha globin chains (numbers 1-5) are known
within the Mus domesticus/M. musculus groups (Chain 6 is found in the
distinct interbreedable species, M. spretus, while chain 5' is the
result of an induced mutation.). The various haplotypes encode these
five chains individually and in various combinations. In some cases,
two haplotypes encode the same chains expressed in different ratios
(see Whitney et al., 1985). One of the difficulties in interpreting
the hemoglobin patterns of wild mice comes from the fact that various
genotypic combinations produce similar patterns (partly because the
hemoglobins with alpha chains 3 and 4 are not resolved by the current
system). For instance, many heterozygous genotypic combinations encode

mixtures of three different major hemoglobins with alpha globin chains 1, 2, and 3 or 4. These include the haplotypes a/b, b/c, c/d, p/d, c/1, p/1, k/d, and k/1. In some cases, the expected amounts of the chains present are quite similar for two different heterozygotes, so breeding studies would be necessary to assign genotypes unequivocally.

DISCUSSION

The mouse alpha globin locus is not found to be polymorphic by the criterion of standard electrophoresis. It is thus like most of the loci tested in the mouse in that it has three or fewer common allelic alternatives detectable by routine methods (Staats, 1980). Loci with many common alleles or haplotypes include the immunoglobulin and histocompatibility loci, but the great majority of the "polymorphic" biochemical genetic loci in the mouse exhibit only two alleles. Almost all of the other polymorphic loci tested have three or four known alleles.

Nonetheless, an extraordinary amount of genetic polymorphism is found at the mouse alpha globin locus by isoelectric focusing in immobilized gradient polyacrylamide gels. It is known that the differences detectable are due to substitutions of neutral amino acids for other neutral amino acids (Popp et al., 1982). Substitutions of this type are not expected to be detected by standard electrophoretic methods.

Alternative Hypotheses

Two dramatically-different alternative explanations for the great heterogeneity found at the Hba locus offer themselves for testing. One is specific and singles out the Hba locus as a special case. The second is more general and has wide-ranging implications.

First, the mouse alpha globin locus may indeed be unusual among biochemical-genetic loci in its having a great number of alternative genotypes (around 13) that encode polypeptides with "silent" substitutions. Some of the special character of the locus could then be explained away by noting that many of the different combinations of alpha globin genes may have arisen by intra-locus recombination or gene conversion between the two adult alpha-globin genes of the Hba complex.

The second possibility is that genetic variants that encode "silent" amino acid substitutions are indeed common and that they have simply been unrecognized in hundreds of routine electrophoretic analyses. That they would have been overlooked is unquestionable. Whether they actually exist has not heretofore been readily testable. If immobilized gradient isoelectric focusing proves capable of revealing as many "silent" substitutions in other proteins and enzymes as have been detected in the alpha globins, then the variety of biochemical genetic variants available for application as markers in different types of biomedical research could easily double by the simple application of this methodology.

Special Characteristics of Immobilized Gradient Isoelectric Focusing

Isoelectric focusing was previously shown to be capable of separating different mouse hemoglobins that differ only by substitutions of neutral amino acids (Whitney et al., 1979). Nonetheless, the separations achieved by standard ampholyte focusing even in "narrow range" gels were not great. Immobilized gradients that can be cast in very small ranges provide several-fold better resolutions of these nearly-identical proteins. A separation of several millimeters is obtained between the hemoglobins with alpha chains 1 and 5, that differ by a glycine for alanine substitution, in the 0.35 unit pH gradient described (Whitney et al., 1985). Gels of a pH span as small as 0.1 unit are said to be possible.

Other special advantages of immobilized gradient isoelectric focusing relative to standard ampholyte focusing include (a) the avoidance of cathodal drift that plagues standard isoelectric focusing, (b) higher load capacities and a tolerance for reasonably high sample ion concentrations, (c) uniform conductivity across the gel and uniform buffering capacity at low concentrations of buffering ions, allowing high voltage gradients, and (d) known and controlled ionic strength in the gels, 100-fold less than in ampholyte gels (Allen et al., 1984). Because very high voltages can be applied without overheating, high degrees of resolution can be achieved (resolution is proportional to the square root of the voltage gradient applied (Allen et al., 1984)). Proteins differing by a pI of 0.001 should be separable from one another on very narrow range gels.

Major disadvantages of immobilized gradients that were considered by Allen et al. (1984) included (a) the necessity to form a gradient for each separation, (b) a "doubtful reproducibility between laboratories," and (c) difficulty in measuring the pH gradient. The requirement for relatively specialized equipment and a long run time may also be restrictive in some contexts. The complexity of preparing thin-layer gradient gels and initially defining suitably-specific pH gradients has certainly dissuaded some potential users of immobilized gradient gels. The possibility of re-using the gradient gels, as described here, overcomes to some extent the first limitation.

Re-use of Immobilized Gradient Isoelectric Focusing Gels

Immobilized pH gradient polyacrylamide gels require a significant initial effort in casting and grooving the gel prior to its first use. When a particularly good separation gel has been created, it is desirable to be able to use it for multiple sets of analyses. Because hemoglobin is visible without staining, no fixation nor staining is necessary before assigning of genotypes, so recycling of the gels is possible by simply eluting the protein prior to the next use of the gel. Since the protein is at its isoelectric point after focusing, its ionic attraction to the medium is at a minimum. In the case of enzymes or other non-hemoglobin proteins, the re-use of separation gels should be feasible if non-destructive methods can be used to reveal the proteins' characteristic pI positions. Where enzyme activity can be visualized without the creation of precipitates, it should be possible to carry out the reactions and then elute both the proteins and reactants following activity detection. Where the products of the visualization reaction are essentially insoluble, it may be necessary to translocate the enzyme from the separation gel prior to its detection via enzymatic activity. Several methods have been described for the transfer of proteins from separation media (for examples, see Righetti, 1983). In this laboratory, nitrocellulose prints of immobilized gradient-resolved hemoglobins have been obtained within a few minutes. Enzymes transferred from ampholyte focusing gels can also be visualized by histochemical means after blotting to nitrocellulose (James E. Carroll and Byron S. McGuire, Jr., Acyl Coenzyme A dehydrogenases; personal communication), and it seems likely that immobilized gradient gels should provide equally good results.

Biochemical Genetics

Immobilized gradient isoelectric focusing promises to have a great impact on the field of population genetics. The measurement of "hidden" genetic variation has been a "central problem of evolutionary genetics" (Lewontin, 1974). As stated by Lewontin (1974), "the possibility of enumerating discrete genotypic classes depends on whether the substitution of one allele for another at a locus leads to a sufficiently large change in phenotype." Because it enables the detection of a large number of previously-undectable variants, immobilized gradient isoelectric focusing can be a valuable technique to provide new markers, readily characterized, to complement those that have recently become detectable only as DNA polymorphisms.

The mouse <u>Hba</u> locus provides a prime example of a locus at which NO variation is observed in natural populations studied at the protein level by standard electrophoretic techniques. Nonetheless, the number of alternative genotypes actually segregating in natural populations proves to be large (Sage et al., this volume). Consequently, many wild individuals tested prove to have heterozygous genotypes, while homozygosity for some genotypes is rarely or never observed.

ACKNOWLEDGEMENTS

This work was supported in part by Biomedical Research Support Grant 2 S07 RR05365-24. This is contribution number 947 from the Department of Cell and Molecular Biology, Medical College of Georgia.

REFERENCES

Allen RC, Saravis CA, Maurer HR (1984) Gel electrophoresis and isoelectric focusing of proteins: selected techniques. de Gruyter, New York, 255 pp
Lewontin RC (1974) The genetic basis of evolutionary change. Columbia University Press, 346 pp
Modiano G, Battistuzzi G, Motulsky AG (1981) nonrandom patterns of codon usage and of nucleotide substitutions in human alpha- and beta-globin genes: An evolutionary strategy reducing the rate of mutations with drastic effects? Proc Natl Acad Sci 78:1110-1114
Popp RA, Bailiff EG, Skow LC, Whitney III JB (1982) The primary structure of genetic variants of mouse hemoglobin. Biochem Genet 20: 199-208
Potter M (1981) Wild mice. Mouse News Letter 64:62-64.
Righetti PG (1983) Isoelectric focusing: Theory, methodology, and applications. Elsevier Biomedical, New York, 386 pp
Staats J (1980) Standardized nomenclature for inbred strains of mice: Seventh listing. Cancer Res 40:2083-2128
Whitney III JB, Copland GT, Skow LC, Russell ES (1979) Resolution of the products of the duplicated alpha-chain loci by isoelectric focusing. Proc Natl Acad Sci 76:867-871
Whitney III JB, Cobb RR, Popp RA, O'Rourke TW (1985) Detection of neutral amino acid substitutions in proteins. Proc Natl Acad Sci 82 (in press)

Ig Heavy Chain

Evolution of the Mouse IgA Gene: Nucleotide Sequence Comparison of IgA in BALB/c and *Mus pahari*

B.A. Osborne, T.E. Golde, R.L. Schwartz, and S. Rudikoff

INTRODUCTION

IgA is the principal antibody of the secretory immune system. It has been found to constitute as much as 80% of the total immuno-globulin found in the fluids secreted by mucous membranes (Kornfeld and Plaut, 1981). The secretory immune system is not only compart-mentalized in distinct regions, but also must perform functionally distinct tasks from other classes of immunoglobulin. It has been clearly demonstrated by a number of laboratories that IgA producing plasma cells lie within the mucousal surfaces of the body that are contiguous with the external environment. Secretory IgA appears to bind to bacteria, viruses, toxins, enzymes and dietary macro-molecules; however, the mechanism through which IgA disposes of antigen is unclear. IgA does not bind completement nor is it opsinized by macrophages. There is convincing evidence that suggests that IgA functions by preventing adherence of bacteria to tissues (Williams and Gibbons, 1972). Since adherence is a prerequisite for infection, this appears to be a reasonable method by which IgA may function in the defense against foreign pathogens.

IgA exists in two forms, a secretory and a serum form. Secretory IgA is a dimeric protein with a molecular weight of about 320,000. The dimer is held together by J chain which attaches to the IgA at the C-terminal of the molecule. Before it is secreted, a glyco-protein secretory component of approximately 55,000 mw is attached via disulfide linkages to the IgA molecule. This secretory component is attached during the transport of the IgA through the epithelial cell layer. Serum IgA, on the otherhand does not contain secretory component and exists in a monomeric form.

In humans, it has been found that there are two subisotypes of IgA, IgA1 and IgA2. IgA1 exhibits the normal immunoglobulin tetrameric structure with the L chains linked to the H chain via disulfide bonds whereas IgA2 has the L chains linked to each other via disulfide linkages, but associated with the H chains by non-covalent inter-actions. The other major difference between these two subisotypes is found in the hinge region where the IgA2 has a deletion of 13 amino acid residues (Putnam, 1977). An elegant hypothesis to explain the differences in the hinge region has been proposed by Capra and coworkers (Plaut et al, 1975). This group has shown that the IgA1 with its extended hinge is more suseptible to bacterial proteases whereas the IgA2 molecule with its shorter hinge is relatively resistent to these proteases. The authors propose that the longer, more extended hinge allows the immunoglobulin more flexibility in binding antigen although rendering the molecule more susceptible to protease cleavage. On the other hand, the smaller hinge of IgA2 protects this molecule from cleavage.

The structure of IgA in mouse has also been determined at both the protein (Robinson and Appella, 1980) and the nucleic acid level (Early et al, 1979; Tucker et al, 1981). Unlike human, there is only one isotype of IgA in the Balb/c mouse. The hinge region has been determined to be of intermediate length between the larger IgAl of human and its smaller counterpart, IgA2. The human IgAl hinge is comprised of four 15bp repeat units. The mouse IgA hinge contains two of these 15bp repeat units and the human IgA2 has only one of the repeat units. Flanagan and colleagues (1984) after determining the nucleotide sequence of human IgAl and two allotypic variants of IgA2 have proposed that the repetitive genetic structure observed in the hinge leads to the rapid rate of evolution that is observed between the human and mouse hinge regions. Tucker et al (1981) proposed that the Balb/c hinge has evolved from a duplication of the pyrimidine rich splice site found immediately 5' to the hinge. This suggestion is supported in the human sequences described by Flanagan et al (1984). Flanagan and colleagues (1984) further conclude that the genetic instability observed in the length of the hinge may be selectively advantageous thus allowing rapid evolution in this region which is crucial in the molecule's functional capability. It must be noted, however, that although the hinge may be evolving rapidly, the accumulated changes are conservative with respect to the 3-dimensional structure of this region. Although there is a large difference between the amino acid structure of IgAl and IgA2, both regions can be expected to be found in a random coil structure typical of all hinges.

We have extended the findings of Tucker et al (1981) and Flanagan et al (1984) by the determination of the nucleotide sequence of the Cα gene from Mus pahari, a genus of Mus which is thought to have evolved from Mus musculus domesticus at least 8-10 MYR ago. Our results are in accordance with both groups in that the Mus pahari Cα gene has a hinge region which is evolving at a much more rapid rate than the rest of the gene and has a repeat structure very similar to that observed in both human and Balb/c. Additionally, we have noted that the rates of substitution between the Balb/c Cα gene and the pahari gene exhibit a mosaic pattern throughout the gene.

MATERIALS AND METHODS

The Mus pahari Cα gene was isolated from a library constructed by partial MboII digestion of pahari liver DNA which was subsequently cloned into the BamHl site of phage λJl. This library was screened with the plasmid pαJ558 (Tucker et al, 1981) and positive clones were isolated, subcloned into pUC8 and further subcloned into Ml3mp9 & 10 vectors. DNA sequence was determined using the method of Sanger et al (1980).

RESULTS AND DISCUSSION

Mus Pahari C α DNA sequence

The sequence of the <u>Mus pahari</u> Cα gene revealed that, as in Balb/c, there are three gene segments CH, Hinge-CH2 and CH3 (Fig. 1). These segments are separated at the DNA level by two introns, 382 and 208 bp in length. The exon/intron junctions conform to the GT/AG rule as proposed by Tucker suggesting that the pahari Cα gene is capable of the proper splicing necessary to form a functional IgA molecule.

The degree of homology at both the nucleotide and amino acid level is shown in Table 1. A number of interesting features can be seen in this table. First of all, the degree of homology found at both the nucleotide and amino acid level varied from one domain to another. We found that the 1st and 2nd domain were 93 and 92% homologous respectively to Balb/c at the nucleic acid level and 92 and 84% homologous at the protein level. In contrast, the 3rd domain of pahari was 98% homologous to Balb/c at both the nucleic acid and protein level. Most striking was the hinge region which differed between the two species by 77% at the nucleic acid level and 66% at the protein level. These data suggested to us that the Cα gene is evolving in a mosaic fashion, that is to say, some portions of the molecule are evolving at a different rate than others. It is quite obvious that the hinge is evolving most rapidly, followed by the 2nd and 1st domains and that the 3rd domain is evolving rather slowly. Although we can not definitively explain these results, it is attractive to speculate that the 3rd domain is evolving most slowly because it is this portion of the gene which encode the portion of the molecule which is inserted in the membrane and provides the attachment sites for both J chain and secretory component.

It is important to note what kind of substitutions are occuring between these two genes. While it is clear that in most comparisons between two genes either within a species, among species or among genuses, the predominant pattern noted is that the overwhelming proportion of substitutions are synonomous or silent in nature. In striking contrast to this observation in other gene systems, we find that the majority of the substitutions found in the pahari Cα gene were replacement site substitutions thus leading to a change at the protein level. More precisely we have observed that of the 54 substitutions in the pahari Cα gene, 36 are replacement (67%) and 18 are synonomous (33%). This is directly opposite to the findings of Lomedico et al (1979) who, when comparing rat preproinsulin I and II, found that of the 23 differences between these two related genes, 65% were synonomous while only 35% were replacement site. Similar results reported by Lomedico (1979) show that of the 84 substitutions between rabbit and mouse β globin genes, 59% were silent and 41% were replacement. Additional data relevant to this issue is found in the elegant study by Kreitman (1983) where ADH genes from eleven different isolates of <u>Drosophila melanogaster</u> were cloned and sequenced. The results from these experiments showed that only 7% of the substitutions in ADH were replacement site while 93% were synonomous. In isolation it would appear as though the situation observed in Cα genes from <u>Mus pahari</u> and Balb/c was uniquely different. However,

144

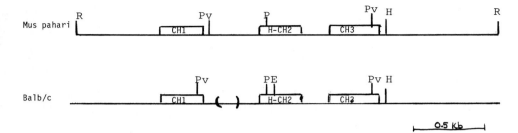

Figure 1. Comparison of Structural Features of the <u>Mus pahari</u>
and Balb/c Cα genes. The ( ) indicates a 140bp insert in
Mus pahari not found in Balb/c in IVS1. R, EcoRl; Pv, PvuII;
P, Pstl; H, HindIII.

Table 1. PERCENT HOMOLOGY BETWEEN THE C-ALPHA GENE
IN BALB/c AND MUS PAHARI

<u>% Homology at the Nucleic Acid Level</u>

	Percentage
1st domain	92.8%
2nd domain (excluding hinge)	92.3%
3rd domain	97.5%
Hinge	77.0%
IVS 1	83.2%
IVS 2	92.7%

<u>% Homology at the Amino Acid Level</u>

1st domain	91.9%
2nd domain (excluding hinge)	84.0%
3rd domain	98.4%
Hinge	66.0%

an examination of the literature reveals that the same skewing toward
replacement site substitutions has been observed between rat and
mouse C-kappa (Shepard and Gutman), amongst C-kappa genes within
the genus Mus (Rudikoff and Marche, this volume), and amongst
V-kappa genes within Balb/c (Joho et al, 1984). Indeed, we have
been unable to find an immunoglobulin gene comparison where the
predominant number of substitutions were synonomous. Table 2
summarizes a portion of this data in a different fashion. As
described by Lomedico et al (1979) these data can best be presented
as a ratio of synonomous to replacement site substitutions. Table
2 shows a sample of such ratios as calculated from evolutionary comparisons found in the literature.

Our interpretation of the apparent tendency of immunoglobulin genes
to collect a preponderance of replacement site substitutions is
that all genes most probably accumulate substitutions randomly and
that approximately 75% of these substitutions should be replacement
and 25% silent. Genes such as ADH in the extreme case and preproinsulin and globin genes in less extreme cases, cannot tolerate
the replacement site changes thus selection operates to eliminate
these changes. Immunoglobulins on the other hand appear to be able
to tolerate such changes in the structure of both the DNA and protein
and selection therefore does not play as large a role in monitoring
the evolutionary end product which we observe today. Although we
can only be observers of the effects of evolution, it is tempting
to speculate that the vertebrate organism is constantly accumulating
variation in immunoglobulins; it is, in fact, the hallmark of many
of the proteins of the immune system. Thus when a substitution
is introduced into such a gene, perhaps selection is less likely
to act upon it.

THE Cα HINGE

As previously stated, the C_α hinge in both human and Balb/c have
been shown to be derived from a 15bp repeat. The various C_α hinge
regions, including that of pahari, are comprised of multiple numbers
of this 15bp repeat. Figure 2 and 3 show an alignment of the
pahari unit 1, unit 2 and splice signal (which is also related to
the 15bp repeat) with either the Balb/c 15bp consensus sequence
(Fig. 2) or with the human 15bp consensus sequence (Fig 3). These
data allow us to conclude that the pahari hinge is almost equally
different from either Balb/c or human hinge segments.

When looking at the intron/exon junction between IVS1 and the
hinge-2nd domain we find that the AG acceptor site necessary for
proper splicing as described by Tucker et al (1979) is found in
the pahari C_α gene. Also in accordance with the data of Tucker
et al (1981), we find an AG dinucleotide precisely at the end of
the hinge and the beginning of the CH2 domain
Therefore as observed in Balb/c (Tucker et al, 1981), pahari has
two tandemly arranged potential RNA splice sites but only the
first is used. The second, if utilized would cause a shift in
translation phase thus causing a premature termination.

Tucker et al (1981) proposed that the C_α hinge has evolved from
a single primordial exon with a single splice site via unequal
crossover between two sister chromatids. They also propose that
this leads to the integration of intronic sequences into the hinge

Table 2. SILENT VS REPLACEMENT SITE SUBSTITUTIONS

Genes	Silent/Replacement Ratio	Reference
Rat preproinsulin I vs II	6.7	Perler et al
Drosophila ADH Genes	44.0	Kreitman
Mouse globin βmajor vs βminor	3.5	Perler et al
Rabbit β globin vs mouse βglobin	4.0	Perler et al
Rat growth hormone vs human growth hormone	4.0	Perler et al
Rat C-Kappa vs Mouse C-Kappa	1.9	Shepard & Gutman
Balb/c C-alpha vs Pahari C-Alpha	1.5	This study

exon. It is their hypothesis that the intervening sequence border
may be a preferential site for mutation, especially those which
lead to incremental changes in the protein. The data from the human
system (Flanagan et al, 1984) supported this hypothesis as does
the sequence data in this paper. Not only is the pahari hinge
different in size (9 amino acids vs 12 in Balb/c) but directly
preceeding the 1st codon in the pahari hinge there is a two nucleotide
substitution as compared to Balb/c.

SUMMARY

When comparing the Cα gene from <u>Mus pahari</u>, we find that the DNA
sequence and in turn, the protein sequence appears to be evolving
in a mosaic fashion with the hinge region evolving most rapidly.
The substitutions observed between Balb/c and pahari are predominately
replacement site in nature in contrast to substitutions observed
between other genes in an evolutionary comparison. We interpret
this to mean that selection is not acting as strongly against these
genes in particular and perhaps against genes encoding certain
molecules of the immune system in general. Lastly, the hinge region
of pahari is quite obviously evolving at a rapid rate supporting
the hypothesis proposed by Tucker that intervening sequence borders
may be preferential sites for mutation thus leading to a rapid rate
of evolution in this region of a particular sequence.

Acknowledgements: We thank Evelyne Marche for the pahari library,
K. Marcu for the pλ J558 plasmid, Richard Goldsby for careful and
critical reading of the manuscript, Julie Fitzgerald for expert
technical help and Lisa Scott for the preparation of this manuscript.
This work was supported by grant #GM36344 from NIGMS and utilized
the services of BIONET (Grant #1 U41 RR-01685-02).

	Sequence	homology to consensus
Balb consensus	TCCTACTACTACTCC	
Balb splice signal	T CTTCTGTTACAGG	8/14
Balb unit 1	TCCTACTCCTCCTCC	13/15
Balb unit 2	TCCTATTACTATTCC	13/15
Pahari splice signal	AC TTCTGTTACAGG	7/14
Pahari unit 1	GCCTCCTCTTCCTCC	10/15
Pahari unit 2	TTCAACAATC-----	5/10

Figure 2. Hinge Region Sequences of Balb/c and Mus Pahari. Sequence differences are indicated by _, gaps by a blank space, and deletions by -.

	Sequence	homology to consensus
Human consensus	TCCCTCAACTCCACC	
Balb/c splice	T CTTCTGTTACAGG	7/14
Balb unit 1	TCCTACTCCTCCTCC	10/15
Balb unit 2	TCCTATTACTATTCC	9/15
Pahari splice	A CTTCTGTTACAGG	6/14
Pahari unit 1	GCCTCCTCTTCCTCC	8/15
Pahari unit 2	TTCAACAATC-----	5/5

Figure 3. Hinge Region Comparison Between Balb/c, Mus Pahari and Human Consensus. Sequence differences are indicated by _, gaps by a blank space, and deletions by -.

REFERENCES

Early P, Davis M, Kaback D, Davidson N, Hood L (1979) An immunoglobulin chain variable region is generated from three segments of DNA: V, D, and J. Proc Natl Acad Sci 76:4240-4244
Flanagan JG, Lefranc MP, Rabbitts TH (1984) Mechanisms of divergence and convergence of the human immunoglobulin 1 and 2 constant region gene sequences. Cell 36:681-688
Joho R, Gershenfeld H, Weissman IL (1984) Evolution of a multigene family of V germ line genes. EMBO J 3:185-191
Kornfeld SJ, Plaut AG (1981) Secretory immunity and the bacterial IgA proteases. Rev Infect Disease 3:521-534

Kreitman M (1983) Nucleotide polymorphism at the alcohol dehydrogenase
    locus of <u>Drosophila melanogaster</u> Nature 304:412-417
Lomedico P, Rosenthal N, Efstratiadis A, Gilbert W, Kolodner R,
    Tizard R (1979) The structure and evolution of the two nonallelic
    rat preproinsulin genes. Cell 18:545-558
Plaut AG, Gilbert JV, Artenstein MS, Capra JD (1975) <u>Neisseria</u>
    <u>gonorrhoeae</u> and <u>Neisseria</u> <u>meningitidis</u>: extracellular enzyme
    cleaves human immunoglobulin A. Science 190:1103-1105
Perler F, Efstratatiadis A, Lomedico P, Gilbert W, Kolodner R,
    Dodgson J (1980) The evolution of genes: The chicken preproinsulin
    gene. Cell 20:555-566
Putnam FW (1977) The plasma proteins. Academic Press, NY pp 1-153
Robinson E, Appella E (1980) Complete amino acid sequence of a mouse
    immunoglobulin chain (MOPC511). Proc Natl Acad Sci 77:4909-4913
Sanger F, Nicklen S, Coulson AR (1977) DNA sequencing with chain-
    terminating inhibitors. Proc Natl Aci 74:5463-5467
Sheppard HW, Gutman GA (1981) Allelic forms of rat chain genes:
    Evidence of strong selection at the level of nucleotide sequence.
    Proc Natl Acad Sci 78:7064-7068
Tucker PW, Marcu KB, Newel N, Richards J, Blattner FR (1979) Sequence
    of the cloned gene for the constant region of murine 2b immuno-
    globulin heavy chain. Science 206:1303-1306
Tucker PW, Slightom JL, Blattner FR (1981) Mouse IgA heavy chain
    gene sequence: Implications for evolution of immunoglobulin
    hinge exons. Proc Natl Acad Sci 78:7684-7688
Williams RC, Gibbons RJ (1972) Inhibition of bacterial adherence
    by secretory immunoglobulin A. Science 177:697-699

Evolution of Immunologically Important Genes in the Genus *Mus*

E. Jouvin-Marche, A. Cuddihy, M. Heller, S. Butler, J. N. Hansen, and S. Rudikoff

INTRODUCTION

It is somewhat surprising, considering the pre-eminent position the laboratory mouse has held in biological research, how little is known about this species as a whole, with the exception of members of the subgenus Mus. Some of the European and Asian subspecies of Mus have been studied by classical morphologic analysis (Marshall and Sage 1981) and biochemical genetics employing protein polymorphisms (Bonhomme 1978a, 1984; Sage 1981). However, there exists to date very little data at the protein or nucleic acid sequence levels to provide information pertaining to actual patterns of gene evolution or relationships between subspecies or subgenera.

We have undertaken an analysis of these questions by employing the wild mouse colony of Michael Potter to approach this problem at the level of gene structure. This wild mouse colony contains members of all subgenera as well as a variety of species and subspecies from the subgenus Mus. Recombinant bacteriophage libraries have been constructed from representatives of the four subgenera and three species of the subgenus Mus presented in Table 1. Members of dif-

Table 1. Origins of wild mice colonies

Species	Sub-Genus	Geographic Origin
M. pahari	Coelomys	Tak Province, Thailand
M. platythrix	Pyromys	Mysore, India
M. minutoides	Nannomys	Nairobi, Kenya
M. cookii	Mus	Tak Province, Thailand
M. spretus	Mus	Azrou, Morocco
M. musculus castaneus	Mus	Thailand
M. musculus domesticus	Mus	U.S.A.

ferent subgenera are both geographically and sexually isolated, providing a unique system to examine the independent evolution of vertebrate genes within a species. The genes we have chosen to characterize are members of the immunological system and encode receptors for B-cells (immunoglobulin) and T-cells. These families are of particular interest in that they contain both single copy genes (i.e., the light chain κ constant region) and multigene

150

families consisting of 2 to >50 members (Cory 1981; Brodeur and Riblet 1984) which encode sets of closely related variable region genes. Both the B and T-cell receptor genes share similar organizational patterns (Fig. 1) in that there exist a series of variable (V) region genes which are 5' to a set of small joining (J) region genes which are in turn separated from the constant (C) region genes (Tonegawa 1983; Hedrick 1984b; Yanagi 1984). In immunoglobulin heavy chains and the T-cell receptor genes an additional gene segment locus, 'D', is found between V and J (Early 1981; Chien 1984). One gene segment from each of these loci is joined by recombination events to produce the expressed gene. In our present studies we have begun analysis of the C_K gene, a V_K multi-gene family, and the constant region for the T-cell β-chain ($C_{T\beta}$).

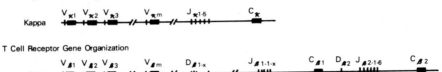

Fig. 1. Schematic representation of the C_K and $C_{T\beta}$ loci. Each locus contains a series of variable (V) genes, several joining (J) genes, and one (C_K) or two (C_β) constant region genes. The $C_{T\beta}$ locus, in addition, contains several diversity (D) genes.

C_K

As might be expected, the C_K gene is highly conserved throughout the genus, and Southern blot analysis (Fig. 2) demonstrates that polymorphism is extremely limited and seen predominantly between subgenera. We have reasoned that since the C_K gene is present as a single copy per haploid genome, it should not be subject to many of the correction mechanisms available to multi-gene families and have chosen to use this gene as a model for single copy gene evolution. The C_K gene has been cloned and sequenced from M. pahari, M. minutoides, M. platythrix, M. cookii and M. spretus.

Analysis of these data indicates that replacement substitutions in the coding region are not scattered throughout, but are localized to regions encoding external bends in the protein structure which are in contact with solvent. The coding regions among members of the different subgenera display similar numbers of substitutions suggesting that the radiation of subgenera may have occurred in a relatively short evolutionary period. All Mus sequences are clearly more related to each other than to Rat, indicating the possibility of a common modern ancestor and establishing a relatedness among subgenera. It remains to be determined whether these subgenera will continue to show more relatedness to each other than to other murids. Several examples are seen in which shared substitutions are found between members of two different subgenera, such as M. pahari and M. platythrix. One of these (M. pahari) may then share an additional

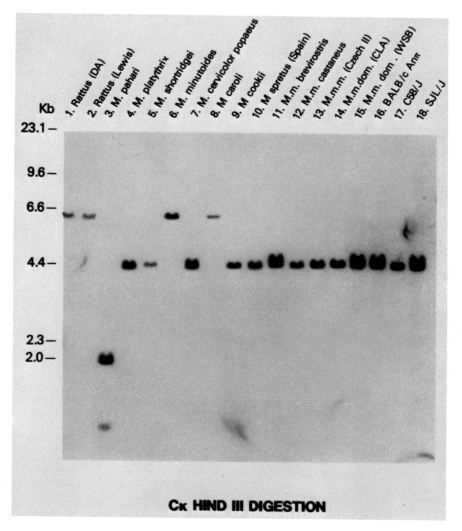

Fig. 2. Southern blot analysis of wild mice DNA using a probe identifying the kappa chain constant region. Blots were washed under
high stringency conditions (65°, 0.1X SSC).

152

set of substitutions with members of a third subgenus such as M.
cookii. This result suggests that either parallel mutations are
occurring at a relatively high frequency during evolution or an
ancestral gene pool with several allelic forms was maintained
throughout the period of subgenus origination. Surprisingly, the
intervening sequence between the J_K and C_K loci is maintained to
nearly the same extent as the coding regions, suggesting the possibility of strong selection on this portion of the DNA sequence.
Furthermore, in the region 5' to the C_K coding region, sequences
corresponding to the light chain enhancer (Emorine 1983) are found
in all subgenera and these sequences are conserved to an even
greater extent than the coding regions.

V_K

To analyze the evolution of a multi-gene family, we have begun to
examine a kappa chain V region subgroup among wild mice. The particular subgroup studied, V_K24, has been characterized in BALB/c mice
and contains at least three presumably functional genes designated
V_K24, V_K24A and V_K24B, as well as a pseudogene (Joho 1984). Using
a cDNA probe corresponding to the V_K24 gene under conditions of high
stringency, a single hybridizing fragment is found in BALB/c. This
gene is also easily identified in all of our wild mice (Fig. 3).
The number of hybridizing bands varies, but most of this variation
is likely due to the fact that the DNA samples are pools of several
individuals, some of which are presumably heterozygotes. The most
obvious exception to this pattern of few hybridizing fragments is M.
platythrix. It is presently unclear whether this species contains
an amplified number of copies of this gene or whether this pattern
results from a partial (although reproducible) digestion of this DNA.
We have begun analysis of this multi-gene family by cloning the V_K24
family from M. pahari believed to be the oldest living member of the
genus. M. pahari displays a single strongly hybridizing fragment
(Fig. 3) with the V_K24 probe, and at reduced stringency several
hybridizing bands are seen as is the case in all species. Five
unique genes were isolated from the M. pahari library, and comparison with the BALB/c genes indicates there are two apparently
non-allelic genes homologous to V_K24, one gene homologous to V_K24A,
one homologous to V_K24B, and a fifth (V_K24C) related to V_K24A but
which is not found in BALB/c. Southern blot analysis using the
individual M. pahari genes as probes reveals that whereas M. pahari
has two copies of the V_K24 gene and one each of V_K24A, V_K24B and
V_K24C, BALB/c has one copy of V_K24 and V_K24A, no copies of V_K24C
and two copies of V_K24B. Thus, there appears to be duplication
and/or deletion occurring at the level of individual genes, but not
at the level of the entire family.

Comparison of the sequences of these genes reveals complex patterns
of evolution which appear to be localized to specific protein segments exemplifying the variable, yet dominant, effect of selection.
This effect is especially pronounced when individual framework and
complementarity determining regions (CDR) are compared. The CDR
regions determine antigen binding specificity and are located at the
bends or tips of protein segments so that they are unlikely to be
subjected to the conformational restraints imposed on the internal
framework segments. Therefore, replacement mutations should accumu-

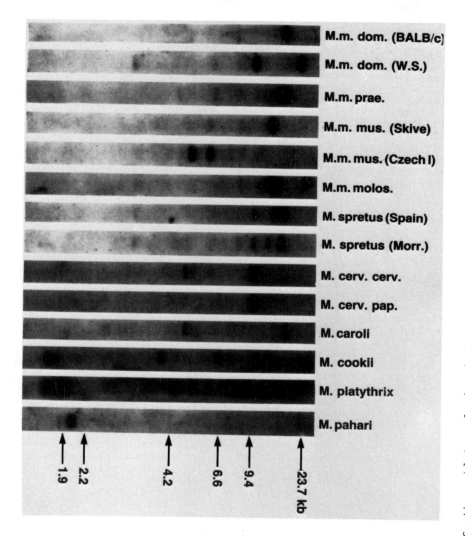

M.m. dom. (BALB/c)

M.m. dom. (W.S.)

M.m. prae.

M.m. mus. (Skive)

M.m. mus. (Czech I)

M.m. molos.

M. spretus (Spain)

M. spretus (Morr.)

M. cerv. cerv.

M. cerv. pap.

M. caroli

M. cookii

M. platythrix

M. pahari

1.9 2.2 4.2 6.6 9.4 23.7 kb

Fig. 3. Southern blot analysis of wild mice DNA hybridized with a probe corresponding to the variable region of MOPC 167, a member of the Vκ24 family. Conditions were as in Fig. 1.

late much more rapidly in these regions and be subject only to environmental selection. Surprisingly, in all comparisons between M. pahari and BALB/c V_K24 family members, the CDR1 region is the most conserved segment with 3 of the light chains showing 100% conservation at the protein level. Sequence homologies are considerably lower in CDR2 and CDR3. Therefore, there appears to be unusually strong selection on CDR1 structure either for conformational reasons or antigen binding specificity. Framework segments, in general, show high degrees of homology (>92%) with the exception of the V_K24B genes where framework homology is only 77%.

Homology patterns in the 5' flanking and leader regions differ significantly from those observed within the coding regions. The V_K24 genes are the most homologous within the coding region yet are among the least homologous 5' to the coding region. In contrast, the V_K24B genes, which show the lowest coding region homology, are among the most homologous in the 5' region. Thus, the 5' regions are clearly diverging at a more rapid rate than the coding regions although there is considerable variation from gene to gene and complex events such as recombination may be contributing to this phenomenon.

$C_T\beta$

The constant region genes for the β-chain of the T-cell receptor fall between the C_K and V_K genes in terms of complexity. There exist two constant region genes, $C_T\beta1$ and $C_T\beta2$, each of which contains 4 exons (Gascoigne 1984, Malissen 1984). The presence of two $C_T\beta$ constant region genes extends quite far back in evolutionary time as humans have the same locus arrangement (Tunnacliffe 1985). Early studies by Mark Davis and colleagues (Gascoigne 1984) demonstrated that only a single nucleotide substitution was found when the exon 1 sequences were compared between $C_T\beta1$ and $C_T\beta2$ from an inbred mouse. This result suggested that a gene correction mechanism had altered these sequences in a manner which minimized divergence. We have, therefore, cloned and sequenced the $C_T\beta1$ and $C_T\beta2$ genes from M. pahari to examine the pattern of evolution in this species. Four nucleotide differences were found between the M. pahari $C_T\beta1$ and $C_T\beta2$ exon 1 sequences which is much less than would be expected considering the time of separation of these two species. Furthermore, the C_K and V_K divergence between M. pahari and BALB/c discussed above would also predict considerably greater divergence than observed. This lack of divergence does not extend to intronic regions or other exons. It thus appears that the M. pahari exon 1 sequences from $C_T\beta1$ and $C_T\beta2$ have been corrected against each other and, based on the sequence patterns, this correction event is clearly independent of that which occurred in the inbred mouse. Similar evidence for $C_T\beta$ gene correction has also been reported in the human indicating that this mechanism is employed frequently in the evolution of the $C_T\beta$ genes although the biological basis for this correction are not known.

CONCLUSION

We have examined genes from the C_K, V_K and $C_{T\beta}$ loci from wild mice
in order to evaluate patterns of gene evolution and establish genealogical relations. Our results suggest that the four murine subgenera
diverged during a relatively short time period in evolution and that
using data from the present studies it should now be possible to
construct more accurate phylogenetic trees describing the evolution
of this species. The pattern of evolution of the three types of
genes examined varied considerably indicating that quite different
mechanisms, in addition to selective pressures, were operating at
the level of the respective genes. This analysis points out the
danger of evolutionary generalizations based on a restricted selection of genes and indicates the need for data derived from multiple
gene types and families before evolutionary questions can be appro-
priately assessed.

REFERENCES

Bonhomme F, Britton-Davidian J, Thaler L, Triantaphyllides C (1978a)
  Sur l'existence en Europe de quatte groupes de Souris (genre Mus
  L.) de rang espece et semi-espece, demontree par la genetique
  biochimique. CR Hebd Seances Acad Sci Ser D 287:631-633
Bonhomme F, Calahen J, Britton-Davidson J, Chapman VM, Moriwaki K,
  New E, Thaler L (1984) Biochemical diversity and evolution in the
  genus Mus. Biochem Genetics 22:275-301
Brodeur PH, Riblet R (1984) The immunoglobulin heavy chain variable
  region (Igh-V) locus in the mouse. I. One hundred Igh-V genes
  comprise seven families of homologous genes. Eur J Immunol 14:
  922-926
Chien Y-H, Gascoigne NRJ, Kavaler J, Lee NE, Davies MM (1984) Somatic
  recombination in a murine T-cell receptor gene. Nature 309:322-326
Cory S, Typer BM, Adams JM (1981) Sets of immunoglobulin V genes
  homologous to ten cloned V sequences: implications for the number
  of germline V genes. J Mol Appl Genet 1:103
Early P, Huang H, Davis M, Calame K, Hood L (1980) An immunoglobulin
  heavy chain variable gene is generated from three segments of DNA:
  V_H, D, and J_H. Cell 19:981
Emorine L, Kuehl M, Weir L, Leder P, Max E (1983) A conserved
  sequence in the immunoglobulin J_K-C_K intron: possible enhancer
  element. Nature 304:447-449
Gascoigne NRJ, Chien Y-H, Becker DM, Kavaler J, Davis MM (1984)
  Genomic organisation and sequence of T-cell receptor β-chain
  constant and joining region genes. Nature 310:387-391
Hedrick S, Nielsen E, Kavaler J, Cohen D, Davis M (1984b) Sequence
  relationships betweenputative T-cell receptor polypeptides and
  immunoglobulins. Nature 308:153-158
Joho R, Weissman IL, Early P, Cole J, Hood L (1980) Organization of
  κ light chain genes in germline and somatic tissue. Proc Natl Acad
  Sci USA 77:1106-1110
Joho R, Gershenfeld H, Weissman TL (1984) Evolution of a multigene
  family of V_K germline genes. EMBO J 3:185-191
Malissen M, Minard K, Mjoisness S, Kronenberg M, Goverman J,
  Hunkapiller T, Prystowsky MB, Yoshikai Y, Fitch F, Mak TW, Hood L

(1984) Mouse T cell antigen receptor: structure and organization
of constant and joining gene segments encoding the β polypeptide.
Cell 37:1101-1110

Marshall JT, Sage RD (1981) Taxonomy of the house mouse. Symp Zool
Soc Lond 47:15-25

Max EE, Seidman JG, Leder P (1979) Sequences of five recombination
sites encoded close to an immunoglobulin κ constant region gene.
Proc Natl Acad Sci USA 76:3450

Sage RD (1981) Wild Mice. The mouse in biomedical research. 1:40-90

Tonegawa S (1983) Somatic generation of antibody diversity. Nature
302:575-581

Tunnacliffe A, Kefford R, Milstein C, Forsta A, Rabbitts TH (1985)
Sequence and evolution of the human T-cell antigen receptor β
chain genes. Proc Natl Acad Sci USA 82:5068-5072

Yanagi, Y, Yoshikai Y, Leggett K, Clark S, Aleksander I, Mak T
(1984) A human T cell-specific cDNA clone encodes a protein having
extensive homology to immunoglobulin chains. Nature 308:145-149

The X-24 VH Gene Family in Inbred Mouse Strains and Wild Mice

A.B. Hartman, L. A. D'Hoostelaere, M. Potter, and S. Rudikoff

INTRODUCTION

The germline content of immunoglobulin (Ig) heavy and light chain variable region genes is one important source of antibody diversity; thus a large germline repetoire of these genes provides a potential capability to respond to a wide variety of antigens independent of subsequent somatic diversification. Immunoglobulin variable region genes appear to have evolved at a more rapid rate than many other proteins (Wilson 1977), which might be expected in a system where selection favors increased diversity. Examining evolutionary changes in immunoglobulin multigene families provides an opportunity to study the rate at which this system is evolving and permits an examination of the relative contribution of point mutations, recombinational events and gene duplications to the generation of germ-line diversity. The Ig repetoire of inbred Mus musculus, which has been extensively studied (for a review, see Honjo 1985, Hood 1985), represents an ideal model for such studies.

One difficulty in studying the evolutionary mechanisms and evolutionary relationships in a particular immunoglobulin gene family arises from the complexities of many of these immunoglobulin families (Brodeur 1984, Cory 1981) and the subsequent difficulties encountered in attempting to trace the evolution of particular genes within the family. In studying the genetic basis for the response of the BALB/c mouse to B-(1,6)-galactan (Hartman 1984), it was discovered that the known antibody repetoire to this antigen (Rudikoff 1983) is encoded by the two genes that comprise the entire X-24 VH (heavy chain variable region) family in the BALB/c mouse. Southern blots of genomic DNA from other inbred strains and many wild mouse species obtained from the wild mouse colony maintained by M. Potter at Hazelton Laboratory in Gaithersburg, MD (under NCI contract #N01-CB-25584) indicate that this VH multigene family is restricted in size throughout the commensal and feral mice tested, thus providing a small subgroup of genes within the VH family suitable for evolutionary analysis.

So far, expression of the X-24 VH family has primarily been restricted to antibodies specific for B-(1,6)-galactan residues, with possible exception of an anti-lysozyme antibody discussed by Brodeur (1984). Galactan antigens are widely distributed in the natural environment of the mouse (Potter 1979) since they are produced by various plants and are also found in wheat germ, which is a constituent of the normal diet of many wild mice. Laboratory mice are continuously exposed to these determinants in both their diet and their cage

bedding, which is made of hardwood shavings that contain arabino-
galactans (Potter 1979). Thus, it is not surprising that inbred
mice normally express antibodies to B-(1,6)-galactan in their serum
(Mushinski 1977). An examination of the evolution of the X-24 VH
gene family thus has the additional advantage of providing an insight into the evolution of VH genes involved in the immune response
to a naturally occurring antigen.

X-24 VH Genes

VH genes of the X-24 family were characterized and isolated using
as hybridizaton probes 500 bp EcoRI restriction fragments (RF)
obtained from genomic BALB/c DNA. One 500 bp fragment contains the
coding region of the X-24 myeloma protein (VHGal 55.1); the other
500 bp fragment contains the coding region of the X-44 myeloma
protein (VHGal 39.1). Both fragments also contain 180 bp of the 3'
flanking region (Hartman 1984). Using Southern transfer techniques
(as in Huppi 1985), EcoRI digests of genomic DNA isolated from
various inbred strains and wild mouse species were surveyed. Most
mice studied revealed only a single EcoRI hybridizing band except M.
platythrix, which has 3 bands, and M. pahari and M. shortridgei,
which are missing the X-24 family altogether. Since the single
EcoRI RF band in the BALB/c mouse represents 2 genes, a different
enzyme, Bgl II (which cuts the coding region of the gene in the
codon for amino acid 83) was used for the survey. Southern blots of
Bgl II digests of genomic DNA revealed that the family is still very
restricted in size and that some inferences as to relationship of
the genes of this family can be made based on RF patterns.

Inbred Strains and Wild Mouse Populations

A survey of several inbred strains of mice (Table 1) reveals 5 Bgl
II RF patterns (Fig. 1). Pattern 4, represented by AKR, CBA and C3H
strains, contains only one gene. The other 4 patterns appear to
have at least two genes. Sequencing of the germline genes from a
strain representing each pattern will be necessary to determine
whether the hybridizing bands correspond to the presence of both the
X-24 and X-44 genes in each strain or whether one of these genes
is deleted and/or the other duplicated.

The results shown in Table 1 indicate that each X-24 VH pattern is
associated with more than one IgCH (heavy chain constant region)
haplotype (allotype) and Igh haplotype (as defined by Brodeur 1984),
except for possibly pattern 2, where only haplotype b has been
identified so far. This finding suggests that recombination events
between CH and VH or between different VH gene families may have
occurred prior to or during the development of inbred strains.
Southern blots of wild mouse genomic DNA digested by Bgl II were
then analyzed for RF patterns. The listing at the end of this
edition gives a description of the trapping locations of the wild
mice used in this study and the number of original breeders. The
current population of each species or subspecies was derived from a
limited number of original breeding pairs, so that the RF patterns
observed probably represent only a sampling of patterns found in the
wild populations. Nevertheless, several interesting observations
can be made based on the data obtained.

159

Table 1.   Bgl II RF patterns found in inbred mouse strains and wild mouse populations

Pattern	Strain	IgCH haplotype[a] (allotype)	Igh haplotype[b]	Wild mouse population
1	BALB/c	a	a	M. m. domesticus (Erfoud, Morocco, formerly M. m. praetextus)
	C57L	a	a	
	NZB	n	n	
	A/He	e	e	
	AL/N	o	o	
	RIII	g	gr	
	P/J	h	*	
	SEA	h or j[+]	*	
2	C57BL/6	b	b	
	SJL	b	b	
3	DBA/2J	c	c	M. m. musculus (Skive, Denmark)
	CE/J	f	f	M. m. domesticus (Centre-ville, MD)
	NH	f	*	M. spretus (Morocco) (1 allele)
4	AKR	d	d	M. hortulanus (Yugoslavia)
	C3H	j	j	M. m. castaneus (Thailand) (1 allele)
	PL/J	j	j	
	CBA/J	j	*	
5	BSVS	g	g	M. musculus (Saqqara, Egypt)
	SWR	p	p	

[a] From Lieberman 1978 and Huang 1983
[b] From Brodeur 1984
[+] SEA is typed as j allotype by Lieberman and h allotype by Huang
[*] Igh haplotypes not tested by Brodeur

160

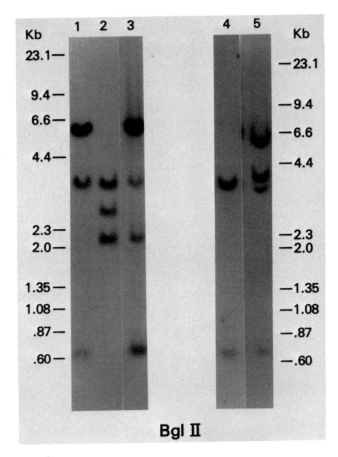

Fig. 1. Restriction fragment (RF) patterns found in Bgl II digests
of genomic DNA from inbred strains of mice. Patterns from left to
right are numbered from 1 through 5. See Table 1 for identification
of inbred strains which possess a particular pattern.

It is apparent that the more distantly related species, such as M.
minutoides, M. platythrix, M. booduga (DNA from M. booduga was
obtained from Dr. T. Sharma, Banaras Hindu University, Varanasi,
India in 1982), M. cervicolor popaeus, M. cervicolor cervicolor, M.
caroli and M. cookii, have little or limited overlap in RF pattern
with each other and with more recently evolved species (data not
shown). The RF patterns shown in Fig. 2 are from more closely
related species of Mus musculus. In these species, more overlap in
RF patterns is found, as exemplified by the shared hybridizing
fragments between M. abbotti (collected by Dr. R. Sage in Yugoslavia,
Macedonia, in fields 6 km northwest of Gradsko in 1979) and M. m.
castaneus and those shared by M. m. molossinus and the Egyptian mouse

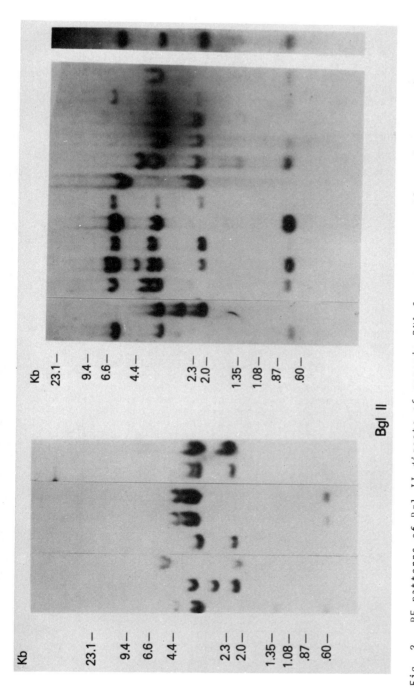

Fig. 2. RF patterns of Bgl II digests of genomic DNA from more recently evolved members of Mus musculus and inbred strains. First panel from left to right: M. m. castaneus, C57BL/6, M. m. poschiavinus, Czech I (M. m. musculus from Morovia), M. abbotti (2 lanes), Czech II (M. m. musculus from Slovakia) (2 lanes). Second panel from left to right: BALB/c, C57BL/6, Egyptian mouse from Saqqara, M. spretus (Morocco), M. spretus (Spain), M. m. domesticus (Erfoud, Morocco, formerly M. m. praetextus), M. m. musculus (Skive, Denmark), M. m. poschiavinus, M. m. molos-sinus, Egyptian mouse from Abu Rawash, Czech I, M. m. domesticus (Azrou, Morocco, formerly M. m. brevirostris), M. hortulanus, M. m. musculus (Vejrumbo, Denmark).

Bgl II

from Abu Rawash. When individuals from M. m. castaneus were
examined for RF pattern (data not shown), two allelic genes were
identified. M. m. molossinus, which is proposed to have arisen
from hybridization of M. m. musculus and M. m. castaneus (Yonekawa,
this edition), appears to have RF bands similar to M. m. castaneus
and the Czech I and Czech II mice (M. m. musculus mice from Studenec,
Morovia and Bratisslava, Slovakia, respectively) in agreement with
the proposed derivation. However, studies of individual mice from
M. m. molossinus would be necessary to compare RF patterns more
precisely, and sequencing of germline genes from each species would
be needed to establish the homologies of the individual genes.

M. spretus (populations from Puerto Real, Spain and Azrou, Morocco)
possess RF patterns more closely resembling those of M. m. domesticus
(Watkins Stars) from Centreville, MD, and M. m. domesticus (formerly
designated M. m. brevirostris) from Azrou, Morocco. When individual members of M. spretus from the Moroccan population were examined,
two sets of allelic genes were found (data not shown). One set
appears to be identical to pattern 3 (Fig. 1), which is also shown by
DBA, CE/J, AL/N and NH inbred strains, as well as the M. m. musculus
mice from Denmark and the Watkins Star A and B lines, in which one
member of chromosome 12 in the Watkins Star mice has been fixed (see
D'Hoostelaere, this edition, for a description of the establishment
of these lines). The Watkins Star heterozygous line is identical in
pattern to M. m. domesticus from Azrou, Morocco. M. m. domesticus
from Erfoud, Morocco (formerly designated M. m. praetextus) has
pattern 1, which is also found in BALB/c, NZB, A/He and other inbred
strains. The pattern shown by C57BL strains has not been identified
in the wild mice surveyed with the X-24 probe, although patterns
found in the Czechoslovakian mice and M. m. molossinus mice have
some similarity to this pattern. Pattern 4 resembles the pattern
shown by M. hortulanus and M. m. castaneus mice homozygous for one
particular chromosome, but further studies are necessary before this
similarity can be confirmed as real or coincidental. Pattern 5,
exhibited by the Swiss inbred mouse strains (BSVS and SWR), is identical to that shown by the wild mice trapped in Saqqara, Egypt (mice
obtained from Dr. H. Hoogstraal in 1981 as frozen tissue samples). It is
Saqqara mice also show patterns 1 and 4 (data not shown). It is
interesting to note that mice trapped in Abu Rawash, Egypt, show a
pattern which is similar to that of the Czechoslovakian mice and
possibly to pattern 4 or to pattern 3 (data not shown) represented
by M. m. musculus mice from Denmark and M. m. domesticus from
Centreville, MD (Abu Rawash is a small rural community about 5 km
north of the Great Pyramid). Again, further studies of individual
Egyptian mice would help to clarify similarity of patterns. In all
cases, comparison of genes on the molecular level is necessary to
determine which genes are most homologous among the RF patterns
found, although the RF patterns suggest potential genetic contributions to inbred laboratory stocks as well as relationships between
various Mus musculus.

Commensal Mice from Restricted Locations

From the above data it is evident that gene number varies in the
X-24 family. This variation is possibly due to both mutations and
recombinational events. To examine more precisely the potential
contributions of these mechanisms, a more controlled survey of gene

Table 2. Distribution of VH haplotype in commensal mice

X-24 genes	Bgl II	Pst I	Hind III	Genes/chromosome
Fixed				
LW	ag or ae*	ag or ae	a	1,2
SN	b	b	a	2
CLA	a	a	a	2
CLB	b	b	a	2
WSA	a	a	a	2
WSB	a	a	a	2
Segregating				
WS	ab	ab	a	2
JJD	b,d	d,bd	a	2
HV	c	c,h**	b	2
TFCS	ag,g	ag,g	a,b	1,2
TFDB	a,ae,e	a,ae,e	a,c	1,2
TFSS	a,c,ac,cg,g,ag	a,ac,ch,ag,g,c	a,b	1,2
TFTS	cf,cg,f,fg,g	hg,fg,hf,cf,f,g	b	1,2

* Bgl II pattern identical to ab, but Pst I pattern like ae or ag. A study of the Pst I patterns of individuals is necessary to determine which pattern is present.
** h - Bgl II pattern identical to c, but Pst I pattern different
LW - Lewes
SN - Sanner's Farm
CLA - Centreville Light, line A
CLB - Centreville Light, line B
WSA - Watkins Star, line A
WSB - Watkins Star, line B
WS - Watkins Star
JJD - J.J. Downs
HV - Haven's Farm
TFCS - Tobacco Farm, Chemical Shed
TFDB - Tobacco Farm, Drying Barn
TFSS - Tobacco Farm, Seed Shed
TFTS - Tobacco Farm, Tool Shed

diversity within a defined population was undertaken. For this purpose, a collection of commensal mice (M. m. domesticus) from 6 different sites in Maryland and Delaware (see D'Hoostelaere, this edition, for a complete description of these mice) was utilized. The mice collected from these populations have been bred in the laboratory by either random or full-sib matings. These mice were used to determine the extent of polymorphic differences found in wild populations and to determine whether these mice would be suitable for studies of mutation and recombination events in the wild mouse genome.

164

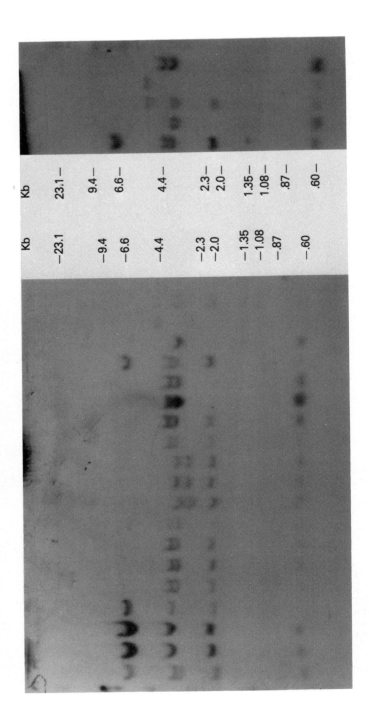

Fig. 3. RF patterns of Bgl II digests of genomic DNA from individual mice from laboratory stocks of commensal mice trapped in Maryland and Delaware. First panel from left to right: Watkins Star, Watkins Star A, Watkins Star B, Centreville Light A, Centreville Light B, Starlight, Starlight, Lewes 12619, Haven's Farm 17498, Haven's Farm 13787, Haven's Farm 13761, Sanner's Farm 13486, J.J. Downs 16755, J.J. Downs 16013, J.J. Downs 7080, Tob. Farm Chem. Shed 14467, Tob. Farm Drying Barn 14498, Tob. Farm Tool Shed 15394, Tob. Farm Tool Shed 14748. Second panel from left to right: Tob. Farm Chem. Shed 14467, Tob. Farm Drying Barn 14498, Tob. Farm Tool Shed 15394, Tob. Farm Tool Shed 14748, J.J. Downs 7080. Allelic patterns represented are WS=ab; WSA,WSB, CLA=a; CLB,SL=b; Lewes=ag or ae (see discussion in Table 2 for explanation of why this pattern is different from ab); HV=c; SN=b; JJ 16755=b; JJ 16013,JJ 7080=d; TFCS 14467=ab; TFDB 14498=e; TFTS 15394=f; TFTS 14748=fg. Pattern g, not shown separately, is identical to the Bgl II pattern of Czech I and appears alone in later generations of Tool Shed and Seed Shed mice. See Table 2 for abbreviations.

Mice tested in these studies were isolated from the laboratory bred stocks, and Tobacco Farm mice tested also included parent-progeny comparisons to allow identification of RF patterns on individual chromosomes. Southern blots obtained from Bgl II digests of genomic DNA isolated from the individual mice showed 7 polymorphic forms of RF patterns (Fig. 3 and Table 2). Pst I digests showed 8 RF patterns, and Hind III digests showed 3 RF patterns (Table 2). Hind III pattern a consists of two bands, a 3.2 kb (kilobase) fragment and a 700 bp fragment, while pattern b contains only the 700 bp (base pair) fragment. Pattern c, which contains only the 3.2 kb fragment and corresponds to Bgl II pattern e, has never been observed in any other inbred or wild mouse tested and may be the product of a recombination event. Other novel patterns that represent possible recombinations or mutations are Bgl II paterns d, f and g. These results suggest that an unexpected diversity of polymorphic RF patterns exists in mice trapped in the same or geographically close locations. For example, the Tobacco Farm mice showed some RF patterns (Bgl II patterns e and f) that were unique to the building in which they were trapped. One can only speculate whether this limited sampling accurately represents the diversity of polymorphic patterns found in the wild and whether the appearance of such a number of possible recombination or mutation events is normal for all immunoglobulin genes or other multigene families. Results from studies of VK genes in these mice (D'Hoostelaere, this edition) indicate that higher than expected alterations in RF patterns by recombination and mutation events may have also occurred in these families. One possible mechanism for increased recombination frequencies could be the presence of disparate numbers of genes on each chromosome (Table 2). The resultant uneven pairing could lead to unequal crossing over, thus producing new RF patterns. One example of such an event may be found in Hind III RF pattern c, where the 3.2 kb gene which had previously only been found linked to the 700 bp gene appears by itself and is found in a unique Bgl II RF pattern. Further investigation using repeated collections of mice from these same locations and controlled matings will be necessary to accurately determine the contribution of mutation and recombination events to this variation in immunoglobulin gene content. Because of its simplicity, the X-24 VH gene family presents an ideal system for such studies.

SUMMARY

Restriction fragment patterns corresponding to the X-24 VH family have been determined for various inbred strains and wild mice species. These studies revealed that for the X-24 VH gene family: (1) allelic patterns represented in inbred strains are found in both M. m. musculus and M. m. domesticus from widely diverse areas; (2) there is no pattern specific for M. m. musculus or M. m. domesticus; (3) in inbred strains, each X-24 VH pattern is associated with more than one IgCH haplotype except possibly pattern 2, where only haplotype b has been identified. These findings imply that these alleles are possibly very ancient and were present prior to the widespread geographic dispersion of Mus musculus. Alternatively, contamination of existing populations by natural processes or by man could lead to the absence of a specific pattern for M. m. musculus or M. m. domes-

ticus. A study of the X-24 gene family in commensal populations
of mice from Maryland and Delaware has revealed a high degree of
polymorphism with a variation in gene copy number. Potential
evidence for a number of recombinational events was detected and the
high number of RF patterns found led to the speculation that recombinational events and mutations within VH families may occur more
frequently within natural populations than would have been expected.

REFERENCES

Brodeur PH, Riblet R (1984) The immunoglobulin heavy chain variable
region (Igh-V) locus in the mouse I. One hundred Igh-V genes
comprise seven families of homologous genes. Eur J Immunol 14:922-
930

Cory S, Tyler BM, Adams JM (1981) Sets of immunoglobulin VK genes
homologous to ten cloned VK sequences: implications for the number
of germline VK genes. J Mol Appl Genet 1:103-116

D'Hoostelaere LA, Potter M (submitted) Igk polymorphism in M. musculus
domesticus populations from Maryland and Delaware. (this edition)

Hartman AB, Rudikoff S (1984) VH genes encoding the immune response to
β-(1,6)-galactan: somatic mutation in IgM molecules. EMBO 3:3023-
3030

Honjo T, Habu S (1985) Origin of immune diversity: genetic variation
and selection. Ann Rev Biochem 54:803-830

Hood L, Kronenberg M, Hunkapiller T (1985) T cell antigen receptors
and the immunoglobulin supergene family. Cell 40:225-229

Huang C-M, Parsars M, Oi VT, Huang H-JS, Herzenberg LA (1983) Genetic
characterizaton of mouse immunoglobulin allotypic determinants
(allotypes) defined by monoclonal antibodies. Immunogenetics 18:
311-321

Huppi K, Jouvin-Marche E, Scott C, Potter M, Weigert M (1985) Genetic
polymorphism at the K chain locus in mice: comparison of restriction
enzyme hybridization fragments of variable and constant region genes.
Immunogenetics 21:445-457

Lieberman R (1978) Genetics of IgCH (allotype) locus in the mouse.
Springer Seminars in Immunopathol 1:7-30

Mushinski EB, Potter M (1977) Idiotypes or galactan binding myeloma
proteins and anti-galactan antibodies in mice. J Immunol 119:
1888-1893

Potter M, Mushinski EB, Rudikoff S, Glaudemans CPJ, Padlan EA, Davies
DR (1979) Structural and genetic basis of idiotypes in the
galactan-binding myeloma proteins. Ann Immunol (Inst Pasteur)
130C:263-271

Rudikoff S, Pawlita M, Pumphrey J, Mushinski E, Potter M (1983)
Galactan-binding antibodies: diversity and structure of idiotypes.
J Exp Med 158:1385-1400

Wilson AC, Carlson SS, White TJ (1977) Biochemical evolution. Ann
Rev Biochem 46:573-639

Yonekawa H, Gotieh O, Tagashira Y, Matsushima Y, Shi L-I, Cho WS,
Miyashita N, Moriwaki K (submitted) A hybrid origin of Japanese
mice "Mus musculus molossinus." (this edition)

Polymorphism and Evolution of Igh-V Gene Families

R. Riblet, A. Tutter, and P. Brodeur

INTRODUCTION

The immunoglobulin heavy chain locus (Igh) is located on chromosome 12 of the mouse. It is a complex locus, containing over one hundred variable region gene segments (Igh-V or Vh), approximately 12 diversity (Dh), 4 joining (Jh) and 8 constant region (Igh-C or Ch) gene segments. Although extensive diversity of antibody structures is generated in the assembly of active variable region genes by fusion of all combinations of V, D and J, it is apparent that there is as well a very high degree of genetic polymorphism at this locus. Examination of a panel of eighteen inbred strains selected to represent a variety of constant region allotypes (Igh-C alleles) revealed correlated allelism of the entire array of Vh and Dh gene segments (Brodeur and Riblet 1984; Brodeur et al. 1984). The extent of this genetic diversity parallels that of the MHC (Klein 1975) consistent with the parallel importance of this locus in protecting an individual from a variable environment. In this study we present further examination of the extent of this polymorphism and some aspects of the evolution of the locus.

Polymorphism of Igh-V

The array of Igh-V, or Vh, gene segments is organized into at least nine Vh gene families (Brodeur et al. 1984; Winter et al. 1985). These gene families range in content from 2 to approximately 60 members, occupy separate regions of the Igh-V locus, and are highly polymorphic. In a survey of common "old inbred" strains polymorphism of each Vh gene family was correlated with the serologic polymorphism - allotypes - of the constant region genes. These polymorphisms defined Vh haplotypes and "complete" (Vh-Ch) Igh haplotypes (Brodeur and Riblet 1984). Table 1 lists these and includes many additional strains which displayed the same allelic arrays of Vh genes. All strains did not possess already identified haplotypic patterns, however. As shown in Fig. 1 new patterns appear in examining further strain panels. The old inbred alleles of the Vh S107 gene family shown in BALB/c (=a), C57BL/6 (=b) and AKR (=d) are seen in 129 and WLL (a) and WC (b); and YBR and YS are the same as DBA (=c, not shown). WB and WK present novel patterns, similar to, but distinguishable from, WC (b). The Connor strains, PAA through PAF, are "new" inbred strains, derived relatively recently from live trapped Mus domesticus (Staats 1981). At least four new patterns, or family alleles, are seen in these strains. This sort of result, defining new alleles and further polymorphism as a consistent part of continuing the study of mouse strains, obtains also when the survey is broadened beyond samples of M. domesticus, represented by inbred strains, to populations of M. musculus or M. castaneus. Mice or DNA samples from these species, obtained from Drs. Verne Chapman and Richard Sage displayed additional variety of Vh haplotypes. In Fig. 2, DNA samples obtained from Dr. Michael Potter representing individuals from an even greater variety of Mus species maintain the same theme: Each Vh gene family is represented, and is of similar size in all species, and displays extraordinary diversity. The extent of polymorphism cannot be estimated from the limited survey accomplished thus far, but it is clearly very large, and transcends the species level, that is, Vh gene haplotypes seen in one Mus species are as different from (or similar to) each other as they are to

168

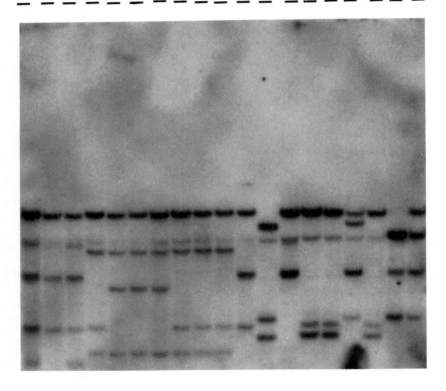

Fig. 1. VhS107 polymorphism in old and new inbred strains. Liver DNA from each mouse strain was digested with EcoRI, "Southern blotted" by electrophoresis through 0.7% agarose in Tris:NaAcetate:EDTA / 40mM:20mM:2mM pH7.8, and transfer to nitrocellulose membranes (BA85). This blot was probed with the S107 Vh gene (Brodeur and Riblet 1984).

Table 1. Inbred strains with "old inbred" Vh haplotypes

Igh Haplotype	Prototype	Other Strains
a	BALB/cAnNIcr	AKR.L-Cha/4Cy, BALB/cByJ, C58/J, C57L/J, DD/HeAf, FB/Ki, HRS, MA/MyJ, NMRI/Navy, RB156BNR, ST/bJ, 129/SvSla
b	C57BL/6NIcr	C57BL/6ByJ, C57BL/6J, CWB-13/Icr, LP/J, RB2BNR, SJL/J, WC
br	SM/J	AE/WfIcr
c	DBA/2AnNIcr	DBA/1J, DBA/2DeJ, DBA/2Ha, DBA/2J*, I/LnJ, RF/J,
d	AKR/NIcr	ACR/A, AKR/J, DBA/LiAf
e	A/HeNIcr	A/BrAf
f	CE/J	PL/J
j	C3H/HeJ	AU/SsJ, CBA/CaJ, CBA/H-T6J, CBA/J, CBA/Ki, C3H.SW, C3HeB/FeJ, C3H/HeSnJ, C3H/HeNIcr, LG/J, Rb1Ald/Rb163H
n	NZB/BlNIcr	NZW

haplotypes in other Mus. As Klein (1975) has argued for H-2 it appears that polymorphism at Igh predates the development of Mus species and may be shared across species divisions. The extent of genetic diversity at Igh is clearly of the same extraordinary magnitude as that at H-2, i.e., Mus domesticus may well have hundreds of independent haplotypes, providing a wealth of genetic potential to ensure the successful defense of the species against all pathogens.

Evolution in Incremental Steps

Early considerations of the modes of evolution of immunoglobulin genes placed emphasis on the multigene family aspect (Hood et al. 1975). Attendant in this were implications of significant expansions and contractions of the number of immunoglobulin V or C genes by unequal crossing over. A more detailed understanding of the genetic structure of the Igh locus places considerable limits on such processes. Different Vh gene families may share sequences which are identical at 50-60% of nucleotides over relatively short regions (300-400 nucleotides); this should make genetic exchange between such families extremely rare. Such exchange, and other intergenic information transfer such as gene conversion, should be limited to occur within single gene families, although such events could well reduce or expand a single family quite significantly. We have searched for such events, by characterizing the Vh haplotypes of large numbers of mouse strains and individual wild mice, and, in a search for recent, well defined, exchanges, we have examined many substrains and their equivalent (for single loci), Recombinant Inbred strains.

A number of instances of evolutionary alteration in family size have been identified. Surprisingly, these are all very limited, resulting in the duplication or deletion of single members of various Vh gene families in a variety of haplotypes. The best defined example is shown in Fig. 3. Of some six strains of DBA mice examined, uniquely DBA/2J, and RI lines derived from it,

170

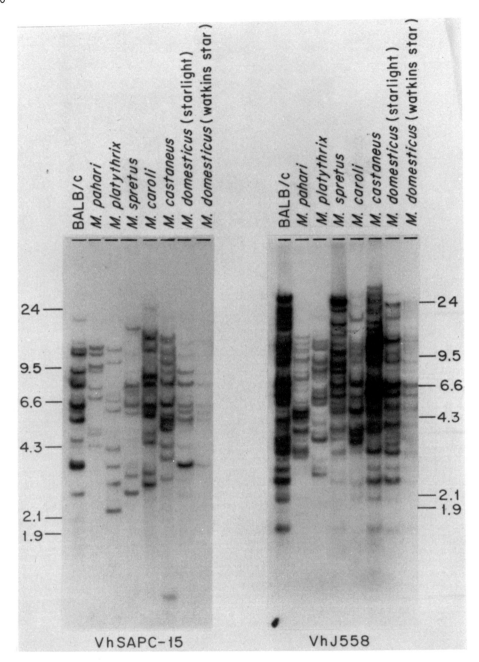

Fig. 2. Vh7183 and VhJ558 gene families in wild mouse species. Analysis was performed as in fig. 1 and probed as indicated. The SAPC-15 Vh gene is a member of the 7183 Vh gene family. Wild mouse DNAs were obtained from Dr. Michael Potter. Size markers (in kilobases) are shown at the sides.

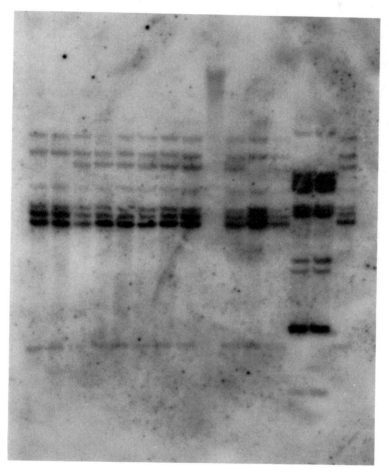

BXD-12
BXD-24
DBA/2Anlcr
DBA/1J
DBA/1J
DBA/2DeJ
DBA/2DeJ
DBA/2Ha

DBA/2Anlcr
DBA/2J
DBA/2J
DBA/LiAf
DBA/LiAf
DBA/2Anlcr

Fig. 3. Loss of a VhQ52N gene in DBA/2J. Liver DNA from various DNA sublines and DBA-derived Recombinant Inbred lines was analyzed as in fig. 1 and probed with the Q52N (nonproductive VDJ rearrangement) Vh gene. The DBA/LiAf substrain is known to be distantly related to other DNA lines and differs from them at other loci (Hilgers 1978). The VhQ52N allele of DBA/LiAf is j (type strain: C3H).

have one fewer members of the VhQ52N family. This reduction event occurred sometime in the last 60 generations of this line, after its divergence from the DBA/2N subline. One such event occurred in the Q52N family in something in excess of 2000 generations of breeding throughout the DBA lineages, and this frequency is probably an overestimate of the true rate of such events. None have been identified in other Vh gene families in the same lineages. Less well defined events have been found. A few mouse strains have Vh haplotypes identical to known haplotypes except for a single duplication/deletion in one Vh gene family. The derivation and timing of these cases cannot even be speculated on, but taken together they do serve to indicate that even within Vh gene families catastrophic contraction or expansion events are not the general mode of change at this locus. Rather, evolution appears to proceed by slow, incremental steps.

Recombination in Igh

In Table 1 SM/J and AE are listed as "br" or b recombinant haplotypes. This haplotype appears to have been generated by recombination between the a and b haplotypes (Brodeur and Riblet 1984). The haplotypes of strains GR and RIII also appear to have arisen from two different recombinations between the a haplotype of BALB/c and the g haplotype of BSVS. The n haplotype of NZB and the o haplotype of AL/N appear to be the result of multiple exchanges among the haplotypes of BALB/c, A, and C3H. These haplotypes may have existed in wild mice but it is likely that at least some of these genetic exchanges occurred during the early years of mouse breeding, in the genesis of these strains. We cannot yet address the question of whether genetic recombination provides a significant degree of haplotype scrambling and generates new combinations of Vh genes. Such recombination clearly can occur in laboratory settings and would be expected in natural populations, but this cannot be documented as yet, so we have no estimation of the contribution of recombination to the evolution of the Igh locus.

ACKNOWLEDGEMENTS

This work was done while the authors were at the Institute for Cancer Research - Fox Chase Cancer Center and the University of Pennsylvania, Philadelphia, PA, and was supported by grants CA06927, RR 05539, T32CA09140 and AI13797 from the National Institutes of Health, IM-362 from the American Cancer Society and an appropriation from the Commonwealth of Pennsylvania. P. Brodeur was a fellow of the Cancer Research Institute, New York.

REFERENCES

Brodeur PH, Riblet R (1984) The immunoglobulin heavy chain variable region (Igh-V) locus in the mouse. I. 100 Igh-V genes comprise 7 families of homologous genes. Eur J Immunol 14:922-930

Brodeur PH, Thompson MA, Riblet R (1984) The content and organization of mouse Igh-V families. In: Cantor H, Chess L, Sercarz E (eds) Regulation of the immune system, Alan R Liss, New York, p. 445

Hilgers J (1978) Mouse News Letter, no. 58, pp. 35-38. Personal communication

Hood L, Campbell JH, Elgin SCR (1975) The organization, expression and evolution of antibody genes and other multigene families. In: Roman HL, Campbell A, Sandler LM (eds) Annual review of genetics, vol. 9, Annual Reviews, Inc, Palo Alto, p. 305

Klein, J (1975) Biology of the mouse histocompatibility-2 complex. Springer-Verlag, New York

Staats, J (1981) Inbred and segregating inbred strains. In: Foster HL, Small JD and Fox JG (eds) The mouse in biomedical research, vol. 1, Academic Press, Inc., New York, p. 177

Winter E, Radbruch, A, Krawinkel U (1985) Members of novel V_H-gene families are found in VDJ-regions of polyclonally activated B-lymphocytes. EMBO J, in press

Ig Kappa

Igk Polymorphism in *M. musculus domesticus* Populations from Maryland and Delaware

L. A. D'Hoostelaere and M. Potter

The genetic locus that codes for Igk light chains in mice is located on chromosome 6 approximately 32 centimorgans from the centromere (Valbuena et al., 1978; Hengartner et al., 1978; Swan et al., 1979; Gibson et al., 1983; Gibson et al., 1984; Gibson and MacLean 1979; D'Hoostelaere et al., 1985). The number of germline sequences for variable kappa (VK) in inbred mice has been estimated to be from 90 to 320 (Cory et al., 1981; Zeelon et al., 1981; Briles and Carroll 1981; Adams et al., 1981; Potter et al., 1982; Gibson 1984; Nishi et al., 1985). Cory et al. (1981) made their estimates on the basis of 7 canonical probes (11 originating from 8 myeloma cell lines). Each canonical DNA probe hybridized with a unique set of VK restriction endonuclease fragments (REFs). The sum of these sets of related VK genes are thought to correspond to a large part but not all of the VK groups identified by partial and complete amino acid sequencing (Potter et al., 1982). Some of the sets are clusters of nearest neighbor genes, e.g., as with VK21 (Heinrich et al., 1984). Clustering must be demonstrated for each canonical set since human VK groups have been found to be interspersed (Jaenichem et al., 1984; Peck et al., 1985).

The molecular probes used in the present study (Table 1) were of two types: 1) approximately 1 kilobase pair (kbp) long cDNA clones which would include sequences for joining (J) and constant (C) kappa regions as well as the desired coding sequence and 2) approximately 1-7 kbp long segments containing the coding sequence and a potentially large flanking region(s) in the germline or rearranged configuration. Using Southern transfer hybridization techniques (as in Huppi et al., 1985) these molecular probes showed under high stringency from 1 to 9 REF in genomic DNA from inbred mice using Bam HI. Although some REF had shared mobility the REF patterns were probe specific and could detect allelic differences among inbred strains (Cory et al., 1981; Huppi et al., 1985).

The commensal mice (Table 2) tested were populations collected in this laboratory over the past 10 years. The populations were trapped in 6 separate locations in Maryland and Delaware and on each occasion the traps were set for only one night. The Maryland Tobacco farm mice came from 4 different builldings on the same farm. The Tobacco, Haven's and Sanner's Farm mice came from a semi-rural district on the western side of the Chesapeake Bay (Fig. 1) and were within 10 miles of each other. The other populations were from the Eastern shore. The Centreville and J.J. Downs locations were 10-15 miles apart. The Lewes location was 45 miles distant from the others. Repeat sampling has not been attempted for any of the locations, and the original trappings were intended to give samples to determine the extent of polymorphism. All of the tested samples were derived from mice bred in the laboratory.

Polymorphisms of VK groups or a canonical set are recognized in inbred mice by differences in the sizes of individual REFs and by the number of REFs (Table 1, Fig. 3). Remarkably only 2 to 4 patterns per probe, a, b, c or d (Table I), were found in the inbred strains so far studied. In the present study we have used 6 of the canonical probes (VK 8,9,10,11,21,24) (Table 1) to study VK polymorphisms in the 10 populations of mice (Table 2, Fig. 1).

We first asked if the inbred patterns a, b, c or d observed in inbred mice existed in these commensal populations. We found one population (Tobacco Farm Seed Shed) which had both of the CK alleles found in inbred mice (Fig. 2). All of the other populations showed only the 12.7 kb REF which is the most common inbred allele. We did not find inbred patterns for VK in some of the wild populations and in others inbred patterns were found (Fig. 3, Table 3). The inbred patterns for VK21 were the most frequent. No alleles of the "a" type were detected (Table 3) for any of the VK groups. In addition, there were a number of patterns that could not be explained as representing one or a combination of inbred patterns (Table 3, Fig. 3). These are potentially new alleles. A new pattern was designated when a novel REF was detected within a set (Table 3). In the majority of cases these are tentative alleles since Igk is known to be segregating and heterozygosity was not established. When an inbred REF pattern was detected in an individual for one canonical set, the patterns for the other gene groups did not necessarily conform to an inbred type.

The mice from the various locations were bred in the laboratory by either full-sib matings or by random matings to maintain the gene pool. In the LW, SF, CNV and HF mice (Tables 2 and 3) the chr 6s appeared to be fixed, and this homozygosity facilitated the identification of allelic canonical phenotypes. All LW and SF mice, though isolated from different sides of the Chesapeake Bay, had identical phenotypes, containing only one inbred allele. In chr 6 segregating populations, typing could only be tentatively made. However, a number of novel phenotypes were found, and individual mice, notably those from the Tobacco Farm within the same barns exhibited multiple different phenotypes (Table 3).

The extraordinary heterogeneity in VK phenotypes in mice caught in the same location is of considerable interest because it reflects aspects of the genetics of immunoglobulin genes. First, there may be a selective advantage for breeding populations to maintain heterogeneity in Ig kappa genotypes. Second, the extraordinary polymorphism may arise from mechanisms that are continuously generating new phenotypes.

These results could have several explanations including migration, mutation and recombination. Population mixing resulting from migrations into a common location cannot be adequately tested in the present samples; however, it should be noted that most of the populations examined were collected in the fall season when migration into dwellings may peak (Rowe et al., 1963) because habitats are disrupted by the harvest or the onset of winter. If migration is the major contributor to the polymorphism detected, most of the mice collected in select Tobacco Farm populations were heterozygous when trapped.

Mutation has been examined for select Ig genes within the genus Mus. The mutation rates are sequence dependent. Constant and variable coding regions have different mutation rates as do regulatory sequences and other regions with unknown function (CK, VK24, Rudikoff and Jouvin-Marche, this edition). These mutation rates (3 to 20% over 10^6-10^7 years) do not reach levels which would account for the total polymorphism observed. Since VK gene groups are linked in inbred mice, and have been shown to yield a very low recombination frequency (Gibson et al., 1983; Gibson et al., 1984) the alteration of linkage patterns displayed here would not be expected. Although recombination frequencies within Igk of the mouse are low; high recombination frequencies have been observed in the MHC multigene family when commensal mice are crossed with domestic mice (Shiroishi et al., 1982; Fischer-Lindahl, this edition; Steinmetz, this edition). It is quite likely that migration, mutation and recombination are all involved in the production of the REF patterns detected.

Since all three possibilities require a different approach we decided to look at recombination first. We selected three mice from the Centreville (CNV) population. One was from the Watkin's Star (WS) population and two mice were from the Centreville Light (CL) population. We produced a series of F_1 and F_2 (first and second filial generations) progeny using the inbred congenic line C.B20. All of the F_1 mice showed identical REF patterns indicating the WS and CL populations had fixed this region of chromosome 6 prior to the separation of these two lines. The F_2 mice did not show the expected distributions (Fig. 4). First, there was a paucity of samples homozygous for the CNV alleles (12.5%). Second was the prodigious number of recombinations (20.8%). These may not be the classical recombination events detected in other systems. The events detected were all unidirectional in that the VK21 pattern was found to be homozygous for the inbred b allele while all the other VK gene groups tested were heterozygous. Since we have not tested for loci outside Igk we cannot be sure that this is the same type of high frequency recombination seen in MHC (Shiroishi et al., 1982; Fischer-Lindahl, this edition; Steinmetz, this edition).

The results obtained from the Tobacco Farm and J.J. Down's populations seem to indicate the Ig genes in nature are in a very dynamic situation. When mice are removed from their natural habitat and subjected to laboratory conditions, different selection factors begin operating. The immune system would be a major selection factor. This selection would have a strong bias since most rodent colonies have a specific set of pathogens; therefore, stagnation could occur resulting in fixation of genes involved in the response to these pathogens. The remaining genes could mutate or be deleted without having a detrimental affect on the population.

We have detected a high degree of polymorphism within and among the 10 commensal populations of mice. Although inbred REF patterns could be found in certain populations, most VK groups had altered REF patterns. The VK21 b allele was found in all but two populations, possibly indicating something special about VK21. All of the VK gene groups examined were present in the commensal mice, and there was evidence for an alteration in gene copy number in VK9, 11 and 24. We also detected a potential recombination hot spot within Igk when commensal mice from Centreville were used in genetic crosses with inbred mice. Again VK21 appeared to be singled out as being important.

REFERENCES

Adams JM, Kemp DJ, Bernard O, Gough N, Webb E, Tyler B, Gerondakis
  S, Cory S (1981) Organization and expression of murine immunoglobulin genes. Immunol Reviews 59:5-32
Briles DE, Carroll RJ (1981) A simple method for estimating the
  probable number of different antibodies by examining the repeat
  frequencies of sequences or isoelectric focusing patterns. Mol
  Immunol 18:29-38
Coleclough C, Perry RP, Karjalainen K, Weigert M (1981) Aberrant
  rearrangements contribute significantly to the allelic exclusion
  of immunoglobulin gene expression. Nature 290:372-378
Cory S, Tyler BM, Adams JM (1981) Sets of immunoglobulin VK genes
  homologous to ten cloned VK sequences: implications for the number
  of germline VK genes. J Mol Appl Genet 1:103-116
D'Hoostelaere LA, Jouvin-Marche E, Huppi K (1985) Localization of
  $C_T\beta$ and $C\kappa$ on murine chromosome six. Immunogenetics 22:277-283
Fischer-Lindahl K (Submitted) Genetic variants of histocompatibility
  antigens from wild mice. (this edition)
Gibson DM (1984) Evidence for 65 electrophoretically distinct groups
  of light chains in BALB/c and NZB myelomas. Mol Immunol 21:421-432
Gibson DM, MacLean SJ (1979) Ef-2: A new Ly-3-linked light-chain
  marker expressed in normal mouse serum immunogloublin. J Exp Med
  149: 1477-1486
Gibson DM, MacLean SJ, Anctil D, Mathieson BJ (1984) Recombination
  between kappa chain genetic markers in the mouse. Immunogenetics
  20:493-501
Gibson DM, MacLean SJ, Cherry M (1983) Recombination between kappa
  chain genetic markers and the Lyt-3 locus. Immunogenetics 18:
  111-116
Heinrich G, Traunecher A, Tonegawa S (1984) Somatic mutation creates
  diversity in the major group of mouse immunoglobulin K light
  chains. J Exp Med 159:417-435
Hengartner H, Meo T, Mullen E (1978) Assignment of genes for immunoglobulin K and heavy chains to chromosome 6 and 12 in mouse. Proc
  Natl Acad Sci USA 75:4494-4498
Huppi K, Jouvin-Marche E, Scott C, Potter M, Weigert M (1985) Genetic
  polymorphism at the K chain locus in mice: comparisons of
  restriction enzyme hybridization fragments of variable and con-
  stant region genes. Immunogenetics 21:445-457
Jaenichen H, Peck M, Lindenmaier W, Wildgruber N, Zachau H (1984)
  Composite human V_K genes and a model of their evolution. Nucl Acid
  Res 12:5249-5263
Nishi M, Kataoka T, Honjo T (1985) Preferential rearrangement of
  immunoglobulin K chain joining region J_K1 and J_K2 segments in
  mouse spleen DNA. Proc Natl Acad Sci USA 82:6399-6403
Peck M, Smola H, Pohlenz H, Straubinger B, Gerl R, Zachau H (1985)
  A large section of the gene locus encoding human immunoglobulin
  variable regions of the kappa type is duplicated. J Mol Biol 183:
  291-299
Perry RR (unpublished) A non-productively rearranged VK11 by DNA
  sequencing. p6684^{K-} is a 4 kbp Hind III fragment. Perry R, ICR,
  Philadelphia
Potter M, Newell JB, Rudikoff S, Haber E (1982) Classification
        of mouse VK groups based on the partial amino acid sequence to the
        first invariant tryptophan: impact of 14 new sequences from IgG
        myeloma proteins. Mol Immunol 19:1619-1630

Rowe FP, Taylor EJ, Chudley AHJ (1963) The numbers and movements of
house-mice (Mus musculus L.) in the vicinity of four corn-ricks.
J Anim Ecol 32:87-97
Rudikoff S, Jouvin-Marche E (submitted) Evolution of CK and VK genes
in wild mice. (this edition)
Selsing E, Storb U (1981) Somatic mutation of immunoglobulin light-
chain variable region genes. Cell 25:47-58
Shapiro M (unpublished) A germline VK10 by DNA sequencing. pC3386
is a 0.9 kbp Eco RI-Hind III fragment. Shapiro M, ICR,
Philadelphia
Shiroishi T, Sagai T, Moriwaki K (1982) A new wild-derived H-2 haplo-
type enhancing K-IA recombination. Nature 300:370-372
Stafford J, Queen C (1983) Cell-type specific expression of a trans-
fected immunoglobulin gene. Nature 306:77-79
Steinmetz M (submitted) Polymorphism and recombination hot spots in
murine MHC (this edition)
Swan D, D'Eustachio P, Leinwand L, Seidman J, Keithley D, Ruddle FH
(1979) Chromosomal assignment of the mouse K light chain genes.
Proc Natl Acad Sci USA 76:2735-2739
Valbuena O, Marcu KB, Croce CM, Huebner K, Weigert M, Perry RP (1978)
Chromosomal location of immunoglobulin genes. Proc Natl Acad Sci
USA 75:2883-2887
Zeelon EP, Bothwell ALM, Kantor F, Schechter I (1981) An experi-
mental approach to enumerate the genes coding for immunoglobulin
variable region. Nucl Acid Res 9:3809-3820

Table 1. Probes for Different Igk Gene Groups

Probe	VK gene group	Source*	Type of Probe	CK +/-	Number of BamHI Restriction Endo-nuclease fragments			
					inbred allele			
					a	b	c	d
M603K2	8	S. Cory	cDNA	+	6	6(1)		
B61K16	21	S. Cory	cDNA	+	8(4)	9(3)	9(3)	8
pC3386	10	M. Shapiro	Germline	-	2(2)	3(3)		
p6684K-	11	R. Perry	Rearranged genomic	+	3(2)	2	2(1)	
MOPC41 5'FL	9	C. Queen	Germline Flanking	-	2	4(2)		
M167VL	24	Selsing & Storb	Germline	-	1(1)	2(2)	2(2)	
pECK		M. Weigert	Germline	+	1(1)	1(1)		

* Cory et al., 1981; Shapiro (unpublished); Perry (unpublished);
  Stafford and Queen 1983; Selsing and Storb 1981; Coleclough et
  al., 1981, for (pECK)
(#) Unique REFs detected within the inbred allele as compared to all
  other inbred alleles.

Table 2. Source of commensal Mus musculus domesticus

Common Name (abbreviations)	Geographic Origin	Description of Populations
Centreville (CNV) Centreville Light (CL) Watkin's Star (WS, WSA, WSB)	Centreville, Queen Anne County, MD	Mice were collected in spring 1975 on one trap night from a single farm. Of the 10 mice trapped, 4 generation zero (G0) mice have passed on genetic information to the current population. Inbreeding was begun after one generation. After 2 inbreeding generations two lines were created based on coat color phenotypes. These lines were named Centreville Light (light agouti coat color) and Watkin's Star (dark agouti coat color with white blaze).
Haven's Farm (HF, HV)	Davidsonville, Anne Arundel County, MD	One pregnant mouse was obtained in the fall of 1982, and the progeny were inbred.
J. J. Downs (JD, JJD)	Ridgely, Queen Anne County, MD	Mice were collected in spring 1981 on one trap night from a single corn crib on J. Downs Farm. Of the 9 mice trapped, 8 G0 mice have passed on genetic information to the current population. These mice are being bred in a semi-random fashion with a bias towards health and reproductive plurality.
Lewes (LW)	Lewes, Sussex County, DE	Trapped by D. Gallahan, Fall 1980. Two G0 mice have passed on genetic information. These mice are being inbred.
Sanner's Farm (SF, SN)	Davidsonville, Anne Arundel County, MD	Mice were collected in fall 1982 in one trap night. Two G0 mice have passed on genetic information to the current population. These mice are being inbred.
Tobacco Farm (TF) Chemical Shed (CS, TFC) Drying Barn (DB, TFD) Seed Shed (SS, TFS) Tool Shed (TS, TFT)	University of Maryland Tobacco Farm, Upper Marlboro, Prince Georges County, MD	Trapped by D. Gallahan, Fall 1982. Mice were collected in one trap night from 4 different buildings. These mice are being bred in a semi-random fashion. Two G0 mice contribute genetic information to current population. Two G0 mice contribute genetic information to current population. Four G0 mice contribute genetic information to current population. Four G0 mice contribute genetic information to current population.

Table 3. Allelic Distribution in Inbred and Commensal Mice

Population	VK21	VK10	VK8	VK9	VK24*	VK11
Inbred						
AKR/N	a	a	a	a	a	a
NZB/J	b	b	b	b	b	b
BALB/c	b	b	b	a	a	a
C58/J	a	a	a	b	b	b
SJL/J	c	b	b	a	a	a
I/LnJ	b	b	b	a	c	c
020/A	d	ND**	c	ND	ND	c
Commensal Igk Fixed						
LW***	b	e	e	e	e	e
SF	b	e	e	e	e	e
CNV	e	e	f	f	f	f
HF	e	b	f	g	g	g
Igk Segregating						
JJD	be	b(f)	f	f	(hij)	(hi)
TFC	b(fi)	e(gikl)	ef(hikln)	e(gjkl)	e	eg
TFD	b	(fjk)	f(hkp)	ef(i)	(k)	fg(h)
TFS	bc(fghi)	(f-l)	(g-m)	eg(ij)	e	cefg(hkl)
TFT	b(j)	e(fi)	f(hknoq)	ef(i)	e	ef

*The exbreeders from the tobacco farm were not tested for VK24
**Not determined
***See Table 2 for abbreviations

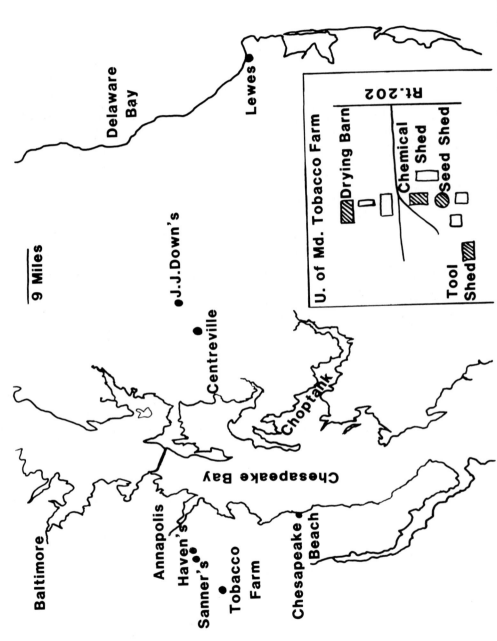

Fig. 1. Map of the trap sites for the commensal populations used in these experiments. The inset shows a schematic of the Tobacco Farm where four of the populations were collected. See Table 2 for a more detailed explanation of these populations.

183

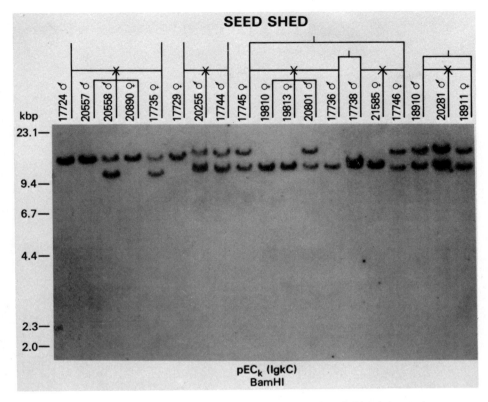

Fig. 2. Segregation of IgCk in Tobacco Farm Seed Shed breeders.
Horizontal lines indicate relationship. X indicates matings.

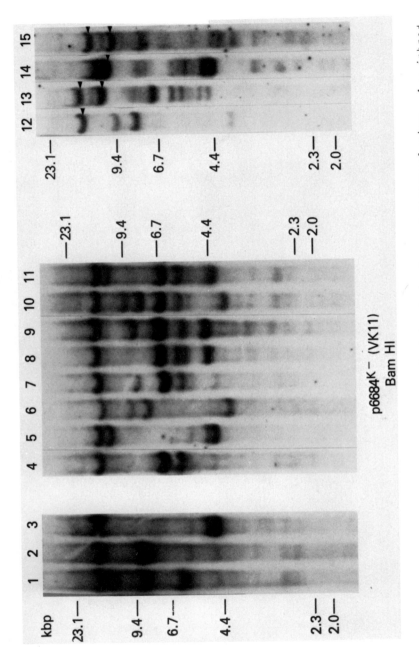

Fig. 3. Allelic differences for VK11 in inbred strains and commensal mice. 1 = inbred a allele; 2 = inbred b allele; 3 = inbred c allele; 4 = CL and WS; 5 = LW, SF and CS; 6 = HF; 7, 8 and 9 = JJD; 10 = DB; 11 = SS and TS; 12, 13, 14 and 15 = SS. (See Table 2 for abbreviations.) Since the p6684K⁻ probe also hybridizes with JK, lanes 1-11 show the 12.7 kb J-CK fragment, and the arrows in lanes 12-15 show the J-CK fragment.

185

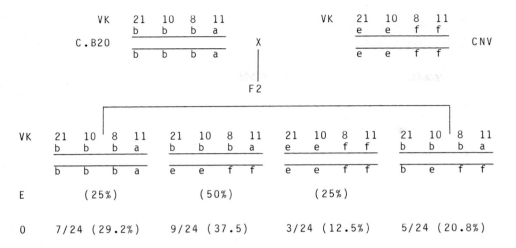

Fig. 4. High frequency recombination within VK of inbred-commensal crosses.

Restriction Enzyme Polymorphisms in V_κ and J_κ Genes of Inbred and Wild Mice

P. D. Gottlieb, R. T. Boyd, P. D. Ponath, and M. M. Goldrick

INTRODUCTION

The existence of phenotypic polymorphisms in immunoglobulin heavy (H) and light (L) chain variable (V) regions suggests that somewhat different repertoires of V regions are expressed by different strains of inbred mice. Southern hybridization analyses of genomic DNA with probes specific for individual $V\kappa$ groups have demonstrated that several of these polymorphisms correlate with inherited differences in V gene segments (Goldrick et al. 1985; Huppi et al. 1985; Moynet et al. 1985). Huppi et al. (1985) also observed $V\kappa$ segment restriction polymorphisms by Southern hybridization that had not been suspected from studies at the protein level. Similarly, though no differences in C_κ regions had been observed among inbred strains, Southern hybridization revealed a restriction polymorphism distinguishing the SJL/J strain from most others tested (Huppi et al. 1985). Use of these restriction polymorphisms and phenotypic markers in genetic experiments will help to determine the long range order of genes in the κ locus. Extension of the analyses to wild mice will give a better idea of the true extent of κ locus polymorphism and help to determine the origin of existing inbred strains.

Expression of two phenotypic markers, the I_B-peptide marker (Edelman and Gottlieb 1970; Gottlieb 1974) and the Efl^a isoelectric focussing marker (Gibson 1976), is known to be due to a group of κ chains ($V\kappa Ser$) that is apparently expressed by some strains of mice and not others (Gottlieb et al. 1981). Southern hybridization of liver DNA from many strains of inbred mice has demonstrated one strongly-hybridizing $V\kappa Ser$-related gene in strains which do and do not express these phenotypic markers (Goldrick et al. 1985). All expressor strains had hybridizing fragments of the same characteristic size with several enzymes. All non-expressor strains tested shared fragments of a different charcteristic size (Goldrick et al. 1985). The present report extends the Southern hybridization analysis of the $V\kappa Ser$ group to several recently inbred wild mouse strains and demonstrates additional $V\kappa Ser$ restriction polymorphisms.

Nucleotide sequence analysis of the rearranged expressed V_k-Ser gene of the myeloma, C.C58 M75, has demonstrated that the region containing the $J\kappa$ gene segments differs somewhat from that of BALB/c described by Max et al. (1981) (Boyd et al. submitted). This suggested that the C.C58 strain, which contains the $V\kappa$ polymorphisms and closely-linked <u>Lyt-2</u> and <u>Lyt-3</u> alleles of C58/J on the BALB/c genetic background (Gottlieb et al. 1980), probably contained the C58/J $J\kappa$ gene segments as well. Comparison of the C.C58 and BALB/c nucleotide sequences suggested the existence of restriction polymorphisms which might be useful in distinguishing $J\kappa$ gene segments of different strains and in genetic analyses. Nucleotide sequence analyses and other details are reported elsewhere (Boyd et al., submitted), but here we describe the $J\kappa$ restriction polymorphisms and their distribution in several recently inbred wild mouse strains.

RESULTS

Southern Hybridization with a V_KSer-specific Probe

Spleen DNA from the inbred descendants of wild mice trapped in widely separated localities was obtained from the Jackson Laboratories (Bar Harbor, Maine) and digested with BamHI. The digests were subjected to agarose gel electrophoresis, transferred to nitrocellulose and hybridized with a V_KSer-specific probe as described by Goldrick et al. (1985). Liver DNA of the C58/J (I_B-positive, Efl[a]-positive) and BALB/c (negative for both markers) strains were included for comparison. As shown in Fig. 1, a single strongly hybridizing fragment was observed in all strains tested. The CAST/Ei and MOLF/Ei strains shared the same size BamHI fragment (3.2 kb) as C58/J, while the hybridizing fragment of the IS/CamEI strain was identical in size (7.8 kb) to that of BALB/c. The PERU/AtteckEi and SF/CamEi DNA contained a hybridizing fragment of 6.6 kb not observed in conventional inbred strains, and the SK/CamRk DNA contained a unique hybridizing fragment of 6.4 kb. The same groupings of strains were observed in Southern hybridizations of HindIII-digested DNA (data not shown), whereas when DNA was digested with EcoRI, the SK/CamRk yielded a fragment identical in size to that of BALB/c and IS/CamEi (Fig. 2). Finally, similar Southern hybridization analysis of liver DNA from the SK/CamEi strain suggest that it falls into the same group as PERU/AtteckEi (data not shown).

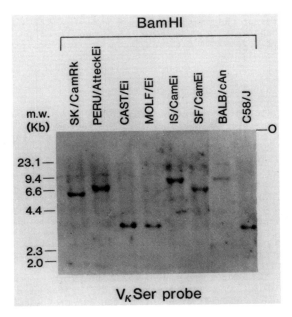

Fig.1. Ten micrograms of DNA from each strain were digested with BamHI and subjected to electrophoresis on an agarose gel. The DNA was transferred to nitrocellulose, hybridized with a radiolabeled V_KSer-specific probe and subjected to autoradiography as described previously (Goldrick et al. 1985).

Our previous results (Goldrick et al. 1985) and those presented here (Figs. 1 and 2) lead us to define four V_KSer haplotypes on the basis of restriction enzyme polymorphisms: that of C58/J, MOLF/Ei and CAST/Ei as Igk-VSer[a], that of BALB/c and IS/CamEi as Igk-VSer[b], that of PERU/AtteckEi, SF/CamEi and SK/CamEi as Igk-VSer[c], and that of SK/CamRk as Igk-VSer[d]. Nomenclature is as suggested by Green (1979).

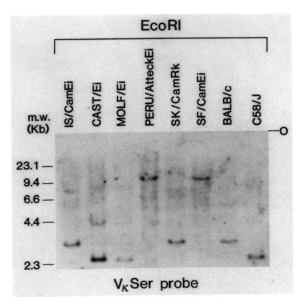

Fig. 2. Ten micrograms of DNA from each strain were digested with EcoRI and subjected to electrophoresis on an agarose gel, transferred to nitrocellulose, and hybridized with a V_KSer-specific probe as previously described (Goldrick et al. 1985).

Southern hybridization with a J_K probe.

Comparison of the nucleotide sequence of the C.C58 M75 myeloma L chain gene with the embryonic J_K sequence of BALB/c suggested that digestion with the restriction enzyme HinfI would yield J_K region fragments of different characteristic size in the C.C58 and BALB/c strains (Boyd et al. submitted). The presence of an extra HinfI site downstream of the C.C58 J_K2 would result in a region represented in BALB/c by an 848 bp fragment being cleaved in C.C58 to fragments of 555 bp and 293 bp. As shown in Fig. 3 for C.C58 and BALB/c, Southern hybridization with a C.C58 M75 probe extending from immediately downstream of J_K1 to a HindIII site in the J_K5 - C_K intron proved this to be the case. Comparison with a panel of inbred, congenic and recombinant inbred strains generally showed linkage of the C.C58-like pattern with the Igk-VSer[a] haplotype and its associated I_B-peptide and Efl[a] phenotypic polymorphisms (Boyd et al., submitted). Of conventional inbred strains which contain the Igk-VSer[b] haplotype and do not express these V_KSer-related phenotypic polymorphisms, only SJL/J (Fig. 3), MA/MyJ and LG/J (data not shown) yielded a HinfI pattern similar to C.C58 (Boyd et al. submitted; Goldrick et al. 1985; Taylor et al. in press). As shown in Fig. 3, Southern hybridization of spleen DNA from the descendants of recently inbred wild mice indicated that MOLF/Ei, CAST/Ei, PERA/Rk (same as PERU/AtteckEi), SF/CamEi and SK/CamEi contained the C.C58-like J_K HinfI pattern, while IS/CamEi and SK/CamRk (data not shown) yielded a pattern identical to BALB/c.

To explore the observed J_K polymorphism further, Southern hybridizations with the same J_K probe were performed with DNA from BALB/c, C.C58, SJL/J and several wild mouse strains which had been digested with the restriction enzyme AccI. Nucleotide sequence comparisons of C.C58 and BALB/c J_K regions had suggested that strain-specific AccI patterns might be observed (Boyd et al., submitted). As shown in Fig. 4 , all strains except BALB/c, SK/CamRk and IS/CamEi contain a strongly hybridizing fragment of 6.75 to 7.0 kb. It is possible that this fragment is slightly larger in MOLF/Ei and C.C58 than in the other strains, but for the moment they will be considered the same. The C.C58, MOLF/Ei and CAST/Ei

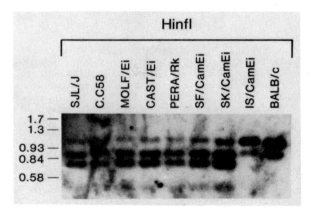

Fig. 3. Ten micrograms of DNA from each strain was digested with HinfI and subjected to electrophoresis on an agarose gel. The DNA was transferred to nitrocellulose, hybridized with a J_K -specific probe (see text and Boyd et al. submitted) and subjected to autoradiography.

strains also contain a hybridizing fragment of 2.0 kb which is absent from SJL/J, PERU/AtteckEi and SF/CamEi (Fig. 4) and from the MA/MyJ and LG/J inbred strains as well (data not shown). The BALB/c and IS/CamEi strains also contain a 2.0 kb hybridizing fragment as well as a second hybridizing fragment of approximately 4.0 kb. The SK/CamRk strain contains a 2.0 kb AccI fragment as well as a unique hybridizing 5.0 kb fragment.

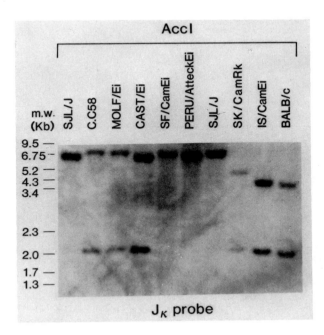

Fig. 4. Ten micrograms of DNA from each strain was digested with AccI and subjected to Southern hybridization with a J_K-specific probe as described in the legend to Fig. 3.

DISCUSSION

Results of the present Southern hybridization studies with V_KSer and J_K probes are summarized in Table 1 along with Efl and Lyt-3 typings reported by Taylor et al. (to be published). Results with the V_KSer probe and BamHI (Fig. 1), EcoRI (Fig.2) and HindIII (data not shown) digests demonstrate the existence of at least four haplotypes defined as Igk-VSer[a,b,c] and [d]. The Igk-VSer[a] haplotype is known to be associated with expression of the Efl[a] and I_B-peptide markers (Goldrick et al. 1985). It is of interest that the Igk-VSer[c] haplotype of SF/CamEi appears to permit expression of the Efl[a] polymorphism while that of PERU/AtteckEi (Table 1) apparently does not (Taylor et al. to be published). This may reflect differences in the V_KSer-related genes of these strains which are not apparent with the particular restriction enzymes employed here. Detailed analysis of these V_KSer-related genes are in progress. Finally, the differences in V_KSer restriction polymorphisms observed between the SK/CamRk and SK/CamEi sublines (see Figs. 1 and 2 and text) must be confirmed, and may reflect initial heterogeneity within the original Skokolm Island isolates.

Table 1. Igk-VSer, Efl[a], Lyt-3[a] and Igk-J Haplotypes of Wild and Inbred Mice

Igk-VSer	Efl	Lyt-3	Igk-J	Strain
a	a	a	a	C58/J, C.C58, MOLF/Ei, CAST/Ei
b	b	b	b	BALB/c, IS/CamEi
b	b	b	c	SJL/J, MA/MyJ, LG/J
c	b	b	c	PERU/AtteckEi
c	a	b	c	SF/CamEi
c	?[b]	?[b]	c	SK/CamEi
d	?[b]	?[b]	d	SK/CamRk

[a] Efl and Lyt-3 alleles are as reported by Taylor et al. (to be published). The Efl[a] allele governs expression of the I_B-peptide and Efl[a] phenotypic polymorphisms.

[b] The SK/CamEi strain has been reported to bear the Efl[b] and Lyt-3[b] alleles (Taylor et al. to be published). However, there is some question as to which SK subline was tested in those studies, and until these typings are repeated for both sublines, the alleles at these loci are treated here as unassigned.

Results of Southern hybridizations with the J_K probe and HinfI and AccI DNA digests define the existence of at least four J_K haplotypes, called Igk-J[a,b,c] and [d] (Table 1).. The Igk-J[b] haplotype gives a unique pattern with both HinfI and AccI (Figs. 3 and 4). Haplotypes Igk-J[a,c] and [d] are indistinguishable by HinfI digestion (Fig. 3) but can be discriminated in Southern hybridizations of AccI-digested DNA (Fig. 4). It is of interest that the SJL/J (Figs. 3 and 4), MA/MyJ and LG/J (data not shown) strains apparently share the Igk-J[c] haplotype of PERU/AtteckEi (PERA/Rk) and SF/CamEi (Table 1). Huppi and coworkers (1985) have reported a C_K polymorphism which is shared by SJL/J, MA/MyJ and PERU/AtteckEi. Since these strains as well as SF/CamEi and SK/CamEi share the

Igk-J^c haplotype, it is likely that the latter two strains will also share the Igk-C^a haplotype defined by Huppi et al. (1985). This is being tested.

It would appear that the Igk-VSer^a - Lyt-3^a - Igk-J^a haplotype combination of MOLF/Ei and CAST/Ei is identical to that of inbred strains like C.C58 and that this haplotype in inbred strains probably owes its origin to Asian mice. It is possible that the slightly smaller J$_K$-related AccI fragment of CAST/Ei (Fig. 4) may eventually prove it to have a unique Igk-J haplotype. The combination of Igk-VSer^b, Lyt-3^b and Igk-J^b haplotypes seen in IS/CamEi is the same as that of BALB/c and most other inbred strains, and this genotype may also have been contributed to inbred strains directly from their wild ancestors. The SJL/J, MA/My and LG/J strains apparently possess the Igk-J^c haplotype similar to that of PERU/AtteckEi (PERA/Rk), SF/CamEi and SK/CamEi but have acquired the Igk-VSer^b haplotype seen in BALB/c. Typing of these recently inbred wild mouse strains at the Lyt-2 locus may help to further delineate the origin of this chromosomal region in the SJL/J, MA/My and LG/J strains (see Table 1). Finally, we are in the process of analyzing the V$_K$Ser genes of the Igk-VSer^c and ^{d} haplotypes observed to date only in the recently inbred wild mouse strains to determine their relationship to those of the Igk-VSer^a and ^{b} haplotypes present in conventional inbred mice (Goldrick et al. 1985).

ACKNOWLEDGMENTS

This work was supported by grants CA-30147 from the National Cancer Institute and CD-218 from the American Cancer Society awarded to Paul D. Gottlieb. We are grateful to Dr. B.A. Taylor, The Jackson Laboratories, Bar Harbor, ME for sending us some of the wild mouse DNA samples.

REFERENCES

Boyd RT, Goldrick MM, Gottlieb, P.D. (submitted) Coding differences and restriction enzyme polymorphisms in J$_K$ gene segments of inbred mice. Immunogenetics

Edelman GM, Gottlieb PD (1970) A genetic marker in the variable region of light chains of mouse immunoglobulins. Proc Natl Acad Sci USA 67: 1192-1199

Gibson D (1976) Genetic polymorphism of mouse immunoglobulin light chains revealed by isoelectric focusing. J Exp Med 144: 298-303

Goldrick MM, Boyd RT, Ponath PD, Lou S-Y, Gottlieb PD (1985) Molecular genetic analysis of the V$_K$Ser group associated with two mouse light chain genetic markers: complementary DNA cloning and Southern hybridization analysis. J Exp Med 162: 713-728

Gottlieb PD (1974) Genetic correlation of a mouse light chain variable region marker with a thymocyte surface antigen. J Exp Med 140: 1432-1437

Gottlieb PD, Marshak-Rothstein A, Auditore-Hargreaves K, Berkoben D.B, August DA, Rosche RM, Benedetto JD (1980) Construction and properties of new Lyt-congenic strains and anti-Lyt-2.2 and anti-Lyt-3.1 monoclonal antibodies. Immunogenetics 10: 545-555

Gottlieb PD, Tsang H C-W, Gibson DM, Cannon, L.E. (1981) Unique V$_K$ group associated with two mouse L chain genetic markers. Proc Natl Acad Sci USA 78: 559-563

Green MC (1979) Genetic nomenclature for the immunoglobulin loci of the mouse. Immunogenetics 8: 89-97

Huppi K, Jouvin-Marche E, Scott C, Potter M, Weigert, M. (1985) Genetic polymorphism at the $_K$ chain locus in mice: comparisons of restriction enzyme hybridization fragments of variable and constant region genes. Immunogenetics 21: 445-457

Max EE, Maizel JV, Leder P (1981) The nucleotide sequence of a 5.5-kilobase DNA segment containing the mouse κ immunoglobulin J and C region genes. J Biol Chem 256: 5116-5120

Moynet D, MacLean SJ, Ng KH, Anctil D, Gibson DM (1985) Polymorphism of variable region (V_K-1) genes in inbred mice: relationship to the Igk-Ef2 serum light chain marker. J Immunol 135: 727-732

Taylor BA, Rowe L, Gibson DM, Riblet R, Yetter R, Gottlieb PD (to be published) Linkage of a 7S RNA sequence and kappa light chain genes in the mouse. Immunogenetics

Ig Lambda

Evidence That Wild Mice *(Mus musculus musculus)* Express Lambda Genes That Differ from Those in BALB/c

L.S. Reidl, B.W. Elliott, Jr., and L.A. Steiner

INTRODUCTION

The immunoglobulin (Ig) λ chains of BALB/c and other common laboratory strains of inbred mice are encoded by a limited number of germ-line genes: there are four $J-C$ segments, only three of which are functional, and two V segments [reviewed by Eisen & Reilly (1985)]. In contrast, many varieties of wild mice, and certain inbred strains derived from such mice, appear to have a greater number of $C\lambda$ genes. Southern-blot analysis of genomic DNA showed that, in some wild mice, as many as 12 restriction fragments cross-hybridized with probes derived from $C\lambda$ genes of BALB/c mice (Scott et al., 1982; Scott & Potter, 1984a; Kindt et al., 1985). However, some of the cross-hybridization could reflect the presence of pseudogenes and it is not known how many of these putative λ genes are actually expressed. The apparent amplification in number of $C\lambda$ genes did not seem to be accompanied by a proportional increase in number of $V\lambda$, although some increase in the number of restriction fragments cross-hybridizing with $V\lambda$ probes was detected in many of these mice (Scott & Potter, 1984b; Kindt et al., 1985). The number of $V\lambda$ genes in wild mice might, however, be underestimated if some of these genes are sufficiently different from $V\lambda1$ and $V\lambda2$ of inbred mice so as not to cross-hybridize with BALB/c $V\lambda$ probes.

We have initiated studies to examine the expression of λ genes in wild mice. Our approach is to prepare hybridomas and to screen them for the production of Igs that contain λ chains. These hybridomas are a source of rearranged λ genes and their corresponding protein products. We report here that a hybridoma from a wild mouse, *Mus musculus musculus*, from Skive, Denmark, produces a light chain that differs from BALB/c $\lambda1$ chains in a few amino acid residues of the constant region and in many residues of the variable region. A preliminary account of these results has been presented (Reidl et al., 1985).

MATERIALS AND METHODS

Wild Mice

Serum samples from four varieties of wild mice [*M. m. musculus* from Skive, Denmark (SD) and Sladeckovce, Czechoslovakia (Czech II); *M. m. domesticus* from Centreville, MD (Centreville Lights); and *M. m. molossinus* from Fukuoka, Kyushu, Japan] were obtained from M. Potter. These mice had been immunized intraperitoneally with 100 μg of alum-precipitated (4-hydroxy-3-nitrophenyl)acetyl (NP)-chicken γ-globulin (CGG) together with 2×10^9 inactivated *Bordetella pertussis*. SD and Czech II mice, which were used for hybridoma production, were from colonies maintained, under National Cancer Institute Contract, at Litton Bionetics, Rockville, MD [for a description of the origin of these mice, see Scott and Potter (1984a)].

Hybridomas

SD and Czech II mice were immunized with NP-CGG; seven days later spleen cells were fused with the non-Ig producing myeloma line X63.Ag8.653, as described by White-Scharf and Imanishi-Kari (1981). The supernatants from wells that contained hybridomas were screened by radioimmunoassay for κ- and λ-containing antibodies. The hybridomas that produced λ chains were subcloned and frozen (10^7 cells/ml 95% fetal calf serum, 5% dimethylsulfoxide). A subclone, SD 9-24-26 (SD-26), was also propagated *in vivo* by injecting 5×10^5 cells in 0.5 ml PBS (0.15 M NaCl, 0.01 M sodium phosphate, pH 7.2) intraperitoneally into BALB/c mice. These mice had been irradiated (∿550 Rads) 24 hr previously and had received 0.5 ml Pristane (Sigma Chemical Company, St. Louis, MO) 3 to 7 days previously.

Antibodies and Radioimmunoassay

The following antibodies were provided by T. Imanishi-Kari: 1) goat anti-κ [prepared against light chains of RPC-5 (γ2a,κ) and absorbed with HOPC-1 (γ2a,λ1)]; 2) rabbit anti-λ (prepared against HOPC-1 and absorbed with RPC-5); these antibodies cross-react with λ2 and λ3-containing Igs; 3) goat anti-λ2 [prepared against MOPC-315 (α,λ2) and absorbed with monoclonal antibody B1-8 (μ,λ1)]; 4) mouse anti-λ1 (a monoclonal antibody, LS136, from SJL mice immunized with B1-8) (Reth *et al.*, 1979); this antibody does not cross-react with λ2 or λ3. Goat anti-κ antibodies were also obtained from Southern Biological Assoc., Birmingham, AL. Antibodies were radiolabeled with ^{125}I by the chloramine-T procedure (Greenwood *et al.*, 1963). The light-chain type of anti-NP antibodies in sera or culture supernatants was determined by radioimmunoassay (Tsu & Herzenberg, 1980). The antigens used in the assay were either (4-hydroxy-5-iodo-3-nitrophenyl)acetyl (NIP)-bovine serum albumin (BSA), donated by T. Imanishi-Kari, or NP-BSA, prepared by coupling the N-hydroxysuccinimide ester of NP to the protein, as described by Wall *et al.* (1983). Plastic wells (Immulon I Removawell strips, Dynatech Laboratories Inc., Alexandria, VA) were saturated with antigen (5 μg/ml PBS), washed, and then coated with 1% BSA. Test samples (dilutions of antisera or undiluted culture supernatants) were added to the wells, followed, after washing, by one of the ^{125}I-labeled anti-light chain antibodies.

Purification of Antibodies and Light Chain SD-26

NP-specific antibodies were purified from ascites by affinity chromatography. An immunoadsorbent was prepared by coupling NP-BSA to Sepharose 4B (March *et al.*, 1974). The bound antibody, which recognizes the phenolate form (pKa∿7.3) of the hapten (Karjalainen *et al.*, 1980), was eluted from the immunoadsorbent with 0.1 M sodium citrate, 0.5 M NaCl, pH 5.4 (Dunham, 1983), concentrated by precipitation with ammonium sulfate, and dialyzed against 0.2 M Tris-HCl, 2 mM EDTA, pH 8.2. The Ig (∿13 mg/ml) was partially reduced with 5 mM dithiothreitol (DTT) and alkylated with [1-^{14}C] iodoacetic acid (Steiner & Lopes, 1979). Heavy and light chains were separated by gel filtration with Sephadex G-100 in 6 M urea-1 M acetic acid. Light chains (400 nmol) in 0.5 M Tris-HCl, 2 mM EDTA, pH 8.2 and 7 M guanidine were completely reduced in 15 mM DTT; 40 nmol of the reduced chains were alkylated with [1-^{14}C] iodoacetic acid and 360 nmol were alkylated with unlabeled iodoacetic acid. Some (150 nmol) of the latter light chains were citraconylated (Steiner *et al.*, 1979).

Isolation and Characterization of Peptides

Completely reduced and carboxymethylated light chains (10 nmol) in
0.05 M ammonium bicarbonate, adjusted to pH 8.4, were digested with
trypsin (2%, w/w) for 4 hr at 37°C, lyophilized, and taken up in 0.1%
trifluoroacetic acid. Tryptic peptides were fractionated by reverse-
phase high-pressure liquid chromatography (HPLC) (Elliott & Steiner,
1984). Citraconylated light chains (90 nmol) in 0.1 M ammonium bicarbonate, pH 8.6, were digested with trypsin (2% w/w) for 1 hr at 37°C,
followed by the addition of soybean trypsin inhibitor (1.5 fold weight
excess). The tryptic digest of the citraconylated light chains was subjected to gel filtration with Sephadex G-50 in 0.05 M ammonium bicarbonate; three peaks were eluted: a large peak at the void volume of the
column and two smaller retarded peaks. Peptides in the pooled fractions
from the two retarded peaks were deblocked by treatment with 5% formic
acid (Steiner et al., 1979) and then fractionated by HPLC. Peptides in
the unretarded peak were deblocked, digested with trypsin (2% w/w) for
2 1/2 hr and subjected to HPLC. Peptide T9 (Table 1) was rechromatog-
raphed in 0.025 M ammonium acetate, as described by Mikoryak et al.
(1986). The procedures for amino acid analysis, automated Edman degradation in a liquid-phase sequencer, the manual micro-dansyl Edman
method, digestion with pyroglutamate aminopeptidase, and electrophoresis
in polyacrylamide slab gels containing sodium dodecyl sulfate have been
described (Elliott & Steiner, 1984; Elliott et al., 1984). The partial
sequence of one peptide was determined in an Applied Biosystems (Model
470A) gas-phase sequencer (Hewick et al., 1981).

RNA Isolation and Nucleotide Sequencing

Total RNA was prepared from SD-26 tumor by the guanidinium isothio-
cyanate/cesium chloride method (Chirgwin et al., 1979). Poly(A)+ RNA
was selected after two passages of total RNA through an oligo(dT)-
cellulose column (Maniatis et al., 1982), followed by rechromatography
of the material eluted by low salt through the same column. The nucleotide sequence beginning at codon 105 and extending in the 5' direction
was obtained from the poly(A)+ RNA by the primer extension method
(Hamlyn et al., 1978). A heptadecadeoxynucleotide primer,
5' dGGCTGGCCTAGGACAGT 3', corresponding to codons 112-107 of λ1 chains,
obtained from E.B. Reilly, was used to prime cDNA synthesis (Reilly
et al., 1984).

RESULTS

Light Chain Types of Serum and Monoclonal Antibodies

Sera from four varieties of wild mice that had been immunized with
NP-CGG were tested to determine the type of light chain (κ or λ)
in the anti-NP antibodies. The results of these assays are summarized
in Fig. 1. In sera from M. m. molossinus, there was a strong reaction
with both anti-κ and anti-λ antibodies, as well as with a monoclonal
antibody highly specific for λ1 chains. It had previously been demonstrated that M. m. molossinus, like the inbred strain C57BL/6, produces
anti-NP antibodies containing λ chains and expressing the NPb idiotype
(Makela et al., 1979). Three other varieties of wild mice produced
mainly κ-bearing anti-NP antibodies, but some λ-bearing ones were also
detected. In the case of Centreville Lights and Czech II, some of the
anti-NP antibodies reacted with anti-λ, but none reacted with specific
anti-λ1 or anti-λ2, suggesting that these mice may produce λ chains
different from those found in inbred mice. In the SD mice, none of the

198

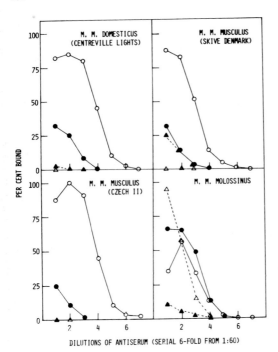

PER CENT BOUND

M. M. DOMESTICUS (CENTREVILLE LIGHTS)

M. M. MUSCULUS (SKIVE DENMARK)

M. M. MUSCULUS (CZECH II)

M. M. MOLOSSINUS

DILUTIONS OF ANTISERUM (SERIAL 6-FOLD FROM 1:60)

Fig. 1. Light chain types of anti-NP antibodies in four varieties of wild mice, as evaluated by a radioimmunoassay with antibodies to mouse κ and λ chains. Mice were bled 2 weeks after immunization with NP-CGG. Diluted antisera were added to microtiter wells containing NIP-BSA. Bound antibodies were detected by reaction with 125I-antibodies to mouse light chains (see text): goat anti-κ, —O—; rabbit anti-λ, —●—; mouse anti-λ1, - -△- -; goat anti-λ2, - -▲- -. The per cent binding is expressed relative to the maximum observed when ascites containing κ, λ1, or λ2 anti-NP antibodies was used as a standard. The results shown are mean values obtained from bleedings of 3 mice in each group.

anti-NP antibodies reacted with the monoclonal anti-λ1, but there was a weak reaction with anti-λ and anti-λ2.

Hybridomas from SD and Czech II mice were screened for the type of light chain in the secreted anti-NP antibodies. Approximately 5 to 10% of these hybridomas produced antibodies containing light chains that reacted with anti-λ, but not with anti-κ antibodies. Five of these hybridomas were subcloned and one, SD-26, was propagated *in vivo* to obtain ascitic fluid and solid tumor. Although the SD-26 monoclonal antibody reacted with anti-λ, it did not react with specific anti-λ1 or anti-λ2, suggesting that its λ chain differed from the λ1 and λ2 chains of BALB/c mice. The λ SD-26 light chain was isolated and characterized, as described below.

Characterization of Light Chain SD-26

The amino acid composition of λ SD-26 was found to differ substantially from that of representative λ1, λ2, and λ3 chains (Elliott *et al.*, 1982) (data not shown). Dansylation of this chain showed that the amino-terminus was blocked, consistent with its identification as a λ chain (Kabat *et al.*, 1983). After treatment with pyroglutamate aminopeptidase, the sequence of the 21 amino-terminal residues of the deblocked chain was determined; this sequence differs markedly from the prototype sequences of λ1 and λ2 chains (Fig. 2).

To obtain information about the internal sequence, the reduced and carboxymethylated λ SD-26 chain was digested with trypsin. In the case of the light chains that had been alkylated with ^{14}C-iodoacetic acid after both mild and complete reduction, it was found that 70% of the radiolabeled material was soluble in 0.1% trifluoroacetic acid. The soluble peptides were subjected to HPLC and selected fractions were analyzed by one or more of the following procedures: determination of the amino acid composition, amino-terminal analysis by dansylation, amino acid sequence analysis. Peptides from citraconylated λ SD-26 were isolated by gel filtration followed by HPLC (in some cases after deblocking lysine residues and further digestion with trypsin) and were characterized in the same way.

The data obtained after analysis of all of the isolated peptides are summarized in Table 1 and Fig. 2. Table 1 shows the amino acid compositions of peptides that were obtained in good yield and that appeared to be reasonably pure. It was evident that eight λ SD-26 peptides (T5 to T12) were similar or identical in composition to segments of the λ1 constant region. The similarity was greater to λ1 than to λ2. Several of

Table 1. Amino acid composition of tryptic peptides[a]

Amino Acid	1-19			20-24			45-63			106-113			114-132			133-152			153-169		
	T1	λ1	λ2	T2	λ1	λ2	T3	λ1	λ2	T4	λ1	λ2	T5	λ1	λ2	T6	λ1	λ2	T7	λ1	λ2
CmCys				0.9	1	1										0.9	1	1			
Asp				0.2			4.9	2	1	0.1			1.2	1	1	2.0	2	1	1.2	1	3
Thr	2.9	5	4				1.0	2	2	0.9	1	1	2.7	2	3	2.8	4	2	3.6	4	4
Ser	4.5	2	2	1.0	1	1	2.8		1	1.0			3.8	5	3	1.3		3	1.2	1	1
Glu	2.3	4	3	0.1			0.2			1.1	1	1	3.3	3	3	0.2			3.3	3	1
Pro	1.2	1	1	0.1			2.1	2	2	1.0	1	1	3.2	3	3	1.1	1	1	1.9	2	2
Gly	1.1	1	2	0.2			1.2	4	4		1	1	0.1			1.2	1	1	2.0	2	2
Ala	0.1	2	2	0.1			0.2	2	1				0.3			1.2	1	2	1.1		1
Val	3.0	3	3	0.1			1.1	1	2	1.0	1	2	1.1	1	1	3.2	4	3	1.7	2	1
Met							0.9													1	
Ile			1				0.9	1	1							0.9	1	1			1
Leu	1.9	1	1	1.0	1	1	0.1	2	2	1.9	2	1	1.9	2	2	1.0	1	2			
Tyr	0.1						1.0									1.0	1				
Phe	1.0							1	1				1.0	1	1	1.2	1	1			
His							0.1														
Lys	1.0			1.0			1.1			1.0	1	1	0.9	1	2	1.1	1	1	1.1	1	1
Arg				0.9	1	1	2.0	2	2				0.2								
% Yield	72			55			46			66			20			42			36		
Dansyl				Leu						Leu											

Amino Acid	153-174			175-186			187-207			208-211			212-215			25-44			1-24		
	T8	λ1	λ2[b]	T9	λ1	λ2	T10	λ1	λ2	T11	λ1	λ2	T12	λ1	λ2	Tx[c]	λ1	λ2	CT1	λ1	λ2
CmCys							1.1	1	1				0.8	1	1				1.4	1	1
Asp	3.4	3	4	0.2		1	0.5		2	0.1			1.1	1		3.3	3	3	2.9	6	5
Thr	3.8	4	4	2.0	2	1	2.7	2	3							1.1	3	3	5.9	3	3
Ser	1.4	2	1	2.0	2	3	2.9	3	2	2.0	2	2	0.9	1		1.6	2	2	5.9	3	3
Glu	4.0	4	2	0.1			4.2	4	4						1	2.3	2	2	2.4	4	3
Pro	1.9	2	2				0.4						0.2			0.1	1	1	1.0	1	1
Gly	2.3	2	3	0.1			1.4	1	1	0.2						3.1	1	1	1.3	1	2
Ala	1.3		1	1.9	2	1	1.0		1	0.1			1.0	1	1	0.4	2	2		2	2
Val	2.1	2	1	0.1			2.0	2	2	0.1						1.1	2	2	2.6	3	3
Met	0.1	1		0.9	1	1	0.1									0.9					
Ile	0.1		1				0.1									1.1			2.5		1
Leu	0.1			2.3	2	2	0.1			1.0	1	1			1	0.3			2.5	2	2
Tyr	0.1			2.0	2		1.0	1								2.7	1	1			
Phe	0.2					2			1							0.4			1.1		
His	0.1					1	2.8	3	2							1.0	1	1			
Lys	1.9	2	2	0.9			1.0	1	1	0.2			0.2				1	1	2.1		
Arg						1	0.1	1	1	1.0	1					1.0			1.2	1	1
% Yield	19			7			18			52			60			7			32		
Dansyl	Ala									Ser			Ala								

[a]The compositions of tryptic (T) peptides from λ SD-26 and a tryptic peptide from citraconylated λ SD-26 (CT1) are compared to the compositions of the matching regions of the prototype λ1 and λ2 chains. The values shown [except S-(carboxymethyl)cysteine (CmCys)] were normalized to the total number of expected residues in each peptide. The amount of CmCys was determined from the specific activity of ^{14}C-iodoacetic acid. Tryptophan residues in the λ1 chain (at positions 37, 151 and 188) were not included in the calculations since tryptophan is not recovered after acid hydrolysis.

[b]The residue at position 173 in λ1 is deleted in λ2.

[c]The amino acid composition of peptide Tx was compared to that of λ1 and λ2 at positions 25-44, but was not assigned a tryptic peptide number since it is a tentative match.

the λ SD-26 peptides were also subjected to sequence analysis. Peptide T12 is probably identical to the carboxy-terminal peptide of the λ1 chain and T11 is identical to a λ1 peptide at positions 208-211. Peptide T8, which appeared to consist of 22 amino acid residues, was placed at positions 153-174. The amino acid sequence of 11 of the first 13 residues of this peptide indicates the presence of two replacements with respect to the homologous λ1 peptide. Another peptide, T5+T6, was isolated in low yield and is probably the result of partial tryptic cleavage. The sequence of its first 11 residues corresponds to positions 114-124 of the λ1 chain; there is one replacement with respect to λ1. Thus, three differences in sequence between the constant regions of λ SD-26 and λ1 have been established (see Fig. 2 and Table 2). From the amino acid compositions it was deduced that there must be *at least* four additional substitutions from the λ1 constant-region sequence. The sequence of the peptide spanning the J-C junction, from positions 106-113, is also shown (Fig. 2, T4); there is a single replacement with respect to λ1, at position 110, the end of the J segment.

```
              1               10                    20
N-term     <E F V L T Q P S T V S T S L G S S V K L X C
T2                                                 L S C K R
BALB/c λ1  - A - V ——— E - A L T ——— P - E T - T - T - R S
BALB/c λ2  - A - V ——— E - A L T ——— P - G T - I - T - R S
Hu λ Mcg   - S A L ——————— P S A - G ——————— Q ——— T I ——— T G

                   50                    60
T3         S P T B M I Y D D N K R P S G V S B R
BALB/c λ1  L F - G L - G G T - N - A P ——— P A -
BALB/c λ2  L F - G L - G G T S N - A P ——— P V -
Hu λ Mcg   A - K V I ——— E V ——————————————— P D -

                110                    120
T4         L T V L S Z P K     T5+T6   T S P(S)V T L F P P S
BALB/c λ1  ——————— G Q ———     λ1      S ———————————————————
BALB/c λ2  V ————— G Q ———     λ2      S T - T L - V ———————
Hu λ Mcg   V ————— G Q ———     Mcg     A N - T ———————————————

                160                      210                    215
T8         A D G T P V T Q X V E X T   T11   S L S R   T12   A B(C.S)
BALB/c λ1  V ——————————— G M - T -     λ1    ———————   λ1    - D ———
BALB/c λ2  - N ——————— I — G - D T S   λ2    ——————— P λ2    - D - L
Hu λ Mcg   ——————— S — K A G —— T -    Mcg   T V A P   Mcg   T E ———
```

Fig. 2. Partial amino acid sequence of λ SD-26 compared to sequences of BALB/c λ1 and λ2 chains (Eisen & Reilly, 1985) and of human λ Mcg (Fett & Deutsch, 1974). Solid lines indicate identity with the sequence of λ SD-26, parentheses indicate tentative assignments, and period (in T12) indicates alignment by homology with BALB/c λ1 and human λ chains. Lambda SD-25 peptides T2, T4, T11 and T12 were subjected to manual dansyl-Edman degradation; peptides T3 and T8, as well as the deblocked intact chain (top line), to automated degradation in the liquid-phase sequencer; and peptide T5+T6 to Edman degradation in the gas-phase sequencer. In some cases, the amino acid compositions of peptides were used to supplement the data obtained by sequence analysis. Single-letter abbreviations for amino acid residues are; A, Ala; B, Asx; C, Cys; D, Asp; E, Glu; <E, pyroglutamic acid; F, Phe; G, Gly; I, Ile; K, Lys; L, Leu; M, Met; N, Asn; P, Pro; Q, Gln; R, Arg; S, Ser; T, Thr; V, Val; X, unknown; Y, Tyr; and Z, Glx. The numbering is based on the λ1 sequence.

Table 2. Comparison of λ SD-26 and other λ chains[a]

	identities/total positions		
λ SD-26 vs:	V	J	C
BALB/c λ1	18/43	4/5	30/33
BALB/c λ2	17/43	3/5	21/33
BALB/c λ3	18/43	3/5	21/33
Human λ Mcg	24/43	3/5	21/33

[a]The partial sequence of λ SD-26 is compared to the sequence of homologous segments of BALB/c λ1, λ2 and λ3 and human λ Mcg. The values are based on data in Fig. 2 and the BALB/c λ3 sequence (Eisen & Reilly, 1985). Tentative assignments were assumed to be correct and it was also assumed that Glx at position 111 of λ SD-26 is Gln and Asx at position 213 is Asp.

It was difficult to assign peptides to the variable region of λ SD-26, presumably because of extensive differences in sequence from either the λ1 or λ2 prototypes. Peptide T2 (Fig. 2) overlaps the amino-terminal sequence. Evidently, only 11 of the first 24 residues in λ SD-26 match residues in the prototype λ1 V region. Peptide T3 was placed, by homology to λ1, at positions 45-63. In this segment of 19 residues, there are only 7 identities with the corresponding λ1 sequence (and only 6 identities with λ2). Peptide Tx has not been sequenced and it could not definitely be placed from its composition, although it may be located at positions 25-44. We did not identify a peptide corresponding to the λ1 sequence from positions 64-105; it may have been in the insoluble tryptic core. In summary, only 18 of 43 identified residues in the V segment of λ SD-26 are identical to homologous positions in λ1 (see Fig. 2 and Table 2).

Partial Sequence of λ SD-26 mRNA

Positions 107-113, spanning the J-C junction, are highly conserved in the λ chains of different species (Kabat *et al.*, 1983). In the corresponding germ-line DNA from the three types of λ chain in BALB/c, there is variation at only one nucleotide position (the third base in codon 110) (see Reilly *et al.*, 1984). The single amino acid substitution in λ SD-26 at position 110 (Ser for Gly) could be the result of a replacement (A for G) in the first position of this codon. A synthetic heptadecadeoxynucleotide primer that had been utilized by Reilly *et al.* (1984) to sequence mRNA of λ3 chains was used to prime cDNA synthesis from the λ SD-26 mRNA. Partial nucleotide sequence was obtained from codon 105 upstream to codon 44. From the alignment of the λ SD-26 and λ1 nucleotide sequences, there appeared to be an insertion of two codons in the region between positions 67 and 71. An insertion of two residues between positions 67 and 68 has been observed in human λVI light chains (Kabat *et al.*, 1983; Frangione *et al.*, 1983). Of the total of 64 codons in this segment, 45 amino acid assignments could be made. Thirteen of these assignments correspond to residues in peptide T3, which had previously been identified by amino acid sequence analysis. When the data obtained by nucleic acid sequencing are combined with the results of amino acid sequencing, it was determined that 29/69 identified residues in V and 9/11 identified residues in the J segment of λ SD-26 are identical with residues in λ1.

SUMMARY AND DISCUSSION

Data obtained in this study from serological analyses of anti-NP antibodies in several varieties of wild mice (Fig. 1) agree with previous evidence (Makela *et al.*, 1979; Amor *et al.*, 1983) that λ chains in wild mice differ from those in the common laboratory strains. These observations are also consistent with reports, at the DNA level, that wild mice, and certain inbred strains derived from such mice, appear to have an increased number of genes encoding λ chains (Scott *et al.*, 1982; Scott & Potter, 1984a&b; Kindt *et al.*, 1985). To examine the expression of these putative λ genes, we prepared anti-NP hybridomas in two varieties of *M. m. musculus:* SD and Czech II. Approximately 5 to 10% of the monoclonal antibodies were typed serologically as containing λ chains. One of these λ chains, from the SD-26 hybridoma, has been characterized in some detail.

The antigenic reactivity of λ SD-26, together with its amino acid composition, suggested that it differed from the λ1, λ2, and λ3 chains of BALB/c mice. More detailed analyses of λ SD-26 were carried out by determination of its amino-terminal sequence, as well as the amino acid composition and the partial or complete amino acid sequence of several tryptic peptides. The results are summarized in Table 1, Table 2, and Fig. 2. The constant region of λ SD-26 resembles that of λ1 chains, although there are at least 7 amino acid substitutions. Three of these (at positions 114, 153 and 162) were established from the amino acid sequence; the composition data indicate that there must be at least four other substitutions. There is less resemblance of λ SD-26 to λ2 or λ3 than to λ1. It is not clear whether the λ SD-26 constant region is an allotypic variant of λ1 or a new isotype. The similarity between the λ SD-26 and λ1 constant regions suggests that their *C* genes would cross-hybridize under reasonably stringent conditions. It is possible, therefore, that the *Cλ* gene expressed in SD-26 is on one of the cross-hybridizing fragments detected in previous studies of *Cλ* genes in wild mice (Scott *et al.*, 1982; Scott & Potter, 1984a; Kindt *et al.*, 1985).

In contrast to the constant region, the V segment of λ SD-26 appears to be substantially different from that of BALB/c λ1 or λ2. Data obtained by amino acid sequence analysis indicate that only 18 of 43 identified residues (at positions 1-24 and 45-63) are identical to residues in λ1 (Fig. 2). Human Vλ belonging to different subgroups are typically more similar to each other at these 43 positions (∿25 to 30 identities) (Kabat *et al.*, 1983). It is extremely likely, therefore, that the V segment of λ SD-26 is the product of a germ-line gene that is different from *Vλ1* or *Vλ2* of BALB/c mice. Such a gene would be unlikely to cross-hybridize, under stringent conditions, with probes derived from inbred mice and would probably not have been detected in studies of *Vλ* genes in wild mice that utilized such probes (Scott & Potter, 1984b; Kindt *et al.*, 1985). We do not presently know whether genes related to SD-26 *Vλ* occur or are expressed in other varieties of wild mice or, for that matter, in inbred strains. If present in BALB/c, such genes would have to be expressed exceedingly rarely as no light chains in myeloma proteins or monoclonal antibodies have been found to have a similar V region.

We were surprised to find that, at the 43 V positions shown in Fig. 2, there are more identities between λ SD-26 and human λ Mcg than between the wild mouse chain and either λ1 or λ2 of BALB/c (see also Table 2). This is largely due to a stretch of five residues that are identical in λ SD-26 and λ Mcg (Fig. 2, positions 54-58). These residues are the last five (of seven) in the second complementarity-determining region, as defined by Kabat *et al.* (1983). It is interesting that this sequence, Asn-Lys-Arg-Pro-Ser, is found not only in λ Mcg but in several other human Vλ belonging to different subgroups [6/41 in the latest compilation of Ig sequences (E.A. Kabat, personal communication)]. The

residues at positions 56-58 are particularly conserved, occurring in
∿75% of human Vλ (Kabat *et al.*, 1983). Thus, in human λ chains, positions 56-58 are not actually "hypervariable". The conservation of such
a segment could be related to structural constraints. However, residues
at positions 54-58 in the Mcg λ dimer are not in β-pleated sheets, nor
do their side-chains line the solvent channel between the V domains that
is thought to represent the binding cavity (Edmundson *et al.*, 1975).
Moreover, the last two residues in this sequence (Pro-Ser), plus the
next five in the adjoining framework segment, are deleted in λ Newm
(Poljak *et al.*, 1973). Although we do not understand the significance,
if any, of this similarity between λ SD-26 and some human λ, it will be
interesting to determine whether these same residues will be found in
other wild mouse λ chains. It is possible that *Vλ* genes containing
these sequences, or elements required for their expression, have been
lost from the laboratory mouse strains.

We have demonstrated here that an unusual Vλ sequence can be identified,
from its association in an Ig chain expressed by a wild mouse, with a
Cλ sequence that closely resembles one of the previously-characterized
Cλ from BALB/c. Conversely, it may be possible to detect additional Cλ
sequences from their association with this or another Vλ. In any case,
it is clear that the identification and characterization of rearranged
genes and/or their protein products is necessary for the estimation of
the full range of V, C and J sequences in diverse mouse populations.
Appropriate nucleic acid probes can then be used to analyze the number
and organization of germ-line λ genes in these mice. Information about
the total number of both *Vλ* and *Cλ* genes is relevant for the evaluation
of models that have been proposed to account for gene duplication in the
λ locus, in particular, whether the unit of duplication includes *V* as
well as *C* genes (Blomberg *et al.*, 1981; Selsing *et al.*, 1982; Scott &
Potter, 1984b; Kindt *et al.*, 1985).

ACKNOWLEDGMENTS

We are indebted to M. Potter for supplying wild mice, for many helpful
discussions, and for his continuing interest in this project. We thank
M. White-Scharf and T. Imanishi-Kari for their generosity in providing
us with antibodies for serological typing and for their help in setting
up the hybridoma technique. We thank V.K. Chang for carrying out serological assays and for preparation of the SD-26 hybridoma, A.W. Brauer
and M.N. Margolies for analyzing peptide T5+T6 in the gas-phase sequencer, L.-P. Li for assistance with amino acid analysis and sequencing,
and M. Bashore for expert typing of this paper. This work was supported
by grants AI-08054 from the National Institutes of Health and IM-369
from the American Cancer Society. L.S.R. was supported by NIH Training
Grant CA-09255 and B.W.E. by NRSA AI-06223.

REFERENCES

Amor, M, Guenet J-L, Bonhomme F, Cazenave P-A (1983) Genetic polymor-
    phism of λ1 and λ3 immunoglobulin light chains in the *Mus* subgenus.
    Eur J Immunol 13:312-317
Blomberg B, Traunecker A, Eisen H, Tonegawa S (1981) Organization of
    four mouse λ light chain immunoglobulin genes. Proc Natl Acad Sci USA
    78:3765-3769

Chirgwin JM, Przybyla AE, MacDonald RJ, Rutter WJ (1979) Isolation of
  biologically active ribonucleic acid from sources enriched in ribo-
  nuclease. Biochemistry 18:5294-5299
Dunham JS (1983) Regulation of murine lambda light chain expression.
  Dissertation (Masssachusetts Institute of Technology) Cambridge, MA
Edmundson AB, Ely KR, Abola EE, Schiffer M, Panagiotopoulos N (1975)
  Rotational allomerism and divergent evolution of domains in immuno-
  globulin light chains. Biochemistry 14:3953-3961
Eisen HN, Reilly EB (1985) Lambda chains and genes in inbred mice. Annu
  Rev Immunol 3:337-365
Elliott BW Jr, Eisen HN, Steiner LA (1982) Unusual association of V, J
  and C regions in a mouse immunoglobulin λ chain. Nature 299:559-561
Elliott BW Jr, Steiner LA (1984) Amino- and carboxy-terminal sequence of
  mouse J chain and analysis of tryptic peptides. J Immunol 132:2968-
  2974
Elliott BW Jr, Eisen HN, Steiner LA (1984) Amino acid sequence diversity
  in mouse $\lambda 2$ variable regions. J Immunol 133:2757-2761
Fett JW, Deutsch HF (1974) Primary structure of the Mcg λ chain. Biochemistry 13:4102-4114
Frangione B, Moloshok T, Solomon A (1983) Primary structure of the variable region of a human λVI light chain: Bence Jones protein SUT. J
  Immunol 131:2490-2493
Greenwood FC, Hunter WM, Glover SS (1963) The preparation of ^{131}I-
  labelled human growth hormone of high specific radioactivity. Biochem
  J 89:114-123
Hamlyn PH, Brownlee GG, Cheng C-C, Gait MJ, Milstein C (1978) Complete
  sequence of constant and 3' noncoding regions of an immunoglobulin
  mRNA using the dideoxynucleotide method of RNA sequencing. Cell 15:
  1067-1075
Hewick RM, Hunkapiller MW, Hood LE, Dreyer WJ (1981) A gas-liquid solid
  phase peptide and protein sequenator. J Biol Chem 256:7990-7997
Kabat EA, Wu TT, Bilofsky H, Reid-Miller M, Perry H (1983) Sequences of
  proteins of immunological interest. US Dept of Health and Human
  Services, Public Health Service, National Institutes of Health,
  Bethesda, MD
Karjalainen K, Bang B, Makela O (1980) Fine specificity and idiotypes of
  early antibodies against (4-hydroxy-3-nitrophenyl)acetyl (NP). J
  Immunol 125:313-317
Kindt TJ, Gris C, Guenet JL, Bonhomme F, Cazenave P-A (1985) Lambda
  light chain constant and variable gene complements in wild-derived
  inbred mouse strains. Eur J Immunol 15:535-540
Makela O, Karjalainen K, Potter M (1979) Evolutionary conservation of a
  gene which controls the VH regions of an anti-hapten antibody (NP).
  Ann Immunol (Inst Pasteur) 130C:215-223
Maniatis T, Fritsch EF, Sambrook J (1982) Molecular cloning, a labora-
  tory manual. Cold Spring Harbor Laboratory, Cold Spring Habor, N.Y. pp
  197-198
March SC, Parikh I, Cuatrecasas P (1974) A simplified method for cyano-
  gen bromide activation of agarose for affinity chromatography. Anal
  Biochem 60:149-152
Mikoryak CA, Elliott BW Jr, Kimball ME, Steiner LA (1986) An extra
  disulfide bridge in the constant domain of *Rana catesbeiana*
  immunoglobulin light chains. J Immunol 136:217-223
Poljak RJ, Amzel LM, Avey HP, Chen BL, Phizackerley RP, Saul F (1973)
  Three-dimensional structure of the Fab' fragment of a human immunoglobulin at 2.8-A resolution. Proc Natl Acad Sci USA 70:3305-3310
Reidl LS, Elliott BW Jr, Chang VK, Steiner LA (1985) A novel immunoglobulin λ chain expressed in wild mice. Fed Proc 44:1317
Reilly EB, Reilly RM, Breyer RM, Sauer RT, Eisen HN (1984) Amino acid
  and nucleotide sequences of variable regions of mouse immunoglobulin
  light chains of the $\lambda 3$-subtype. J Immunol 133:471-475

Reth M, Imanishi-Kari T, Rajewsky K (1979) Analysis of the repertoire of anti-(4-hydroxy-3-nitrophenyl)acetyl (NP) antibodies in C57BL/6 mice by cell fusion. II. Characterization of idiotypes by monoclonal anti-idiotype antibodies. Eur J Immunol 9:1004-1013

Scott CL, Mushinski JF, Huppi K, Weigert M, Potter M (1982) Amplification of immunoglobulin λ constant genes in populations of wild mice. Nature 300:757-760

Scott CL, Potter M (1984a) Polymorphism of Cλ genes and units of duplication in the genus *Mus*. J Immunol 132:2630-2637

Scott CL, Potter M (1984b) Variation in Vλ genes in the genus *Mus*. J Immunol 132:2638-2643

Selsing E, Miller J, Wilson R, Storb U (1982) Evolution of mouse immunoglobulin λ genes. Proc Natl Acad Sci USA 79:4681-4685

Steiner LA, Lopes AD (1979) The crystallizable human myeloma protein Dob has a hinge-region deletion. Biochemistry 18:4054-4067

Steiner LA, Pardo AG, Margolies MN (1979) Amino acid sequence of the heavy-chain variable region of the crystallizable human myeloma protein Dob. Biochemistry 18:4068-4080

Tsu TT, Herzenberg LA (1980) Solid-phase radioimmune assays. In: Mishell BB, Shiigi SM (eds) Selected methods in cellular immunology. WH Freeman and Company, San Francisco, CA, pp 382-388

Wall KA, Frackelton AR Jr, Reilly EB, Azuma T, Chang T-W, Eisen HN (1983) Quantitation of anti-NP (4-hydroxy-3-nitrophenyl)-acetyl idiotype expression on spleen and thymus cells. Eur J Immunol 13:441-448

White-Scharf ME, Imanishi-Kari T (1981) Characterization of the NP[a] idiotype through the analysis of monoclonal BALB/c anti-(4-hydroxy-3-nitrophenyl)acetyl (NP) antibodies. Eur J Immunol 11:897-904

A Comparative Analyis of the Anti-Phosphorylcholine Response of CLA and BALB/c Mice

D. M. Hilbert and M. P. Cancro

INTRODUCTION

Wild mice have been used in basic research as a source of new genetic material and in the generation of a Mus phylogenetic tree. Studies of this nature have used morphologic and chromosomal polymorphisms to define the genealogic relationship of various Mus species, as well as to define the origins of inbred laboratory mice. It is now clear that the common inbred strains of mice are derived from a small number of progenitors (Marshall, 1981; Yonekowa, 1980; Ferris, 1982). Given the limited genetic pool from which inbred mice have been derived, the question arises whether the immune phenomena described in inbred mice accurately reflect those found in more distantly related populations of mice. Therefore, comparison of inbred immune responses with those observed in outbred populations of mice may foster an understanding of the processes which shape an individual's immune repertoire.

We report here a comparative analysis of the anti-phosphorylcholine (PC) response of an outbred population of mice, CLA, with that observed in inbred BALB/c mice.

CLA mice were derived from mouse stocks trapped on the Delmarva Penninsula by Michael Potter. Subsequently, Leiberman (1983) found CLA mice to be non-responders or very low responders to the antigen PC. This finding raises several questions: First, do CLA mice produce primary B-cells capable of responding to the PC determinant? Second, do CLA mice have structural genes capable of generating PC-binding antibodies, and if so, are these similar to those commonly used by inbred strains? Finally, if PC-specific responses are necessary for pathogen resistance, (Briles, 1981, 1982) how have CLA populations survived exposure to PC-bearing pathogens?

This report describes CLA derived B-cell hybridomas which produce PC-binding antibody. These antibodies: a) exhibit high affinity for PC ($KA > 10^5 M^{-1}$); b) do not react with antisera which recognizes the T15 idiotype or its allelic forms; c) utilize lambda light chains which, by nucleotide sequence are identical to the lambda-2 light chains of inbred mice; and d) utilize a heavy chain variable region gene which is distantly related to the T15 V_H gene family, and which exists within inbred laboratory strains but has gone undetected by the previously available molecular probes.

RESULTS AND DISCUSSION

Can CLA mice produce PC responsive B-cells?

To determine whether CLA mice produce primary B-cells capable of responding to the PC determinant we generated B-cell hybridomas (Kohler, 1975). The resulting hybridomas were assayed for PC-binding activity by radioimmunoassay. Several fusions yielded 230 proliferating hybrids, 38 of which bound the hapten PC.

The specificity of two CLA PC-binding antibodies, 1C4 and 6G8, was further assessed by affinity measurements (Fig. 1). The association constants of 1C4 and 6G8 were found to be 5.47 x 10^5 M^{-1} and 8.96 x 10^5 M^{-1}, respectively. These values are comparable to those previously reported for inbred anti-PC antibodies (Rodwell, 1983).

These results indicate that CLA mice can produce B-cells capable of secreting antibodies which bind PC with affinities comparable to those produced by most inbred mice in response to PC-bearing antigens.

Which CLA structural genes encode the PC-specific antibodies?

The humoral response of inbred mice to PC is dominated by antibodies bearing the T15 idiotype (Lieberman, 1974). This idiotype is encoded by a single heavy chain variable region gene whose product associates with the V_{K22} light chain (Crews, 1981). Two additional PC binding myelomas from inbred mice have been described, M603 and M167, which utilize somatic variants of the T15 prototype heavy chain gene, but whose light chains are members of the V_{K8} and V_{K24} subgroups, respectively (Rudikoff, 1981, 1983). The limited number of genes used in the inbred response to PC has led to considerable speculation about the selective pressures which control antibody responses to environmental antigens (Dzierzak, 1985).

To determine if the CLA PC-specific antibodies bear the T15 idiotype, a competitive inhibition assay was established. Figure 2 demonstrates that T15 idiotype bearing antibodies (T15 and HPCM-2), as well as the T15 allelic idiotype antibody (CBBPC3), inhibit the binding of a radiolabeled T15 by an anti-T15 antisera. In contrast, neither 1C4 nor 6G8 inhibit T15 binding, even at concentrations where T15$^+$ antibodies would inhibit greater than 60-80% of the radiolabeled species binding. Thus, the CLA PC--specific hybridomas do not bear the T15 idiotype.

The absence of the T15 idiotype in the CLA antibodies suggests that CLA mice use V_H and V_L gene combinations not commonly associated with PC-specific antibodies among inbred mice.

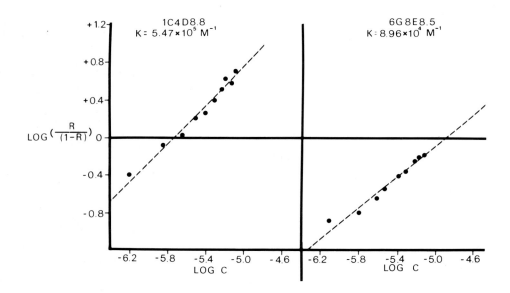

Figure 1: Sips plots derived from fluorescence quenching analysis studies of PC-binding CLA hybridoma proteins: The affinities of purified PC-binding CLA hybridoma proteins were assessed by fluorescence quenching analysis according to the method of Rodwell (1983) using dinitrophenyl-phosphorylcholine (DPPC) at 1.86×10^{-5} M as the free hapten species. The left panel shows the results obtained for CLA hybridoma 1C4 using an initial antibody combining site concentration of 1.03×10^{-6} M. In this plot the heterogeneity index is 1.0006, and the least squares correlation coefficient is 0.9869. The right panel represents the plot of data obtained for CLA hybridoma 6G8 using an initial antibody combining site concentration of 1.02×10^{-6} M. In this plot the heterogeneity index is 1.006, and the least squares correlation coefficient is 0.9954. R = the fraction of antibody sites bound and C = the free concentration of ligand.

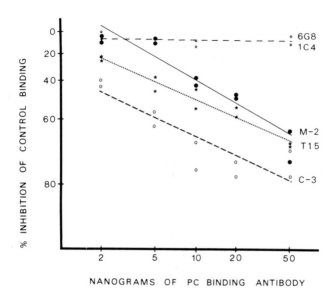

Figure 2: CLA hybridoma proteins 1C4 and 6G8 were tested for
expression of the T15 idiotype in a competitive inhibition assay.
Various PC-binding proteins were incubated with a fixed amount of
radiolabeled T15 protein (specific activity = 15 uCi/ug) in 96-well
polyvinyl plates, to which A/He anti-T15 antisera had been
adsorbed. After incubation, the plates were washed and bound
radioactivity counted. Control proteins include T15 and HPCM-2
which are of BALB/c origin and T15 idiotype positive; and CBBPC3, a
C.B20 myeloma protein which expresses the IgH^b allele of T15.

To characterize further the immunoglobulin heavy chains from the
CLA hybridomas, Northern blot analyses of total cytoplasmic RNA
were performed using a panel of C_H and V_H specific probes
(Leharach, 1977; Goldberg, 1979). The left panel of Figure 3 shows
the hybridization of a Cu probe to total cytoplasmic RNA from 27B4,
1C4, and 6G8. These results confirm the serologic data that 1C4
and 6G8 are IgM antibodies. Furthermore, it shows that the mRNA
encoding the Ig heavy chain is of the expected size and is present
in approximately equal quantities in all samples. The right panel
shows the same samples hybridized with S107, a $T15V_H$ family
probe. As expected, 27B4 hybridizes strongly, while 1C4 and 6G8
hybridize poorly. These results suggest that CLA mice express PC-
specific clonotypes which use a V_H gene distantly related to the
$T15V_H$ predominantly expressed among laboratory inbred mice.

210

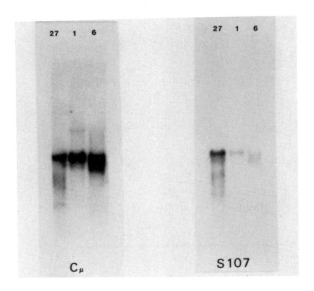

Figure 3: Northern blot hybridization of CLA cytoplasmic RNA with Cu and S107 cDNA probes. Cytoplasmic RNA was prepared, electrophoresed in agarose, and blotted to nitrocellulose filters. The bound RNA was hybridized to either a Cu probe (left gel) or the S107 probe (Crews, 1981) which detects the T15 gene family, (right gel). In each gel, RNA from three cell lines were run. From left to right on each gel, these are: 27B4D6 a C57BL/6 PC-binding hybrid which expresses the CBBPC3 idiotype;, 1C4D8.8, and 6G8B8.5.

To understand the nature of the 1C4 V_H, a cDNA was synthesized (5B6) (Estratiatis, 1979; Rowekamp, 1979). The hybridization patterns of ^{32}P labeled Cu, 5B6, and T15V_H (Southern, 1975) were compared on restriction enzyme digests of CLA and BALB/c liver DNA (Fig. 4). Using the S107 probe, it is clear that CLA mice have a unique T15 V_H family, since a 4.7kb band is present in EcoR1 digested CLA liver DNA but not in BALB/c liver DNA. Further, the 5B6, 1C4 cDNA probe not only hybridizes with the same fragments as the T15V_H probe, but also hybridizes weakly with a 4.7kb fragment in BALB/c DNA. This fragment corresponds to the strongly hybridizing, unique, CLA fragment, suggesting that BALB/c mice have a previously undetected member of the T15V_H family. The existence of this gene suggests that the number of genes visualized within a V_H family may be dictated by the probe used. If this is true then the estimates of the number of total V_H genes may be underestimated.

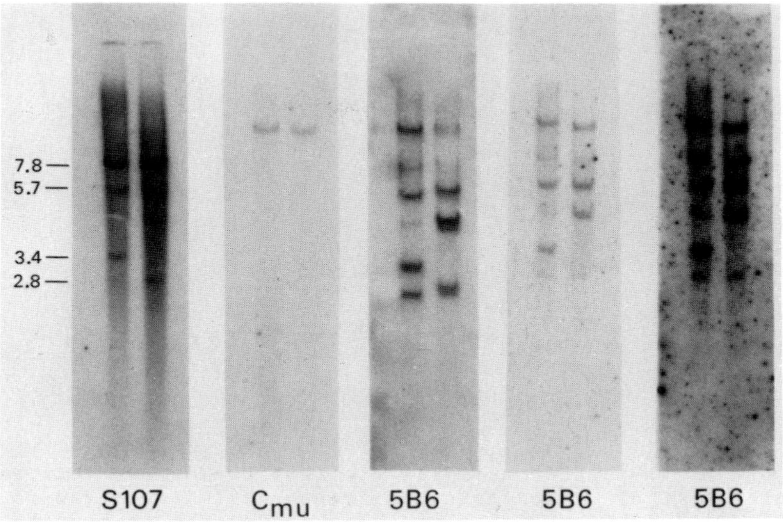
7.8
5.7
3.4
2.8
S107
Cmu
5B6
5B6
5B6

Figure 4: Standard Southern blot analyses were performed on EcoR1 digested BALB/c (left lane in each gel) and CLA (right lane of each gel). The left most gels were hybridized to a S107 V_H specific probe. The middle set of gels was hybridized to the p3741 (Marcu, 1980) a Cu specific, probe. The right most gels were hybridized to 5B6 (1C4 heavy chain cDNA). Note the 4.7kb band in BALB/c DNA which corresponds with the strongly hybridizing CLA 4.7kb band.

We are currently sequencing the 1C4 heavy chain cDNA to determine its degree of homology with previously described members of the $T15V_H$ gene family. Sequence analysis will allow comparison of the antigen-antibody interaction which occurs in inbred anti-PC antibody molecules with those of CLA anti-PC antibodies.

Light Chain Analysis

The nature of the variable portion of the light chain used by CLA PC-specific antibodies was also studied. Northern blot analyses using $C_{\lambda 1}$, $C_{\lambda 2-3}$, and V_{λ} specific probes, demonstrated that 1C4 and 6G8 are homologous to the $C_{\lambda 2-3}$ and V_{λ} genes (Fig. 5).

212

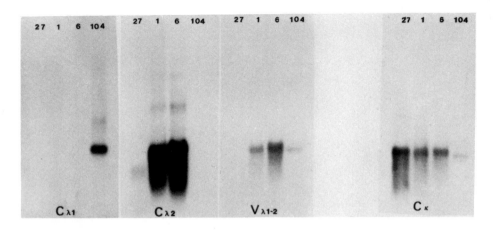

Figure 5: Northern blot analysis of light chains from CLA anti-PC
antibodies. Total cytoplasmic RNA from 4 cell lines; 27B4D6,
1C4D8.8, 6G8E8.5 and MOPC104E was electrophoresed in agarose,
blotted to nitrocellulose filters, and hybridized with several
probes. The left most group of 3 gels were hybridized to a $C_{\lambda 1}$-,
$C_{\lambda 2}$- and V_λ -specific probe respectively. These probes were
provided by Dr. Cynthia Scott (N.I.H. Bethesda, MD).

Southern blot analysis of the lambda family in CLA and BALB/c mice
was carried out using $C_{\lambda 2}$, V_λ and the 1C4 light chain cDNA as
hybridization probes. Restriction fragment analysis of BamHl (Fig.
6) and Bgll digests of CLA and BALB/c liver DNA reveal that: 1.)
CLA mice carry the known $C_{\lambda 2}$ and $C_{\lambda 3}$ genes and, 2.) CLA mice have
an additional $C_{\lambda 2}$ gene not present in inbred mice. EcoRl digests
of the same DNA do not delineate the novel CLA C gene indicating
that is is closely linked to either $C_{\lambda 2}$ or $C_{\lambda 3}$ (Fig. 7).

Although CLA mice have an expanded C_λ family, we have been unable
to detect additional V_λ genes in these mice. Hybridization of a
labeled V_λ specific probe to EcoRl digests of CLA and BALB/c DNA
reveals identical 3.9kb and 4.9kb restriction fragments. It is,
however, interesting to note that in CLA mice, these fragment sizes
are identical to those which hybridize to a $C_{\lambda 2-3}$ specific probe.
One possible explanation for this finding would be that V_λ and C_λ
are coincidentally located on different restriction fragments of
the same sizes. Alternatively, V_λ and C_λ genes may be closely
linked, resulting in two restriction fragments each containing a

C_λ and a V_λ gene. We are currently expanding our restriction enzyme analyses to determine the relative position of V_λ and C_λ genes in CLA mice.

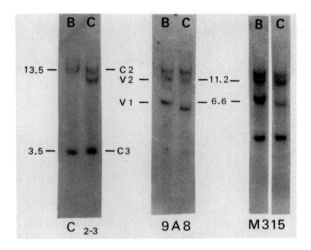

Figure 6: <u>Southern analyses of BamHl digested BALB/c (left lane of each gel)</u> and CLA (right lane of each gel) liver DNA. The left most gels were hybridized to a $C_{\lambda 2-3}$ probe. The middle set of gels were hybridized to 9A8 (1C4 light chain cDNA). Finally, the right most gels were hybridized to M315, a full-length cDNA of inbred lambda light chain. The CLA genome clearly contains an additional $C_{\lambda 2-3}$ homologous gene at approximately 11.2 kb.

214

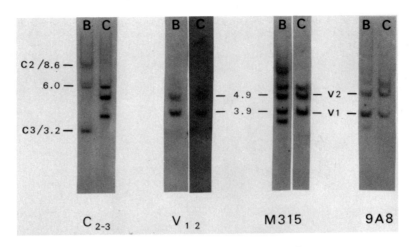

Figure 7: Southern analyses of EcoRl digested BALB/c (left lane of each gel) and CLA (right lane of each gel) liver DNA. From left to right, the gels were hybridized with a, $C_{\lambda 2-3}$ probe, $V_{\lambda 1-2}$ probe, M315 and 9A8, a IC4 light chain cDNA. The unique CLA C^{λ} gene is not seen in EcoRl digested CLA DNA indicating that it may be closely linked to one of the known $C_{\lambda 2-3}$ genes in CLA mice. The 6.0 kb band in both CLA and BALB/c lanes is a partial digest as reported by Tonegawa (1984).

The data presented above differs from those reported by Scott (1983a,b). Their studies reported 5-7 V_{λ} and an equal number of C_{λ} genes in DNA samples from CLA mice of the first few brother by sister matings. In contrast, our studies of individual CLA mice from the 11th through 17th filial generation have revealed two V_{λ} and three C_{λ} genes. This discrepancy may be explained in two ways. First, a dramatic loss of lambda genes may have occurred between the 6th and 11th generations of CLA inbreeding. It remains unclear whether this loss would be the result of a single catastrophic deletion or multiple lambda gene deletions.

Alternatively, the small size of the CLA colony and the large number of genomic screenings necessitated pooling DNA from several CLA mice. Estimates of the number of CLA lambda genes may reflect polymorphism rather than the number of lambda genes per haploid genome. Further analyses of CLA lambda genes and gene products may be useful in delineating these possibilities, as well as in understanding antibody structure-function correlates.

Our analysis of the 1C4 light chain cDNA (9A8) has revealed only
six nucleotide differences between it and the germline lambda 2 C_λ,
$V\lambda$, and $J\lambda$ genes in inbred mice (Tonegawa, 1978; Wu, 1982;
Bloomberg, 1982). It remains unclear whether these differences are
germline encoded or the result of somatic mutation.

The use of the CLA lambda 2 gene in a PC binding antibody raises
several questions. First, why do Balb/c mice lack detectable
lambda 2 bearing anti-PC antibodies? Most likely, inbred mice fail
to use their lambda repertoire in an anti-PC response because they
lack the appropriate V_H gene which when associated with a $V_{\lambda 2}$ gene
can generate a PC-binding antibody. The necessary V_H may be the
4.7 kb gene which, in inbreds, has evolved away from the T15 family
due to the preferential use of the V_1 (TI5 prototype) gene in
response to PC. The divergence of the novel Balb/c V_H gene does
not preclude its association with a V_K or V_λ but the resultant
antibody may not bind PC.

Alternatively, inbred mice may have retained a PC-specific $V_H V_L$
combination, but fail to express it as part of the anti-PC
response. For example, the environmental form of PC is a T-cell
independent antigen, resulting in only primary B-cell activation.
Since newly emerging B-cells may preferentially rearrange their
kappa genes first, and only attempt lambda rearrangements after
abortive rearrangements on both kappa-bearing homologues
(Coleclough, 1981) most PC-specific responses of inbred mice will
be dominated by $V_H V_K$ pairs. Only in those cases where the
appropriate V_K gene could not be found will lambda-bearing PC-
reactive B-cells be present in high enough frequency to be readily
observed. In this way, inbred mice would maintain a V_K dominant
PC-specific B-cell pool which is reflected in their serum
responses.

Similarly, the use of the lambda family in CLA anti-PC responses
may be the result of CLA structural gene deficiencies in either the
T15V_H family or the kappa genes necessary for production of a kappa
bearing anti-PC antibodies (Rudikoff, 1983).

Finally, the use of the lambda family in CLA mice would explain the
PC low responder phenotype simply because very few lambda bearing
B-cells emerge from the bone marrow. The low frequency of lambda
bearing, PC responsive B-cells in the periphery of CLA mice may be
sufficient to protect them from PC bearing pathogens, but incapable
of producing high serum levels of PC-specific antibody.

ACKNOWLEDGEMENTS

We would like to thank the following people for their help in
preparing this manuscript. Dr. Cynthia Scott for her direction in
the cDNA syntheses; Dr. Fred Karush for his help in the affinity
measurements, Dr. Martin Weigert for the Cu probe, Dr. Michael
Potter for the original CLA breeding pairs. Finally we greatly
appreciate the expert manuscript preparation of Debbie Rupp and Val
Rementer.

REFERENCES

Blomberg B, Tonegawa S (1982) DNA sequences of the joining regions of mouse lambda light chain immunoglobulin genes. Proc Natl Acad Sci USA 79:530

Blomberg B, Trounecker A, Eisen H, Tonegawa S (1981) Organization of four mouse lambda light chain immunoglobulin genes. PNAS 76:3765

Briles DE, Forman C, Hudak S, Claflin JL (1982) Anti-phosphorylcholine antibodies of the T15 idiotype are optimally protective against Streptococcus pneumoniae. J Exp Med 156:1177

Briles DE, Nahm M, Schroer K, Davie J, Baker P, Kearney J, and Barletta R (1981) Anti-phosphocholine antibodies in normal mouse serum are protective against intravenous infection with type III Streptococcus pneumoniae. J Exp Med 153:694

Claflin JL, Hudak S, Meddalena A, Bender T (1985) Antigen specific anti-phosphocholine antibodies: binding site studies. J Immunol 134:2536

Coleclough C, Perry RP, Karjalainen K, Weigert M (1981) Aberrant rearrangements contribute significantly to the allelic exclusion of immunoglobulin gene expression. Nature 290:372

Cory S, Adams JM (1980) Deletions are associated with somatic rearrangement of immunoglobulin heavy chain genes. Cell 19:37

Crews S, Griffen J, Huang H, Calame K, Hood L (1981) A single V_H gene segment encodes the immune response to phosphorylcholine. Cell 25:59

Davis MM, Calame K, Early PW, Livant DL, Joho R, Weissman IL, Hood L (1980) An immunoglobulin heavy chain gene is formed by at least two recombinational events. Nature 283:733

Dzierzak EA, Brodeur P, Marion T, Janeway CA, Bothwell A (1985) Molecular characterization of antibodies bearing Id-460, II. Molecular basis for Id-460 expression. J Exp Med 162:1494.

Ferris SD, Sage RD, Wilson AC (1982) Evidence from mtDNA sequences that common laboratory strains of inbred mice are descended from a single female. Nature 295:163

Ferris SD, Sage RD, Prager EM, Ritte U, Wilson AC (1983) Mitochondrial evolution in mice. Genetics 105:681

Efstratiadis A, Villa-Komaroff L (1979) Cloning of double stranded DNA. In: Stelow JK, Hollaender A (ed) Genetic engineering, Plenum Press, New York

Goldberg ML, Lefton RP, Stark GR, Williams JG (1979) Isolation of specific RNAs using DNA covalently linked to diazyloxylcellulose on paper. Methods in Enzymology 68:206

Honjo T, Nakai S, Nishida Y, Kataoka T, Yamawaki-Kataoka Y, Takahashi N, Obata M, Shimizu A, Yaoita Y, Nikaido T, Ishida N (1981) Rearrangements of immunoglobulin genes during differentiation and evolution. Immunological Rev 59:33

Kohler G, Milstein C (1975) Continuous cultures of fused cells secreting antibody of predefined specificity. Nature 256:695

Leder P, Seidman JG, Max E., Nishioka Y, Leder A, Norman B, Nau M (1979) The arrangement, rearrangement and origin of immunoglobulin genes. In: From gene to protein: informational transfer in normal and abnormal cells. Academic Press, New York, p 133.

Leharach H, Diamond D, Wozney JM, Boedtker H (1977) RNA molecular
    weight determinations by gel electrophoresis under denaturing
    conditions, a critical reexamination. Biochemistry 16:4743
Lieberman R, D'Hoostelaere LA, Humphrey, Jr, Nishinarita S, Potter
    M (1983) An allotype linked gene that is associated with a
    negative or very low anti-phosphorylcholine (PC) phenotype in
    wild mice (CNV). J Immunol 131:1570
Lieberman R, Potter M, Mushinski EB, Humphrey W, Rudikoff S (1974)
    Genetics of a new IgV$_H$ (T15 Idiotype) marker in the mouse
    regulating natural antibody to phosphorylcholine. J Exp Med
    138:983
Maki R, Traunecker A, Sakano H, Roder W, Tonegowa S (1980) Exon
    shuffling generates an immunoglobulin heavy chain gene. Proc
    Natl Acad Sci USA 77:2138
Marcu KB, Banerji J, Penncavage N, Lang R, Arnheim N (1980) 5'
    Flanking region of immunoglobulin heavy chain constant region
    genes displays length heterogeneity in germlines of inbred mouse
    strains. Cell 22:187
Marshall JT, Sage RD (1981) Taxonomy of the house mouse. Symp Zool
    Soc Lond 47:15
Rigby PWJ, Dickerman M, Rhodes C, Berg P (1977) Labeling
    deoxyribonucleic acid to high specific activity in vitro by nick
    translation with DNA polymerase. J Mol Biol 113:237
Rodwell JD, Gearhart JP, Karush F (1983) Restriction in IgM
    expression IV. Affinity analysis of monoclonal anti-PC
    antibodies. J Immunol 130:313
Rowekamp W, Firtel RA (1979) Isolation of developmentally regulated
    genes from Dictyostelium. Dev Biol 79:409
Rudikoff S (1983) Immunoglobulin structure-function correlates:
    antigen binding and idiotypes. Contemporary Topics in Molecular
    Immunology 9:169
Scott CL, Mushinski JD, Huppi JF, Weigert M, Potter M (1982)
    Amplification of immunoglobulin constant genes in populations of
    wild mice. Nature 300:757
Scott CL, Potter M: (1984) Polymorphism of C genes and units of
    duplication in the genus Mus. J Immunol 132:2630
Scott CL, Potter M (1984) Variation in V genes in the genus
    Mus. J Immunol 132:2638
Southern E (1975) Detection of specific sequences among DNA
    fragments separated by gel electrophoresis. J Mol Biol 98:503
Tonegawa S, Maxam AM, Tizard R, Bernard O, Gilbert W (1978)
    Sequence of a mouse germ-line gene for a variable region of an
    immunoglobulin light chain. Proc Natl Acad Sci USA 75:1485
Wu GE, Govindji N, Hozumi N, Murialdo H (1982) Nucleotide sequence
    of a chromsomal rearranged $_2$ immunoglobulin gene of mouse.
    Nucleic Acid Res 10:3831
Yonekawa HK, Moriwaki O, Gotoh J, Watanabe JI, Hayashi N, Miyashita
    ML, Petras ML, Tagashira Y (1980) Relationship between laboratory
    mice and the subspecies Mus musculus domesticus based on
    restriction endonuclease cleavage patterns of mitochondrial
    DNA. Jpn J Genet 55:289

λ1 Bearing Antibodies Against the α(1-3) and α(1-6)Glycosidic Linkages of the B1355 Dextran in Wild Mice

D. Juy, J.L. Guénet, F. Bonhomme, and P.-A. Cazenave

The immune response to the α(1-3) glycosidic linkage of the dextran (Dex) B1355 has been shown to be linked to the Igh locus (Blomberg et al. 1972, Riblet et al. 1975). In laboratory strains only mice with the Igh^a allotypic haplotype produce anti-α(1-3) Dex antibodies. This response is characterized by antibodies bearing the λ1 light chain (Carson and Weigert, 1973). The majority of these antibodies express a recurrent idiotypic specificity (IdX) present on both J558 and M104 myeloma proteins in addition to either IdI 558 or IdI 104 recurrent individual idiotypic specificities (Hansburg 1977, Clevinger et al. 1980, Stohrer et al. 1983^a). At the clonal level, IdI 558 and IdI 104 determinants were not found to be present on the same molecule (Clevinger et al. 1980, Kearney et al. 1983).

In this study we have investigated at first the expression of the λ1 light chain, secondly the Igh haplotype from wild mice of different origins and thirdly their response to a single injection of B1355 Dex.

Expression of the λ1 light chain

Before studying the anti-α(1-3) Dex response of 18 different inbred or partially inbred wild derived strains we analyzed the nature and the level of expression of their λ1 light chains. To this aim two radioimmunoassays (RIA) based on the inhibition of the binding of ^{125}I-labelled anti-λ1 antibodies to insolubilized λ1 bearing monoclonal immunoglobulins (Ig) (558=IgA,λ1 and TNP15=IgM,λ1) were used. The first RIA was performed with purified polyclonal rabbit anti-λ1 antibodies which slightly cross-react with the λ2 and λ3 isotypes (Sanchez et al. 1984). In the second RIA a ^{125}I-labelled monoclonal SPE anti-λ1 antibody (MS40) was used. MS40 has been shown to be specific for the λ1 light chain isotype of all laboratory mouse strains tested including SJL (Cazenave and Mazié, unpublished). As shown in Table 1 although most wild mouse strains expressed "normal" levels of λ1 bearing Ig, six of the 18 strains studied were characterized by low levels of circulating λ1 isotype. These strains were classified into four groups. WGQ expressed low levels of λ1 isotype detected by both rabbit polyclonal and MS40 monoclonal anti-λ1 antibodies, as did the inbred strain SJL. MAI and DFL probably possess another allotypic form of λ1 because this isotype was recognized by the rabbit anti-λ1 antibody but its amount could not be quantified because the slope of its inhibition curve was very different from those of J558 or TNP15. BNC could express a third allotypic form which cross-reacts with both rabbit polyclonal and MS40 monoclonal antibodies. Concerning PWK and XBZ, their λ1 chains were normally recognized by the rabbit antibodies but failed to react with MS40 monoclonal antibodies, suggesting that either those mice do not synthesize the λ1 isotype (but rather λ2 and/or λ3 cross reactive with rabbit anti-λ1 antibodies), or, more likely, produce a different allotype. Finally, in the serum of one strain, ULA, the λ1 isotype is not detectable with the antibodies used. Work is in progress to determine the nature of the λ1 expression defect observed in these different strains and its relationship with the well known defect in the SJL strain (Geckeler et al. 1978, Sanchez et al. 1984).

Table I. Expression of λ1 light chain.

Strain	Biochemical group	Igh-1 allele	Radioimmunoassay with	
			Rabbit anti-λ1*	MS40 mAb**
BALB/c	Mus 1	a	+++	+++
SJL	Mus 1	b	±	±
DBP	Mus 1	not a	+++	+++
WLA	Mus 1	a	+++	+++
BFM	Mus 1	a	+++	+++
WBG	Mus 1	a	+++	+++
38 CH	Mus 1	not a	+++	+++
BNC	Mus 1	not a	NQ	NQ
WMP	Mus 1	not a	+++	+++
DFL	Mus 1	not a	NQ	+
WGQ	Mus 1	a	+	+
ULA	Mus 1	not a	-	-
C.B20	Mus 1	b	+++	+++
MAI	Mus 2	not a	NQ	-
MBT	Mus 2	not a	+++	+++
CALIF	Mus 2	not a	+++	+++
PWK	Mus 2A	a	+	-
MBB	Mus 2A	not a	+++	+++
MBK	Mus 2A	not a	+++	+++
MPW	Mus 2A	not a	+++	+++
XBZ	Mus 4A	not a	+	-

The dosage of λ1 bearing Ig was performed in a RIA based on inhibition of the fixation of ^{125}I-labelled rabbit anti-mouse λ1 purified antibodies to insolubilized TNP15 protein (IgM λ1) (*) or of ^{125}I MS40 purified anti-λ1 monoclonal antibodies to insolubilized J558 protein (IgA λ1) (**) +++: >150 μg/ml in RIA (*) and >100 μg/ml in RIA (**); +: 25 μg/ml; ±: 1-10 μg/ml; -: λ1 not detected; NQ: λ1 is expressed but not quantifiable because its inhibition curve slope was very different from those of J558 or TNP15.
The determination of the Igh-1 allele was carried out in a RIA based on the inhibition of the fixation of ^{125}I monoclonal anti-allotypes to insolubilized allotypes.

TABLE 2. λ bearing anti-α(1-3) and anti-α(1-6)Dex responses of different strains and expression of IdX, IdI558, IdI104 idiotopes.

Strain	Igh-1 allele	λ bearing anti-α (1-3) response (a)	λ bearing anti-α (1-6) response (a)	Anti-α(1-3)Dex associated idiotopes (b) IdX			IdI104			IdI558	
				CD (●)	E1 (○)	E7 (○)	E6 (○)	E3 (○)	18-1 (○)	EB (●)	558-1 (○)
BALB/c	a	10/10 +++	–								
C.B20	b	10/10 –	–								
DBP	not a	2/5 +	–								
WLA	a	10/10 +++	–								
BFM	a	–	–								
WBG	a	8/12 +++	4/12 +++								
MAI	not a	–	–								
MBT	not a	–	–								
38 CH	not a	–	–								
PWK	a	–	–								
MBB	not a	–	–								
CALIF	not a	3/6 ++	3/6 +								
BNC	not a	10/10 +++	–								
WMP	not a	3/5 +++	–								
MBK	not a	8/15 +++	–								
DFL	not a	2/6 ++	1/6 +								
XBZ	not a	3/6 +++	–								
WBQ	a	–	–								
MPW	not a	11/11 +++	4/11 +++								

a) The detection of λ bearing anti-α(1-3) or anti-α(1-6)Dex antibodies was carried out in a sandwich RIA. Plates were coated with 1 μg/ml 1355-BSA, 1 μg/ml 512-BSA or BSA for 1 h at 20°C, then washed, incubated 30 min at 20°C with 0.5% BSA in PBS. Thereafter serial dilutions of the sera to be studied or of J558 or M104 (used as controls) were incubated 4 h at 20°C. The plates were then washed and incubated 18 h at 4°C with either ^{125}I-labelled MS40 or ^{125}I-labelled rabbit anti-λ1 antibodies according to the data presented in Table I.

b) The detection of IdX, IdI558, IdI104 bearing anti-α(1-3)Dex antibodies was performed in a sandwich RIA. Plates were coated with the different monoclonal anti-idiotypic antibodies for 1 h at 20°C and the assay was carried on as described in Fig.1a a part that ^{125}I-labelled 1355-tyramine was used instead of ^{125}I-labelled anti-λ1 antibodies. (■) positif, (□) not done. (●) Stohrer 1983b, (○) Weiler et al. 1984.

The $\lambda 1$ bearing anti-$\alpha(1-3)$ dextran antibody response

Ten days after a single injection of 100 µg of B1355 antigen emulsified in Complete Freund's Adjuvant (CFA), mice were bled and their serum screened for the presence of $\lambda 1$ bearing anti-$\alpha(1-3)$ Dex and anti-$\alpha(1-6)$ Dex antibodies. The response was tested either with MS40 for MS40 positive strains or with the rabbit anti-$\lambda 1$ antibodies for the MS40 negative strains. As shown on Table 2 two strains (WLA and WBG) with the Igh^a haplotype (as determined using a series of anti-allotypic mAb) responded to B1355 by the production of high levels of anti-$\alpha(1-3)$ linkage-specific antibodies. These data are in agreement with the known Igh^a linkage of the $\lambda 1$ anti-$\alpha(1-3)$ antibody response (Blomberg et al. 1972, Riblet et al. 1972). On the other hand, BFM, PWK and WGQ mice, while also Igh^a, failed to produce significant amounts of anti-$\alpha(1-3)$ Dex antibodies. However, PWK and WGQ were shown (Table I) to express low amount of $\lambda 1$ (Ig). We are now studying whether the anti-$\lambda 1$-LPS treatment described by Primi et al. (1984) will permit the detection of anti-$\alpha(1-3)$ Dex antibodies in these strains. The fact that BFM mice, which synthesize normal levels of $\lambda 1$ bearing Ig, failed to produce an anti-$\alpha(1-3)$ Dex response suggests that there may be either recombinations within the VH segments or an association between VH^{Dex} and a preferential CH gene segment. As expected, 4 wild mouse strains (MAI, 38CH, MBB and MBT) with a Igh$^{not\ a}$ haplotype failed to produce $\lambda 1$ bearing anti-$\alpha(1-3)$ Dex antibodies. On the other hand WMP, DFL, BNC, MBK, XBZ and MPW mice were able to synthesize high amounts of these antibodies, suggesting recombinations between the IghV^a and the IghC$^{not\ a}$ loci or within the IghV locus itself. Alternatively, it is possible that these strains use VH segments other than those used by Igh^a positive laboratory strains in their $\lambda 1$ positive anti-α (1-3) Dex antibody response.

Idiotypy of the $\lambda 1$ bearing anti-$\alpha(1-3)$Dex antibodies

The anti-$\alpha(1-3)$Dex positive sera were screened for the presence of IdX, IdI558 or IdI104 idiotypic determinants using a sandwich RIA as described in Table II. As shown on the right part of this table all anti-$\alpha(1-3)$Dextran positive sera except those of CALIF contained significant amounts of IdX, IdI558, and IdI104 idiotopes. CALIF was the only strain to synthetize antibodies which bound to insolubilized B1355 but failed to express any IdI or IdX idiotopes, suggesting that these antibodies in fact recognized the $\alpha(1-6)$ linkage of the 1355 antigen (see next section).

It is worth noting that the IdX and IdI idiotopes appear to be quite conserved in the Mus genus since they are expressed in Mus 1, Mus 2 and Mus 4 mice independently of the Igh haplotype.

It might also be noted that the WLA inbred strain, which has a $\lambda 1$ allotype different from that found in $\alpha(1-3)$ Dex high responder laboratory strains (Amor et al. 1983 and Cazenave, unpublished), is able to express high levels of anti-$\alpha(1-3)$dex antibodies bearing IdX and IdI idiotopes.

The $\lambda 1$ bearing anti-$\alpha(1-6)$ antibody response

The B1355 Dex is composed of 35% $\alpha(1-3)$, 5% $\alpha(1-4)$ and 60% $\alpha(1-6)$ glycosidic linkages. In spite of its herogeneity, a single injection of this antigen emulsified in CFA led to the production by Igh^a mice of only $\lambda 1$ bearing anti-α (1-3)Dex antibodies (Blomberg et al. 1972). On the other hand some Igh$^{not\ a}$ mice gave rise to anti-$\alpha(1-6)$Dex antibodies characterized exclusively by this light chain isotype (Juy and Cazenave, 1985). Because of the high polymorphism present within the wild mouse population, we decided to look for the presence of λ1 bearing anti-α(1-6) Dex antibodies in the serum of mice injected with B1355 Dex. Surprisingly, as shown on Table 2, some mice among the WBG, CALIF, DFL and MPW strains gave rise to λ1 bearing anti-α(1-6)Dex antibodies. These results are illustrated in Fig.1.

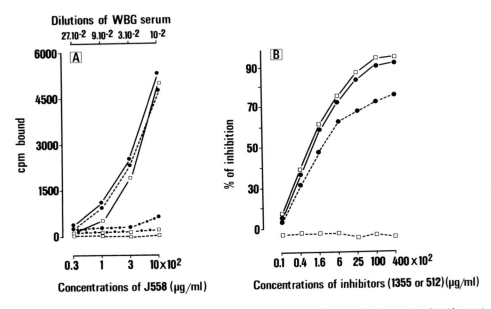

Fig. 1. λ1 bearing α(1-6) Dex activity. 1A: Detection of λ1 anti-α(1-3) and anti-α(1-6)Dex antibodies. The binding of J558 (□) or of WBG antibodies (●) on 1355-BSA (—), on 512-BSA (--) or on BSA (-●-) coated plates was revealed by ^{125}I-MS40 as described in Table 2. 1B: Study of the specificity of the binding of anti-α(1-3) and of anti-α(1-6) Dex antibodies. It was studied in a RIA based on the inhibition of the binding of J558 (□) or of WBG antibodies (●) on 1355-BSA coated plates by 1355 (—) or by 512 (--) Dextran. Same RIA as in Fig. 1A a part that J558 and WBG sera were incubated together with soluble 1355 or 512 Dextran.

Fig.1A shows that WBG #4 produced λ1 bearing antibodies which bound to both 1355- and 512-coated plates with roughly the same efficiency. Fig.2B shows that the binding of WBG anti-Dex antibodies to 1355- coated plates could be inhibited by 1355 as well as by 512. By contrast, the binding of 558 was inhibited by 1355 but not by 512.

It should be noted that inhibition of the binding of WBG antibodies with 512 was incomplete, suggesting the presence of anti-α(1-3) in addition to anti-α(1-6) antibodies. In fact, WBG mice did synthesize anti- α(1-3) antibodies, as IdX, IdI104, IdI558 molecules were found (Table 2) in the serum of such immunized mice. Lambda 1 bearing anti-α(1-6)Dex antibodies were never found in the serum of any B1355-immunized laboratory mice tested. Interestingly, Southern blot ana-lysis of the genomic DNA of wild mice (Scott and Potter, 1984; Kindt et al. 1985) showed that some mice displayed three restriction fragments (after either Hind III or EcoRI enzymatic digestion) which strongly hybridized with a Vλ1 probe derived from BALB/c. In the wild-type WBG strain, two of these fragments were of size similar to those obtained with BALB/c. It will, therefore, be of interest to know whether WBG mice used a third Vλ gene for the anti-α(1-6) activity, and these experiments are currently in progress in our laboratory.

An anti-α(1-3)Dex antibody which expresses both the IdI558, and the IdI104 idiotopes in addition to the IdX.

By fusion of spleen cells from WLA mice immunized with B1355 Dex emulsified in CFA we obtained an hybridoma, named WLA8, which synthesizes a λ1 protein with anti-α(1-3) Dex activity.

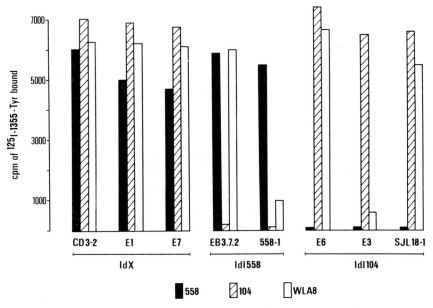

Fig. 2. Expression of IdX, IdI104, IdI558 one the same molecule. The detection of the IdX, IdI104, IdI558 has been performed in a sandwich RIA described on Table 2.

In Fig.2 the idiotypic profiles of WLA8, J558 and M104 are compared using a sandwich radioimmunoassay (for details, see Table 2 legends). As can be seen, WLA8 expresses the CD3-2, E1 and E7 IdX idiotopes as well as J558 and M104. In addition to IdX, WLA8 expresses the EB-3-7-2 idiotope (IdI558) and probably an idiotope closely related to the 558-1 idiotope. This antibody also expresses the E6 and SJL 18-1 idiotopes (IdI104) and probably an idiotope cross reactive with the E3 idiotope, which is also an idiotope of the IdI104 series.

This hybridoma protein is the first antibody described to express, in addition to IdX, both IdI558 and IdI104 idiotopes. Interestingly, WLA belongs to that group of mice from which Southern blot analysis reveals three bands which cross-hybridize with the BALB/c Vλ1 probe. Experiments in progress in our lab will determine whether the third Vλ gene (the one not found in BALB/c) is used by WLA8 to express both IdI104 and IdI558. Furthermore, it should be emphasized that the λ1 light chain of M104 and J558 as well as those of 10 anti-α(1-3)Dex monoclonal antibodies have been shown to be identical (Clevinger et al. 1980). After sequencing the 120 first amino acids of these antibody heavy chains the same authors have suggested that IdI determinants may correlate with the D segment variations. Consequently IdI104 and IdI558 would not be expressed together on the same protein. Therefore we are now sequencing the RNA's coding for the λ1 light and the μ heavy chains in order to understand the structural basis of these two idiotopes.

CONCLUSION

The data reported in this paper show that three groups of mice can be grouped according to their $\lambda 1$ expression. In the first group, the $\lambda 1$ chain is expressed as it is in laboratory strains. The second group may be considered as $\lambda 1$ low producer and third group appears to produce new allotypic forms of the $\lambda 1$ chain. The data concerning the anti-1355 response shows clearly that some Igh[a] as well as some Igh[not a] wild derived strains are able to produce $\lambda 1$ bearing anti-α(1-3) antibodies which express the IdX, IdI104 and IdI558 idiotypes. This suggests that recombinations may have occured in these strains between IghV and IghC genes or within the IghV locus itself. Unlike the laboratory strains, some wild mice, following an immunization with the B1355 antigen, are able to synthesize $\lambda 1$ bearing anti-α(1-6) antibodies. Finally, a hybridoma is described which expresses, in addition to IdX, both the IdI558 and the IdI104 idiotopes.

Acknowledgments

We are indebted Dr. S.Hauser for proofreading the manuscript and to Dr. P.Sanchez for his helpful discussions. We are grateful to Dr. Slodki for his generous gift of Dextran B1355, and to Drs J.F.Kearney and E.Weiler for their generous gift of monoclonal anti-idiotype antibodies. We thank Ms A.M.Drapier and D.Voegtle for their excellent technical assistance and Mrs M.Berson for her kind and efficient secretarial help.

REFERENCES

Amor M, Guenet JL, Bonhomme F, Cazenave PA (1983) Genetic polymorphism of $\lambda 1$ and $\lambda 3$ immunoglobulin light chains in the mus subgenus. Eur J Immunol 13:312-317

Blomberg B, Geckeler WR, Weigert M (1972) Genetics of the antibody response to Dextran in mice. Science 177:178-181

Carson D, Weigert M (1973) Immunological analysis of the cross-reacting idiotopes of mouse myeloma proteins with anti-Dextran activity and normal anti-Dextran antibodies. Proc Natl Acad Sci USA 70:235- 239

Clevinger B, Schilling J, Hood L, Davie J (1980) Structural correlates of cross-reactive and individual idiotypic determinants on murine antibodies to α(1-3)Dextran. J Exp Med 151:1059-1070

Geckeler W, Faversham J, Cohn M (1978) On a regulatory gene controlling the expression of the murine $\lambda 1$ light chain. J Exp Med 148:1122-1136

Hansburg D, Briles DE, Davie J (1977) Analysis of the diversity of murine antibodies to Dextran B1355. II.Demonstration of multiple idiotypes with variable expression in several strains. J Immunol 119:1406-1412

Juy D, Cazenave PA (1985) Igh restriction of the anti-α(1-3)Dextran response: polyclonal B cell activators induce the synthesis of anti-α(1-3)Dextran antibodies in lymphocytes from Igh[a] mice only. Eur J Immunol 135:1239-1244

Kearney JF, Pollock BA, Stohrer R (1983) Analysis of idiotypic heterogeneity in the anti-α(1-3)Dextran and anti-phosphorylcholine responses using monoclonal anti-idiotype antibodies. "Immune networks" Ed C. Bona and H. Kohler. Annals of the NY Acad of Scicnes 418:151-170

Kindt TJ, Gris C, Guenet JL, Bonhomme F, Cazenave PA (1985) Lambda light chain constant and variable gene complements in wild-derived inbred mouse strains. Eur J Immunol 15:535-540

Primi D, Sanchez P, Cazenave PA (1984) Selective and polyclonal induction of high level of $\lambda 1$ light chain-bearing immunoglobulins in BALB/c and SJL mice. Eur J Immunol 14:1159-1162

Riblet R, Blomberg B, Weigert M, Lieberman R, Taylor BA, Potter M (1975)
    Genetics of mouse antibodies. I.Linkage of the Dextran response locus VH-Dex
    to allotype. Eur J Immunol 5:775-777
Sanchez P, Primi D, Levi-Strauss M, and Cazenave PA (1985) The regulatory locus
    rλ1 affects the level of λ1 light chain synthesis in lipopolysaccharide-acti-
    vated lymphocytes but not the frequency of λ1-positive B cell precursors. Eur
    J Immunol 15:66-72
Stohrer R, Kearney JF (1983[a]) Fine idiotype analysis of B cell precursors in
    the T-dependent and T-independent responses to α(1-3)Dextran responses in
    BALB/c mice. J Exp Med 158:2081-2094
Stohrer R, Lee MC, Kearney JF (1983[b]) Analysis of the anti-α(1-3)Dextran
    response with monoclonal anti-idiotype antibodies. J Immunol 131:1375-1380
Scott CL, Potter M (1984) Variation in Vλ genes in the genus Mus.
    J Immunol 132:2638-2643
Weiler E, Lehle G, Wilke J, Weiler YJ (1984) Isogeneic anti-idiotype repertoire
    and modulation of idiotype expression in the anti-Dextran system. In "Idiotypy
    in Biology and Medicine" 12:203-218

Lymphocyte Alloantigens

Polymorphism of Lymphocyte Antigens-Encoding Loci in Wild Mice

F. Figueroa, H. Tichy, I. McKenzie, U. Hämmerling, and J. Klein

Wild mice presumably colonized western Europe over the last 10,000 years, the Americas during post-Columbian times, and Australia over the last 200 years (for a review, see Klein 1975). The colonization probably occurred gradually, hand in hand with the spread of humans through the world. The migration patterns that established the present-day distribution of wild mice are conceivably still reflected in the distribution of alleles and in the allelic frequencies of different mouse populations. Tracing these patterns may be useful, not only for the understanding of the population biology of the mouse, but also for tracing the main migration routes of early humans in Eurasia.

In humans, blood groups have been very useful for defining relationships among populations. In the mouse, at least seven erythrocyte antigens have been identified (Klein 1975) but the defining reagents are not easily available and they have therefore not been used in population studies. There are, however, at least 20 antigens that are predominantly expressed on lymphocytes and that are therefore referred to as Ly antigens (McKenzie and Potter 1979). These can potentially be used to trace the origins of the individual mouse populations. Here, we report preliminary results on the feasibility of such a study.

We have selected 17 lymphocyte antigens for which monoclonal antibodies are available (Table 1). Most of the antigens are expressed on T cells but some are also expressed on B lymphocytes and a few other cells. They could all be detected on lymphoid cells by using the complement-dependent cytotoxic assay. In our version of the assay, we used single cell suspensions prepared from spleen and lymph nodes. We removed erythrocytes and dead cells by fractionation on a Ficoll Paque column, and then carried out the test in Terasaki microplates (see Zaleska-Rutczynska et al. 1983 for details). The complement was a 1:1:4 mixture of rabbit normal serum, guinea pig normal serum, and Hanks' balanced salt solution. The cytotoxicity was evaluated automatically by the propidium iodide method of Bruning and his colleagues (1982).

All the Ly antigens we have tested were originally detected in inbred mouse strains using allogeneic antibodies. Their strain distribution is given in Table 2. The antigens are encoded in 12 separate loci. At most of the loci, two alleles have been identified which code for the antithetically distributed antigens 1 and 2. At some of the loci, only

Table 1. Antigens tested and antibodies used to detect them

Antigen	Antibody	Reactivity of antibody with	Reference
Thy-1.1	HO-22.1	T cells	Marshak-Rothstein et al. (1970)
Thy-1.2	5032-1.3	T cells	McKenzie IFC (unpublished data)
Ly-1.1	7.20.6/3	T cells	Hogarth et al. (1982)
Ly-1.2	C3PO	T cells	Mark et al. (1982)
Ly-2.1	49-11-1	T cells	Hogarth et al. (1982)
Ly-2.2	19-178	T cells	Hämmerling U (unpublished data)
Ly-6.2 A	S8.106	T and B cells	Kimura et al. (1984)
Ly-6.2 C	SK 142.446	T and B cells	Kimura et al. (1984)
Ly-6.2 F	TU 192.2.10	T and B cells	Klein D et al. (unpublished data)
Ly-10.1	T18/870	T cells, some B cells	Kimura et al. (1980)
Ly-15.2	8.6.2	T cells	Potter et al. (1981)
Ly-18.2	S8.261	T and B cells	Kimura et al. (1981a)
Ly-17(20).2	K9-361	T and B cells	Kimura et al. (1981b)
Ly-19.2	K10.6	B cells	Tada et al. (1981)
Ly-22.2	T281/596.6	T cells	Tada et al. (1983)
Ly-28.2	5075-12.1	T and B cells	Hogarth et al. (1984)
B2m	S19/8	T and B cells	Tada et al. (1980)

Table 2. Strain distribution pattern of Ly alloantigens in the mouse

Mouse strain	Thy-1	Ly-1	Ly-2	Ly-6	Ly-10	Ly-15	Ly-17	Ly-18	Ly-19	Ly-22	Ly-28	β_2m
C57BL/6	2	2	2	2	-	2	2	2	2	2	2	2
C57L	2	2	2	2	1	2	2	2	2	2	2	2
C57BR/cd	2	2	2	2	1	2	2	2	2	2	2	2
C58	2	2	1	2	-	1	2	2	2	-	-	-
A	2	2	2	1	-	1	1	-	2	-	-	-
BALB/c	2	2	2	1	-	1	2	-	2	2	-	-
NZB	2	2	2	1	-	1	.	.	2	-	-	.
SJL	2	2	2	2	-	1	1	2	-	-	2	-
SWR	2	2	2	2	.	1	1	-	2	-	2	-
129	2	2	2	2	-	1	1	-	2	2	2	-
LP	2	2	2	1	.	2	.	.	2	2	2	-
C3H/HeJ	2	1	1	1	-	2	1	-	2	2	-	-
CBA/J	2	1	1	1	1	2	1	-	2	2	-	-
CE	2	2	1	1	-	2	1	2	-	.	-	-
DBA/1	2	1	1	1	1	2	2	2	2	-	2	-
DBA/2	2	1	1	2	1	2	2	2	2	-	2	-
AKR	1	2	1	2	-	1	2	-	-	2	2	-
PL	1	2	1	2	-	.	-	.	2	2	2	-
RF	1	2	1	2	.	2	1	-	-	-	2	-
BDP	2	2	1	2	.	.	1	.	-	-	.	-
RIII	.	2	2	1	.	.	.	.	2	.	.	-

Numbers in the body of the table are the determinants defined by antibody. "-" means that no serologically detected determinant has been defined for the indicated strain. "." = not determined.

one allele is known to code for an identifiable antigen; the other
allele is either silent or codes for an as yet unidentified antigen.

Using the antibodies listed in Table 1, we tested 122 wild mice, all
except two belonging to the species Mus domesticus (these two were of
the M. musculus species). The mice represented 17 different populations
from West Germany, Switzerland, Italy, Spain, Czechoslovakia, Israel,
Costa Rica, Venezuela, and Australia. Although the samples from the
individual populations were relatively small, they revealed certain
tendencies in the distribution of some of the antigens (Table 3).

According to Kurihara and his colleagues (1985), all M. musculus mice
express the Thy-1.1-encoding allele (Thy-1^a), whereas all M. domesticus
mice express the Thy-1.2-encoding allele (Thy-1^b). We confirm this observation but find one exception to this rule: two of the eight domesticus mice from Costa Rica expressed the Thy-1^a allele; they did not
express the Thy-1^b allele. The difference between the two antigenic
forms of the Thy-1 molecule is known to be in a single amino acid substitution at position 89 (Williams and Gagnon 1982). The two exceptional animals could therefore have been the progeny of a mouse in
which a recurrent mutation caused the Thy-1.2 $\longrightarrow$ Thy-1.1 conversion.
If this were the case, however, the mutation would have had to occur a
number of generations back, otherwise the mice would have been heterozygous at the Thy-1 locus. The homozygosity could have been achieved by
inbreeding within a deme. Alternatively, however, the exceptional mice
may signal the existence of Thy-1 polymorphism that may turn out to be
present in some populations of M. domesticus. Only through more extensive sampling will it be possible to distinguish between these two
possibilities. Clearly, however, the presence of the Thy-1^a allele in
some inbred mouse strains does not necessarily indicate that the laboratory mice derive from a mixture of M. domesticus and M. musculus.
The Thy-1 typing also indicated that at least some of the Australian
mice belong to the species M. domesticus -- a conclusion compatible
with the general morphology of these animals. (As far as we are aware,
the species of the Australian wild mice has previously not been identified.) This identification supports the hypothesis that most Australian mice derive from stowaway founders brought into the country by
British settlers from areas occupied by M. domesticus.

The Ly-1 typing revealed that most of the wild mice populations are
fixed for the Ly-1^b allele which codes for the Ly-1.2 antigen, while
others contain this allele at a relatively high frequency. Many of
the populations that are fixed for the Ly-1^b allele lack the Ly-1.1-
encoding (Ly-1^a) allele altogether. In most other populations, the
Ly-1^a allele is present at a relatively low frequency. The Ly-1
antigens are therefore good markers for small mouse populations; they
may prove to be ideal for determining the migration rates between
local populations. Since some of the wild mice did not react with
either the Ly-1.1-specific or with the Ly-1.2-specific antibodies, it
appears that there is at least one other allele at the Ly-1 locus
which again could either be silent or code for an as yet unidentified
Ly-1.3 antigen.

The situation with regard to the Ly-2 locus is similar to that at
the Ly-1 locus. Here, too, most populations are fixed for one allele
(Ly-2^a coding for the antigen Ly-2.1) and several populations lack the
second allele (Ly-2^b, coding for the antigen Ly-2.2). In these populations, the Ly-2 locus, like the Ly-1 locus, could therefore serve as
an excellent marker in genetic and ecological studies. The occurrence
of wild mice that do not express either the Ly-2.1 or the Ly-2.2
antigen again suggests the presence of a third allele at the Ly-2

Table 3. Frequency of Ly antigens in different populations of wild mice

Population	No. of animals tested	Thy-1.1	Thy-1.2	Ly-1.1	Ly-1.2	Ly-2.1	Ly-2.2	Ly-6.2A	Ly-6.2C	Ly-6.2F	Ly-10.1	Ly-15.2	Ly-18.2	Ly-19.2	Ly-17	Ly-22.2	Ly-28.2	β_2m
								Antigen frequency										
Tübingen (Germany)	9	0	1.0	0	1.0	1.0	0.55	0	0	0	0	0	0	1.0	0	0	0	1.0
Laubach (Germany)	12	0	1.0	0	0.83	0.33	0.41	0	0	0	0	0	0	0.33	0	0	0	0.41
Vohl (Germany)	13	0	1.0	0.10	0.80	0.80	0.50	0	0	0	0	0.23	0	0.92	0.07	0	0	0.30
Kampenbruck (Germany)	4	0	1.0	0.25	1.0	1.0	0.25	0	0	1.0	0	0.07	0	0.25	0	0	0	1.0
Helgoland (Germany)	7	0	1.0	0.42	0.85	1.0	0.57	0.57	0.57	0.14	0	0	0	0.85	0	0	0	0
Freiburg (Switzerland)	4	0	1.0	0	1.0	0	1.0	0	0	0	0	0	0	0	0	0	0	0
Pisa (Italy)	7	0	1.0	0.16	1.0	0.66	1.0	0	0	0	0.28	0.14	0	0.57	0	0	0	0.42
Grosseto (Italy)	4	0	1.0	0	0.50	0.50	0	0	0	0	0	0	0	0.25	0	0	0	0
Bozen (Italy)	4	0	1.0	0	1.0	1.0	0	0	0	0	0	0	0	0.75	0	0	0	0.25
Penedes (Spain)	15	0	1.0	0	1.0	0.60	0.40	0.26	0	0	0.26	0.06	0	0.92	0	0	0	0.73
Mallorca (Spain)	5	0	1.0	0	1.0	1.0	0.40	0	0	0	0	0.20	0	0.80	0	0	0	0.80
San José (Costa Rica)	8	0.28	0.71	0.14	1.0	1.0	0.28	0	0	0	0	0	0	0.62	0	0	0	0
Caracas (Venezuela)	2	0	1.0	0.50	1.0	1.0	0.50	0	0	0	0.50	0	0	1.0	0	0	0	0.50
Victoria (Australia)	4	0	1.0	0.33	1.0	1.0	0	0	0	0	0	0	0.50	0.50	0.25	0	0	0.25
L.Habashan (Israel)	13	0	1.0	0.16	0.83	0.25	0.75	0	0	0	0	0	0	0.15	0	0	0	0.23
Yitav (Israel)	8	0	1.0	0.14	0.71	0.71	0.71	0	0	0	0	0	0	0.62	0	0	0	0
Prague (Czechoslovakia)	2	1.0	0	0	1.0	1.0	0	1.0	0	1.0	1.0	1.0	1.0	1.0	0	0	0	1.0

locus. Neither the Ly-1 nor the Ly-2 typing reveals, however, any trends in geographical distribution which would be indicative of gross migration patterns in the colonization of Europe by wild mice.

The Ly-6 is a complex antigen which may consist of several antigenic determinants detected by various antibodies. We used three different antibodies, two of which gave a similar distribution of reactivity (the discrepancies might have been caused by false negativities due to the weakness of one of the antibodies), whereas the third gave a different pattern. Most of the wild mice failed to react with any of the three antibodies, however, indicating that the "null" allele is more common than the antigen-encoding allele. Only in one population of M. domesticus might the antigen-encoding allele have been fixed, but the tested sample was too small to allow a firm conclusion on this point.

One of the antibodies which was originally thought to define the Ly-11 antigen in actual fact defines a variant at the β_2-microglobulin locus (the $B2m^b$ allele) which codes for one of the two chains of the class I Mhc molecules. The antibody specific for this variant reacts with in-bred strains derived from Little's original No. 57 female (see Klein 1975) and with no other inbred strains. Robinson and his coworkers (1984) have reported that the $B2m^b$ allele is present in M. musculus and absent in M. domesticus which carries the $B2m^a$ allele. It came therefore as a surprise to us that almost half of the wild M. domesticus mice in our collection reacted with the β_2m-specific antibody; in some of the populations, this allele even appeared to be fixed. There are two possible explanations for this discrepancy between our results and those of Robinson and his colleagues. First, the discrepancy is caused by a crossreaction of our antibody with unidentified antigens. This possibility seems unlikely because Robinson and his colleagues used in part the same antibody to determine the distribution of B2m alleles in their mouse samples. They did, however, use a different technique for testing the reactivity of this antibody. Second, the M. domesticus mice tested by Robinson and his colleagues by chance all carried the $B2m^a$ allele. The discrepancy will need to be resolved by further testing. If, however, M. domesticus populations carry the $B2m^b$ allele, there would again be no need to postulate that its presence in laboratory mice is caused by M. musculus admixture in the colonies of the early mouse breeders.

The typing for the remaining Ly antigens revealed that the alleles coding for the Ly-22.2 and Ly-28.2 antigens are absent in our collection of wild mice; that alleles coding for the Ly-15.2, Ly-18.2, and Ly-17.2 antigens are very rare; and that, by contrast, the Ly-19.2-encoding allele is very common.

An interesting situation occurs on the island Helgoland in the North Sea. Mhc typing of mice trapped on this island indicates the presence of only two major H-2 haplotypes -- a very unusual situation for wild mice (Figueroa et al. 1986). The population therefore appears to be quite homogeneous. By contrast, the Ly typing reveals polymorphism at several of the Ly loci.

In summary, we have shown that it is feasible to type wild mice for Ly antigens and that some of the antigens could be used as markers in genetic and ecological studies of small populations. We have also demonstrated that the $Thy-1^a$ allele does occur in M. domesticus; that the sampled Australian mice are of the M. domesticus species; that a good proportion of the M. domesticus mice reacts with an antibody which presumably detects the $B2m^b$ allele; and that isolates relatively homogeneous at the Mhc loci can be polymorphic at their <u>Ly</u> loci.

ACKNOWLEDGMENTS

We thank Dr. J. Vives, Hospital Clinico y Provincial (Barcelona,
Spain), Dr. F. Merino, Instituto Venezolano de investigaciones
Cientificas, Caracas, Venezuela, Dr. Uzi Ritte, Genetic Department,
Hebrew University of Jerusalem, Israel, for help in the trapping of
wild mice.

REFERENCES

Bruning JW, Claas FHJ, Kardol MJ, Lansbergen Q, Naipol AM, Tanke HJ
  (1982) Automated reading of HLA-A,B,C typing and screening. The
  propidium iodide method. Hum Immunol 5:225-231
Figueroa F, Tichy H, Berry RJ, Klein J (1986) Mhc polymorphism in
  island populations of wild mice (this volume)
Hogarth PM, Potter TA, Cornell FN, McLaughlin R, McKenzie IFC (1980)
  Monoclonal antibodies to murine cell surface antigens. I. Lyt-1.1
  J Immunol 125:1618-1624
Hogarth PM, Edwards J, McKenzie IFC, Goding JW, Liew FY (1982) Mono-
  clonal antibodies to murine Ly-2.1 cell surface antigen. Immunology
  46:135-144
Hogarth PM, Houlden BA, Latham SE, Sutton VR, McKenzie IFC (1984) Def-
  inition of a new alloantigen encoded by genes in the Ly-6 complex.
  Immunogenetics 20:57-69
Kimura S, Tada N, Hämmerling U (1980) A new lymphocyte alloantigen
  (Ly-10) controlled by a gene linked to the Lyt-1 locus. Immunogenet-
  ics 10:363-372
Kimura S, Tada N, Liu Y, Hämmerling U (1981a) A new mouse cell-surface
  antigen (Ly-m18) defined by a monoclonal antibody. Immunogenetics
  13:547-554
Kimura S, Tada N, Nakayama E, Liu Y, Hämmerling U (1981b) A new mouse
  cell-surface antigen (Ly-m20) controlled by a gene linked to <u>Mls</u>
  locus and defined by monoclonal antibodies. Immunogenetics 14:3-14
Kimura S, Tada N, Liu-Lam Y, Hämmerling U (1984) Studies of the mouse
  Ly-6 alloantigen system. II. Complexities of the Ly-6 region. Immuno-
  genetics 20:47-56
Klein J (1975) Biology of the mouse histocompatibility-2 complex.
  Springer, New York
Kurihara Y, Miyashita N, Moriwaki K, Petras ML, Bonhomme F, Cho WS,
  Kohno S (1985) Serological survey of T-lymphocyte differentiation
  antigens in wild mice. Immunogenetics 22:211-218
Mark C, Figueroa F, Nagy ZA, Klein J (1982) Cytotoxic monoclonal anti-
  body specific for the Lyt-1.2 antigen. Immunogenetics 16:95-97
Marshak-Rothstein A, Fink P, Gridley T, Raulet DH, Bevan MJ, Gefter
  ML (1979) Properties and applications of monoclonal antibodies
  directed against determinants of the Thy-1 locus. J Immunol 122:
  2491-2497
McKenzie IFC, Potter T (1979) Murine lymphocyte surface antigens. Adv
  Immunol 27:179-338
Potter TA, Hogarth PM, McKenzie IFC (1981) <u>Ly-15</u>: A new murine lymphocyte alloantigenic locus. Transplantation 31:339-342
Robinson PJ, Steinmetz M, Moriwaki K, Fischer-Lindahl K (1984) Beta-2
  miocroglobulin types of mice of wild origin. Immunogenetics 20:655-
  665

Tada N, Kimura S, Hatzfeld A, Hämmerling U (1980) Ly-m11: The H-3 region of mouse chromosome 2 controls a new surface alloantigen. Immunogenetics 11:441-449

Tada N, Kimura S, Liu Y, Taylor BA, Hämmerling U (1981) Ly-m19: The Lyb-2 region of mouse chromosome 4 controls a new surface alloantigen. Immunogenetics 13:539-546

Tada N, Kimura S, Liu-Lam Y, Hämmerling U (1983) Mouse alloantigen system Ly-m22 predominantly expressed on T lymphocytes and controlled by a gene linked to Mls region on chromosome 1. Hybridoma 2:29-38

Williams AF, Gagnon J (1982) Neuronal cell Thy-1 glocoprotein: homology with immunoglobulin. Science 216:696-703

Zaleska-Rutczynska Z, Figueroa F, Klein J (1983) Sixteen new H-2 haplotypes derived from wild mice. Immunogenetics 18:189-203

t-Haplotypes and H-2

On the Origin of *t* Chromosomes

J. Klein, M. Golubić, O. Budimir, R. Schöpfer, M. Kasahara, and F. Figueroa

The t chromosomes are the curse of wild mice. Some of the mutant genes they carry serve no apparent purpose except that of propagating themselves and disseminating through the population -- superb examples of selfish DNA. They may have prevailed on the population long before a house mouse became a house mouse and they will most likely hold fast on it until this species becomes extinct. The two reasons for the perseverance of t chromosomes in wild mouse populations are the ability to sway their own transmission into the progeny of male parents strongly in their favor and the power to keep the genetic elements responsible for this segregation distortion together by the suppression of crossing-over in a kind of "frozen linkage group". All other characteristics of the t chromosomes (male sterility, lethality, influence on embryonic development, omnipresence in natural populations; for review see Klein 1975) are probably secondary tack-ons to these primary qualities; they are inconsequential for the conquest of the population by selfish DNA.

The nature of the segregation distorters remains a total mystery. The best bet at the moment is that they represent a foreign DNA that was somehow inserted into and has since taken hold of the normal chromosome (Sandler and Golic 1985). If Fred Hoyle knew about the t chromosomes, he might wish to speculate that the distorters come from outer space but for those of us who are less inclined to mix science with science-fiction, the postulate of a viral origin might suffice. The important point of such a speculation is that there may not be non-mutant counterparts of this foreign DNA in the non-t chromosomes. By the same token, there may not be a counterpart of the segregation distorters in other species (including the human) except those species in which systems similar to the t complex have been described. In drosophila, in which segregation distorters resemble t distorters very closely, a pretty good case has been put forward for the extraneous origin of the selfish DNA (Sandler and Golic 1985). The segregation distorters may not actually be transcribed and translated. It may therefore be futile to search for the products of the segregation distortion genes: one should perhaps concentrate on differences in DNA between the t and non-t chromosomes.

As for the suppression of crossing-over -- the second of the two defining properties of the t chromosome -- the evidence is accumulating that it is caused by a much more mundane mechanism than the distortion of transmission ratios. Several investigators have now reported that the t chromosomes contain at least one and probably more than one inversion -- a classical suppressor of recombination (Artzt et al. 1982b; Artzt 1984; Shin et al. 1984; Pla and Condamine 1984; Condamine et al. 1983). The identified inversion apparently includes the H-2 complex on the turned-over chromosomal segment. Inversions are also known to hold together the segregation disorters on chromosome 2 in drosophila (Sandler and Golic 1985).

If the hypothesis claiming an extraneous origin of the segregation distorters were correct, one would expect the events that led to the generation of the t chromosomes to be extremely rare. In fact, it is very unlikely that these events would happen more than once in any species; probably they would happen only in certain species. One could therefore further expect all the t chromosomes present in the house mouse to be related to one another and the relatedness to be a reflection of their common origin from a single ancestral chromosome which was, a long time ago, raided by the extraneous elements.

These deductions seem to be contradicted by the polymorphism of the t chromosomes. Until recently, only two or three different t chromosomes were known to occur frequently among wild mice (Bennett 1975), but this knowledge was based largely on sampling of North American wild mice which may be -- because of their recent origin from a few founders -- more homogeneous than mice in other parts of the world. Indeed, our sampling of European and Asian wild populations has revealed the presence of at least 16 different t chromosomes, all occurring in appreciable frequencies (Klein et al. 1984). The indications are that this number is not all there is to t-chromosome heterogeneity. Is this heterogeneity incompatible with the origin from a single ancestral chromosome? We think not, because the heterogeneity lies largely in the lethality genes which, as previously mentioned, may be just one of the adjunct phenomena associated with the distorters. Because of the high ratios at which t chromosomes are transmitted onto progeny, natural selection is virtually powerless against any deleterious mutation that occurs in the genes on these chromosomes. As a result, the t chromosomes accumulate lethal mutations and, since there are many genes on any chromosome which can cause lethality when inactivated and when present in a homozygous state, the road is open for the diversification of the t chromosomes. The reason why most of the lethal genes on the chromosomes disturb embryonic development may simply be that many genes on any chromosome are required during embryogenesis. The genes themselves may have nothing to do with regulating differentiation and may be totally unrelated to the distorters. The distorters themselves may remain -- despite all this variability of the chromosomal genes -- largely invariable. Whatever the mechanism by which they cause the distortion in transmission ratios, it must be dependent on a certain integrity and invariability of the distorting elements. Too much variation in the distorters may cost them their ability to perpetuate themselves and may consequently cost them their existence. Hence, while most genes on the t chromosomes are allowed to vary freely, certain portions of the chromosome related to the segregation distortion and to suppression of crossing-over must remain relatively constant. That there are, indeed, regions in the t chromosomes that vary very little, if at all, is indicated by recent studies on the restriction fragment length polymorphisms (RFLPs) using DNA probes specific for the centromeric portion of chromosome 17 (Röhme et al. 1984; Fox et al. 1985; L.M. Silver, H. Lehrach, and J. Klein, unpublished data). However, the most convincing evidence for the common origin of all t chromosomes has been provided by our studies of the H-2 genes residing in these chromomosomes.

Because of its extensive polymorphism, the H-2 complex is uniquely suited for the study of chromosomal ancestry (Klein and Figueroa 1981). The alleles that occur at the H-2 loci in any randomly chosen sample of wild mice are normally quite far apart in terms of evolutionary distance, most of them differing in as much as 20-30% of their nucleotide sequence (Klein 1986). Furthermore, the alleles at different loci frequently dissociate and reassociate in new combinations. Therefore, when one finds H-2 alleles that are clearly closely related and that only

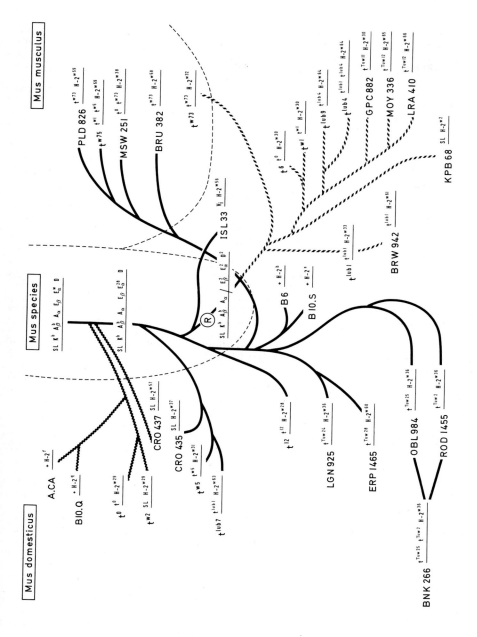

Fig. 1. The genealogical tree of t chromosomes.

occur in certain combinations, in a particular sample of chromosomes, one can deduce that the chromosomes have shared a common ancestor which was different from the ancestors of other chromosomes. We have documented this situation in regard to the t chromosomes.

We have analyzed the products of the class I and class II loci serologically (Sturm et al. 1982, Ni* žetić et al. 1984) and we have determined the restriction fragment length polymorphism of the class II loci, as well as the loci coding for the complement component 4 (located between the class I and the class II loci within the H-2 complex) (Figueroa et al. 1985; Golubić et al. 1985). All the generated data are consistent with the division of the t chromosomes into three groups as depicted in Figure. 1. The t chromosomes within each group are very clearly related to one another in terms of their H-2 genes. The products of these genes give identical or very similar patterns of serological reactivity and their RFLPs differ only slightly, if at all. The chromosomes differ in the lethality genes they carry, in the slight variations of their H-2 genes, or in the combinations of the H-2 genes. The chromosomes within a group can therefore be derived from a single ancestral chromosome by mutations and through recombination. Representatives of at least two of these groups (depicted as different branches on the genealogical tree in Figure 1) have been extracted from both Mus domesticus and M. musculus, the two species of the house mouse believed to have been separated genetically for at least one million years (Yonekawa et al. 1980). This observation suggests that the origin of each of these two branches goes back for at least this much time.

The serological and RFLP analyses, however, failed to clearly establish the relationship among the three branches of the tree. Although there were obvious indications that the branches are related to one another, it was impossible to deduce how they might have arisen. In the hope that some light could be shed on the origin of the branches by analyzing the structure of some of the H-2 genes, we have sequenced DNA stretches of the A_β genes from representatives of the three branches. A full account of the data will be given later; here, we merely wish to point out that the data have indeed allowed us to work out a scheme showing how the H-2 haplotypes in each branch might have arisen from a common ancestral haplotype (Fig. 2). Here again, the only mechanisms required to explain these derivations are mutations and crossing-over. Both mechanisms have been documented as occurring within the t chromosomes. Although the frequency of recombination within the suppressed region is greatly reduced in t/+ heterozygotes (Artzt et al. 1982a), a number of crossovers have been obtained in the laboratory. The products of these recombinations have retained some of the t-complex genes and have lost others (Lyon and Meredith 1964ab). Through the additional loss of mutant genes from these derived "partial" t haplotypes, it is possible to restore normal gene order on the recombinant chromosomes. Furthermore, double crossing-over involving two strands within the inverted region could restore the standard gene order as well. Finally, crossing-over within the t complex occurs with normal or even increased frequency in heterozygotes carrying two t chromosomes with complementary lethal genes (Silver and Artzt 1981). All these considerations indicate that genes can be exchanged between t chromosomes carrying different lethality genes, as well as between t and non-t chromosomes. Hence, all the events postulated in Figure 2 are completely feasible.

In our version of how the t complex originated, we envision an ancestral chromosome 17 which carried three copies of the C4 gene and class II H-2 genes related to the contemporary $H-2^b$ genes. Its $H-2K$ gene was similar to the corresponding gene in the contemporary $H-2^k$ haplotype.

243

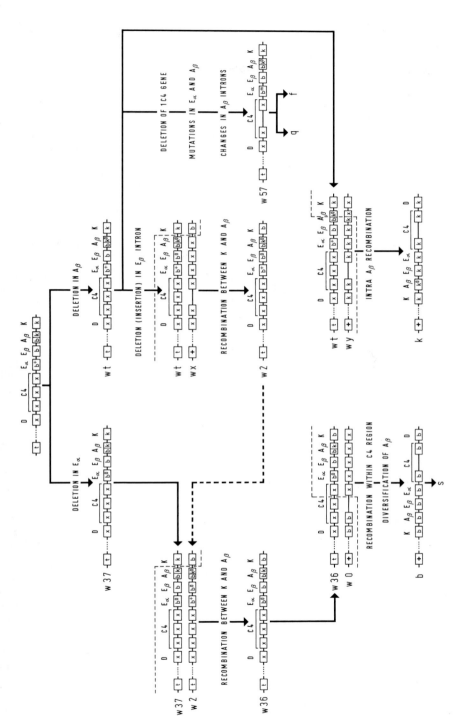

Fig. 2. Postulated events in the evolution of the H-2 complexes borne by <u>t</u> chromosomes.

(The origin of the D gene could thus far not be determined.) It was this ancestral chromosome that was invaded by the extraneous genetic elements. Its H-2 complex then diversified in two ways. In one of the primitive t chromosomes a mutation occurred which deleted the promoter region in the E_α gene (Dembić et al. 1985). As a result of this deletion, the E_α gene fails to be transcribed and expressed. The deletion is still present in about half of the t chromosomes currently present in wild mice. The branch represented by t^{Tuw7} and carrying the $H-2^{w37}$ haplotype might be closest to this ancestral chromosome. The group represented by the t^{Tuw2} and the $H-2^{w36}$ haplotype might have arisen from t^{Tuw7} by an intra-H-2 recombination between $H-2^{w37}$ and $H-2^{w2}$, and the $H-2^{w36}$ might have been the progenitor of the $H-2^b$ haplotype which in turn may have contributed the defective E_α gene to the $H-2^s$ haplotype.

In the t chromosomes lacking the E_α deletion another mutation occurred which deleted two codons within the A_β gene. The gene remained functional and, luckily for us, became a good marker for the other main branch of the evolutionary tree. In one of the secondary branches of this main branch an as yet unidentified mutation changed the size of an intron in the E_β gene and so dramatically altered the RFLP pattern of this gene. The resulting hypothetical t chromosome was then involved in an intra-H-2 crossing-over with a non-t chromosome, and this event gave rise to the contemporary t^{Tuw10} chromosome carrying the $H-2^{w2}$ haplotype. In another secondary branch, a deletion of one of the three C4 genes and mutation in the E_β gene gave rise to the t^{Tuw8} chromosome carrying the $H-2^{w57}$ haplotype. The mutation is responsible for a defect in splicing of the E_β mRNA and hence for the lack of translation of the messenger into a protein. Non-t $H-2^q$ and $H-2^f$ haplotypes may derive from this t chromosome. The progenitor of this secondary branch may have been involved in an intra-H-2 recombination with a non-t chromosome which gave rise to the extant $H-2^k$ haplotype.

The genealogy in Figure 2 has been deduced according to the assumption that the H-2 complex is inverted in all the t chromosomes, as the accumulating evidence seems to suggest (Artzt et al. 1982; Pla and Condamine 1984). It should be pointed out, however, that an even simpler tree can be constructed which is based on the assumption that the H-2 complex is not inverted in the t chromosomes.
The fact that the branches of the genealogical tree have split before the separation of M. domesticus and M. musculus, as well as the number of nucleotide substitutions which have occurred in the introns of the alleles at the class II loci suggest that the events establishing the ancestral t chromosome occurred more than one million years ago. Sequencing of additional H-2 genes and perhaps of other genes on the t chromosome might be necessary to determine the age of the t chromosomes more precisely. The observation that M. castaneus and M. molossinus apparently lack t chromosomes may be regarded as an indication that the creation of the t chromosome occurred after these two species separated from the ancestor they had in common with M. musculus and M. domesticus. It is, however, also possible that M. castaneus and M. molossinus escaped the curse of the t chromosomes through a founder effect: the population that gave rise to these species might have been small enough for it to lack by chance the t chromosomes present in other ancestral populations. So far, it seems that only M. domesticus and M. musculus have had a visitation from the t curse. However, considering the wide distribution of these two species, the curse does not seem to have done them much harm.

ACKNOWLEDGMENTS

The experimental work cited in this communication has been supported
in part by grant A14736 from the National Institutes of Health,
Bethesda, Maryland, and by a grant from the Deutsche Forschungsgemein-
schaft.

REFERENCES

Artzt K (1984) Gene mapping within the $\underline{T/t}$ complex of the mouse. III.
t-lethal genes are arranged in three clusters on chromosome 17. Cell
39:565-572
Artzt K, McCormick, P, Bennett D (1982a) Gene mapping within the $\underline{T/t}$
complex of the mouse. I. $\underline{t}$-lethal genes are nonallelic. Cell 28:
463-470
Artzt K, Shin, HS, Bennett D (1982b) Gene mapping within the $\underline{T/t}$ complex of the mouse. II. Anomalous position of the $\underline{H-2}$ complex in $\underline{t}$
haplotypes. Cell 28:471-476
Bennett D (1975) The T-locus of the mouse. Cell 6:441-454
Condamine H, Guenet JL, Jacob F (1983) Recombination between two mouse
$\underline{t}$ haplotypes $(\underline{t^{w12}tf}$ and $\underline{t^{lub-1}})$. Segregation of lethal factors
relative to centromere and tufter ($\underline{tf}$) locus. Genet Res (Camb)
42:335-344
Dembić Z, Ayane M, Klein J, Steinmetz M, Benoist CO, Mathis DJ (1985)
Inbred and wild mice carry identical deletions in their E_α MHC
genes. EMBO J 4:127-131
Dembić Z, Singer P, Klein J (1985) E^α: A history of a mutation EMBO J
3:1647-1654
Figueroa F, Golubić M, Nizetić D, Klein J (1985) Evolution of mouse
major histocompatibility complex genes borne by $\underline{t}$ chromosomes.
Proc Natl Acad Sci USA 82:2819-2823
Fox JS, Martin GR, Lyon MF, Herrmann B, Frischauf A-M, Lehrach H,
Silver LM (1985) Molecular probes define different regions of the
mouse $\underline{t}$ complex. Cell 40:63-69
Golubić M, Figueroa F, Tosi M, Klein J (1985) Restriction fragment
length polymorphism of $\underline{C4}$ genes in mice with $\underline{t}$ chromosomes. Immuno-
genetics 21:247-256
Klein J (1975) Biology of the mouse histocompatibility-2 complex.
Springer-Verlag, New York
Klein J (1986) Natural history of the major histocompatibility complex.
Wiley and Sons, New York
Klein J, Figueroa F (1981) Polymorphism of the mouse $\underline{H-2}$ loci. Immunol
Rev 60:23-57
Klein J, Sipos P, Figueroa F (1984) Polymorphism of t complex genes
in European wild mice. Genet Res (Camb) 14:39-46
Lyon MF, Meredith R (1964a) Investigations of the nature of $\underline{t}$-alleles
in the mouse. I. Genetic analysis of a series of mutants derived
from a lethal $\underline{t}$ allele. Heredity 19:301-312
Lyon MF, Meredith R (1964b) Investigations of the nature of $\underline{t}$-alleles
in the mouse. II. Genetic analysis of an unusual mutant allele and
its derivatives. Heredity 19:313-325
Nizetić D, Figueroa F, Klein J (1984) Evolutionary relationships be-
tween the $\underline{t}$ and $\underline{H-2}$ haplotypes in the house mouse. Immunogenetics
19:311-320
Pla M, Condamine H (1984) Recombination between two mouse $\underline{t}$ haplo-
types $(\underline{t^{w12}tf}$ and $\underline{t^{lub1}})$: Mapping of the $\underline{H-2}$ complex relative
to centromere and tufter ($\underline{tf}$) locus. Immunogenetics 20:277-285

Röhme D, Fox H, Herrmann B, Frischauf A-M, Edström J-E, Mains P, Silver LM, Lehrach H (1984) Molecular clones of the mouse t complex derived from microdissected metaphase chromosomes. Cell 36:783-788

Sandler L, Golic K (1985) Segregation distortion in Drosophila. Trends Genet 1:181-185

Shin HS, Bennett D, Artzt K (1984) Gene mapping within the T/t complex of the mouse. IV. The inverted MHC is intermingled with several t-lethal genes. Cell 39:573-578

Silver LM, Artzt K (1981) Recombination suppression of mouse t haplotypes due to chromatin mismatching. Nature 290:68-70

Sturm S, Figueroa F, Klein J (1982) The relationship between t and H-2 complexes in wild mice. I. The H-2 haplotypes of 20 t-bearing strains. Genet Res (Camb) 40:73-88

Yonekawa H, Moriwaki K, Gotoh O, Watanabe J, Hayashi J, Miyashita N, Petras ML, Tagashira Y (1980) Relationships between laboratory mice and th subspecies Mus musculus domesticus based on restriction endonuclease cleavage patterns of mitochondrial DNA. Jap J Genet 55:289-296

Amplification and Rearrangement of DNA Sequences During the Evolutionary Divergence of t Haplotypes and Wild-Type Forms of Mouse Chromosome 17

J. Schimenti and L. M. Silver

INTRODUCTION

The most proximal portion of mouse chromosome 17 occurs in a variant form known as a t haplotype, which is present at a high frequency in wild populations of mus domesticus and mus musculus. While t haplotypes have been studied by a number of investigators over the last 50 years, it is only within the last 5 years that we have begun to appreciate the true nature of these unusual genetic elements (for a recent review, see Silver, 1986). A large body of new data from a number of laboratories indicates that all naturally occurring t haplotypes are closely related to each other with a characteristic genomic organization that differs from the wild-type organization of this chromosomal region. (The "wild-type chromosome 17" refers to the non-t-haplotype form normally found in mus domesticus or mus musculus). Within the structurally variant region that defines t haplotypes (approximately 20-30,000 kb of DNA encompassing the T locus and the entire MHC), are many normally functioning genes interspersed with a number of independent "mutant loci" that mediate the characteristic t haplotype effects on fertility and development.

The t haplotype maintains itself as a well-defined genomic entity by suppression of recombination with wild-type along its length, and it propagates itself through mouse populations by means of a male-specific transmission ratio distortion (TRD) in its favor. Wild males that are heterozygous for a t haplotype can transmit it to nearly all (over 99%) of their offspring. A synthesis of recent work from several laboratories indicates that the physiological basis for TRD lies in the ability of t-carrying haploid germ cells to functionally inactivate their meiotic partners during spermiogenesis (Silver and Olds-Clarke, 1984; Olds-Clarke and Peitz, 1986).

The question of why t haplotypes exist has been an enigma to workers in the field for many years. In light of the currently available data, the simplest answer to this question is that t haplotypes are selfish chromosomes or genomic parasites present within wild populations of mus domesticus and mus musculus. A t haplotype does not appear to confer any selective advantage on individual animals. Instead, it appears that a single founder t chromosome acquired a set of properties (most importantly, TRD and recombination suppression) that allowed it to infiltrate the collective genomes of wild mice present throughout the world today.

To gain a better understanding of the evolution of t haplotypes into selfish chromosomes, we have begun a comparative analysis of DNA sequences present in t haplotype and wild-type forms of mouse chromosome 17. The implications of these results on the evolution of t haplotype structure is presented in this report.

MATERIALS AND METHODS

All genomic DNA isolations and recombinant DNA protocols were performed as described in previous publications (see Silver, 1982). The t complex probe T66 was obtained by direct cloning of genomic sequences from microdissected fragments of the proximal region of a wild-type form of chromosome 17 (Rohme et al., 1984; Fox et al., 1985). This probe was used to identify bacteriophage lambda clones from a homozyogous t haplotype library, and the T66-alpha clone was derived as a 3.4 kb Eco RI fragment from one such lambda clone.

RESULTS AND DISCUSSION

t Haplotype DNA is Rearranged Relative to Wild-type

The discovery that all t haplotypes could undergo normal recombination with all other t haplotypes provided initial insight into the structure of t haplotypes and their close relationship to each other (Silver and Artzt, 1981). In further studies, Artzt and her colleagues (1982) used this observation as a genetic tool for the demonstration of an inversion over the distal portion of t haplotypes, encompassing the tufted locus and the MHC (see Fig. 1).

With the identification and generation of a large number of molecular probes to the t complex (Silver et al., 1983; Rohme et al., 1984; Fox et al., 1984), it has become possible to determine and compare the structures of t and wild-type forms of chromosome 17 in great detail (Fox et al., 1985). These data have led to the identification and characterization of a second inversion of genetic material within t haplotypes relative to wild-type (Herrmann et al., 1986; Sarvetnick et al., 1986). This proximal inversion encompasses the loci of T and qk, and together with the distal inversion, it accounts for suppression of recombination over nearly the entire length of t haplotypes (Fig. 1). The structure of a small central region of t DNA not located within these major inversions remains to be determined – a third smaller inversion can not be ruled out.

All t Haplotypes Derive from a Recent Founder Chromosome

The accumulated data demonstrate that all naturally occurring t haplotypes share the same overall genomic structure. In addition, genomic analyses of a variety of independently-derived t haplotypes indicate that they are all highly homologous to each other at the actual level of primary DNA sequence (Fox et al., 1984; 1985). A variety of molecular probes to different t complex regions readily detect restriction fragment polymorphisms between different inbred strains of mice. However, none of these probes (with the exception of those derived from the MHC region) detect any polymorphisms between different t haplotypes. Furthermore, whereas the MHC region is highly polymorphic among different strains of mice, the level of intra-t MHC polymorphism is greatly restricted (Shin et al., 1982; Silver, 1982; Nizetic et al., 1984).

The simplest interpretation of these data is that all t haplotypes were derived from a common ancestor that existed relatively recently in evolutionary terms. However, the results presented in this report indicate that this common t-ancestor is the end-product of a longer period of divergent evolution from the wild-type chromosome.

Amplification of the T66 region during the evolution of t haplotypes

The genomic sequence called T66 was obtained as an insert within a random clone derived by the microdissection cloning procedure (Roehme et al., 1984). We have used this clone to probe the structures of the central t complex region present in different animals. This clone identifies a locally dispersed family of DNA elements with approximately 6 to 9 members located in the middle of t haplotypes in and around the proximal inversion. Preliminary cosmid analysis indicates that the size of the actual genomic region that has been amplified is at least 35 kilobases in length. The products of rare recombination events within t haplotypes have been used as genetic tools to dissect this genetic region into three subregions - called 66A, 66B and 66C - each of which contains several copies of the T66 element (Fig. 1; Fox et al., 1985). Since the rat genome carries only a single weakly hybridizing copy of the T66 element (unpublished data), it would appear that a series of tandem duplications of T66-containing sequences have occurred along the evolutionary line leading to t haplotypes.

An analysis of the wild-type form of the t complex with the T66 clone shows a very different picture from that observed in t haplotypes. First, the number of T66 elements present in wild-type chromosomes is much less (3 to 5) than the number present in t haplotypes. This result implies that an initial amplification of T66 elements occurred subsequent to the divergence of rat and mus, and that a further amplification of T66 elements occurred within the line leading to t haplotypes subsequent to the divergence of this line from the common ancestor leading to the wild-type mus chromosome.

Inversion within the T66 region during the evolution of mus domesticus/musculus

A second result from this analysis is that a portion of the T66 region is clearly displaced to a more proximal location on the wild-type chromosome (Herrmann et al., 1986). This result strongly suggests that the relative inversion of the proximal regions of wild-type and t chromosomes is a consequence of an actual inversion that occurred within the evolutionary line leading to the wild-type chromosome subsequent to the divergence of wild-type and t chromosomes from a common ancestor. A schematic diagram of these two lines of evolutionary divergence is presented in Fig. 1.

We have obtained support for this view of evolutionary divergence between t and wild-type in studies with a second generation T66-region probe (derived as a 3.2 kb subclone from a T66-containing phage clone). This clone detects only a single T66 element within wild-type chromosomes and three elements within t haplotypes (Fig. 2). The sub-family of T66 elements detected by this clone are called T66-alpha. Each of the t haplotype subregions, 66A, 66B & 66C contain

one of the T66-alpha elements along with other more divergent T66
elements. This conclusion is based on an analysis of the T66 elements
present in a series of different partial t haplotypes (Fox et al.,
1985).

The t haplotype genomic arrangement can be explained through the
triplication of an original set of T66 elements (called alpha, beta
and gamma) present within the common ancestor to t and wild-type. The
wild-type line maintained the original set of T66 elements but
diverged from a common ancestor through an inversion, with one
breakpoint located within the T66 region, causing the displacement of
the single T66-alpha element to a more proximal position on the
chromosome.

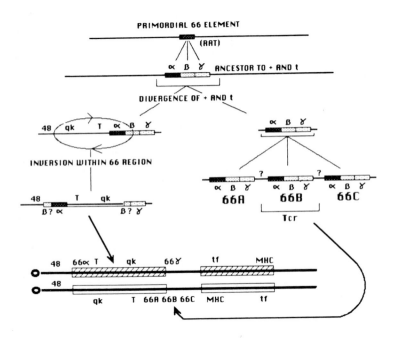

Fig. 1. A working hypothesis for the divergent evolution of t
haplotypes and wild-type (domesticus/musculus) forms of chromosome 17.
The evolutionary scheme is described in the text. The T48 element is
located between the centromere and the proximal inversion (Herrman et
al., 1986; Sarvetnick et al., 1986).

Implications for the Origin of t Haplotypes

The data presented here have several major implications. First,
wild-type and t chromosomes appear to have undergone quite separate
modes of evolution for a long period of time. The line leading to t
haplotypes must have split from the wild-type line prior to the

divergence of mus musculus and mus domesticus (between 1 and 2 million years ago), since these animals carry wild-type forms of chromosome 17 that share the same proximal inversion. However, closely homologous t haplotypes exist in both domesticus and musculus populations (Nizetic et al., 1984). This observation implies that an introgression of t haplotypes must have occurred from one of these species to the other, subsequent to the establishment of the original founder t chromosome.

The relative inversion in the proximal region of the t complex represents one of the crucial components of the mechanism by which t haplotypes maintain their separate identity, and this inversion appears to have occurred in the wild-type chromosome. Where was the primordial t chromosome located when the wild-type inversion occurred? Was it present as a polymorphism within the same population of mice or was it derived from another species of mus (see Silver, 1982; 1986)? An analysis of the organizations of chromosome 17 in other species could be informative.

The major genetic component of the t-specific property of transmission ratio distortion is a locus called Tcr (Lyon, 1984). The Tcr locus is present within the T66B subregion. It is possible that one of the repetitive elements identified by T66 evolved into the Tcr function after the triplication event in an ancestor to t haplotypes. If this is true, there may not be any formal wild-type analogue of the t-specific Tcr locus.

REFERENCES

Fox H, Silver LM, Martin GR (1984) An alpha globin pseudogene is located within the mouse t complex. Immunogenetics 19:125-130
Fox H, Martin G, Lyon MF, Herrmann B, Frischauf A-M, Lehrach H, Silver LM (1985) Molecular probes define different regions of the t complex. Cell 40:63-69
Herrmann B, Bucan M, Mains P, Frischauf A-M, Silver LM, Lehrach H (1986) Analysis of the proximal portion of the mouse t complex: Evidence for a second inversion within t haplotypes. Cell, in press.
Lyon MF (1984) Transmission ratio distortion in mouse t-haplotypes is due to multiple distorter genes acting on a responder locus. Cell 37:621-628
Nizetic D, Figueroa F, Klein J (1984) Evolutionary relationships between the t and H-2 haplotypes in the house mouse. Immunogenetics 19:311-320
Olds-Clarke P, Peitz B (in press) Fertility of sperm from t/+ mice: Evidence that +-bearing sperm are dysfunctional. Genetical Research
Roehme D, Fox H, Herrmann B, Frischauf A-M, Edstrom J-E, Mains P, Silver LM, Lehrach H (1984) Molecular clones of the mouse t complex derived from microdissected metaphase chromosomes. Cell 36:783-788
Sarvetnick N, Mann E, Mains P, Elliott R, Silver LM (1986) Nonhomologous pairing in mouse t haplotype heterozygotes can produce recombinant chromosomes with adjacent duplications and deletions.
Shin H-S, Stavnezer J, Artzt K, Bennett D (1982) The genetic structure and origin of t-haplotypes of mice, analysed with H-2 cDNA probes. Cell 29:969-976
Silver LM (1982) Genomic analysis of the H-2 complex region associated with mouse t haplotypes. Cell 29:961-968
Silver LM (1986) Mouse t haplotypes. Ann. Rev. Genet. 19:179-208

Silver LM, Olds-Clarke P (1984) Transmission ratio distortion of mouse
    t haplotypes is not a consequence of wild-type sperm degeneration.
    Develop. Biol. 105:250-252
Silver LM, Uman J, Danska J, Garrels JI (1983) A diversified set of
    testicular cell proteins specified by genes within the mouse t
    complex. Cell 35:35-45

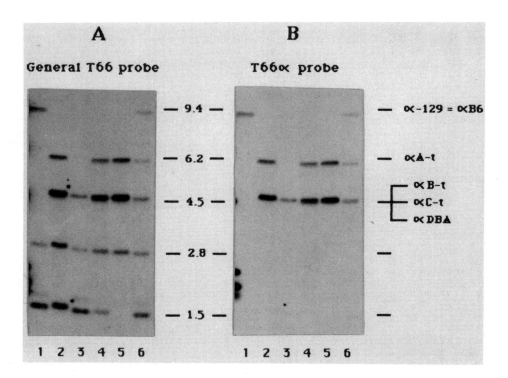

Fig. 2. Genomic analysis with a general probe for all T66 elements
(A) and a more specific probe for the T66-alpha elements (B). The
same blot was probed in sequence with the two clones. Lane 1 is
129/SvJ; lanes 2 & 4 are from animals homozygous for complete t
haplotypes; lane 3 is DBA/2J; lane 5 is from an animal heterozygous
for a partial t haplotype which is missing non-alpha elements; lane 6
is from an animal heterozygous for a t haplotype and a wild-type
chromosome. The 4.5 kb fragment is conserved among the alpha-B-t,
alpha-C-t and alpha-DBA elements.

H-2

Genetic Diversity of Class II Genes in Wild Mice: Definition of Five Evolutionary Groups by RFLP Analysis of A_α and A_β

E.K. Wakeland, R.A. McIndoe, and T.J. McConnell

INTRODUCTION

The class II genes of the murine major histocompatibility complex (H-2) are a tightly linked cluster of highly polymorphic genes which encode molecules involved in the recognition of antigen by T lymphocytes. Biochemical analyses of class II molecules have identified two molecules, designated I-A and I-E, which are expressed on the surfaces of antigen presenting cells and B lymphocytes (Cullen et al. 1976; Uhr et al. 1979). Both molecules are integral membrane glycoproteins and each is a heterodimer formed by noncovalent interactions between an alpha (α) and beta (β) subunit.

The molecular cloning and sequencing of a large portion of the murine $\underline{I}$ region has supplied extensive information on the organization of the murine class II genes and the structures of the molecules they encode (Steinmetz et al. 1982; Choi et al 1983). The $\underline{A_\alpha}$, $\underline{A_\beta}$, $\underline{E_\alpha}$, and $\underline{E_\beta}$ genes are single-copy genes present on a segment of about 100 kilobases (kb) of DNA in the $\underline{I}$ region of the $\underline{H-2}$ complex. Each class II gene consists of at least 5 exons and occupies more than 5 kb of genomic DNA. $\underline{A_\alpha}$, $\underline{A_\beta}$, and part of $\underline{E_\beta}$ are located within a portion of the $\underline{I}$ region which exhibits extensive sequence polymorphism. This region, which has been termed a "polymorphic tract", extends 5' from a recombinational hot spot located within the central intron of $\underline{E_\beta}$ (Steinmetz et al. 1984). The $\underline{E_\alpha}$ gene is located 3' to $\underline{E_\beta}$ in a "conserved tract" of the $\underline{I}$ region and exhibits much less polymorphism than $\underline{A_\alpha}$, $\underline{A_\beta}$, or $\underline{E_\beta}$.

We have been studying the genetic polymorphism of class II genes in wild mouse populations (Wakeland and Klein 1983; Wakeland and Darby 1983; McConnell et al 1986). One goal of these studies has been to determine the evolutionary relationships of $\underline{I-A}$ alleles present in a collection of mouse strains derived from wild mouse stocks obtained from Dr. Richard Sage. Dr. Sage's breeding stocks included wild mice representative of 6 separate sub-species of $\underline{Mus}$ (Sage 1980). We have produced a total of 25 $\underline{H-2}$ homozygous mouse strains which carry these wild-mouse-derived $\underline{H-2}$ haplotypes. We are in the process of genetically characterizing the $\underline{I}$ region alleles present in these new mouse strains and comparing them with the alleles found in the $\underline{H-2}$ haplotypes of standard laboratory mice and the B10.W lines which were produced predominantly from North American wild mice by Jan Klein (Klein 1975).

DEFINITION OF EVOLUTIONARY GROUPS BY RFLP ANALYSIS

The analysis of restriction fragment length polymorphisms (RFLP) detected by Southern blot hybridization with DNA probes specific for $\underline{A_\alpha}$ and $\underline{A_\beta}$ can be used to compare the genomic structures of the $\underline{I-A}$ alleles in our collection of $\underline{H-2}$ haplotypes. We have compared the

restriction fragment (RF) genotypes of 32 I-A alleles digested with
7 restriction endonucleases (Eco RI, Hind III, Bam HI, Sac I, Pst I,
Pvu II, and Kpn I). This RFLP analysis defined 26 A_β alleles and 24
A_α alleles. These findings indicate that the genomic structures of
alleles at each of these loci are highly polymorphic in natural
mouse populations, an observation consistent with the extensive
structural variability of the Aα and Aβ subunits they encode.

The DNA sequence homology among these alleles can be quantitatively
estimated by calculating the fraction homologous (F) value as
defined by Nei and Li (1979). The F value is the fraction of
restriction fragments which two alleles have in common when compared
with a battery of restriction enzymes. F values can vary from 0 to
a maximum of 1.0 with larger values representing greater sequence
homology between the compared alleles. The evolutionary relationships of the A_α and A_β alleles in our panel were determined by
analyses of the F values calculated from pairwise comparisons of all
their RF genotypes. The results indicate that the 26 A_β alleles can
be organized into 5 evolutionary groups while the 24 A_α alleles can
be organized into 2 groups. The mean F values calculated by allelic
comparisons within and between these evolutionary groups are
presented in Table 1.

TABLE 1. Statistical analysis of the F values defining the
evolutionary groups detected by RFLP analysis of A_α and A_β

| Locus | Group | Mean F value + S.D. | |
		Within same group	Between different groups
A_β	1	.63 + .09	.13 + .08
	2	.66 + .14	.14 + .08
	3	.61	.13 + .08
	4	.64	.21 + .10
	5	.78 + .19	.24 + .11
A_α	1	.58 + .16	.31 + .13
	2	1.0	.31 + .13

The comparison of RF genotypes of alleles in the same evolutionary
group yield F values in excess of 0.6 while RF comparisons of
alleles in separate groups generally yield F values below 0.2.
These results indicate that alleles in separate evolutionary groups
have distinct genomic structures which differ in excess of 10% of
their sequence, while alleles within the same evolutionary group
often differ by less then 2%. These estimates are consistent with
previous reports which have indicated that I-A[wr7], I-A[k], and I-A[d]
differ extensively in the non-coding regions flanking these A_α and
A_β alleles (Steinmetz et al 1984). From our analysis, these 3
alleles are in evolutionary groups 2, 5, and 1 respectively and
consequently would be predicted to exhibit very distinct genomic
structures.

A_β evolutionary group 1 contains 7 of the 20 Mus m. domesticus A_β
alleles and all the alleles from the other Mus sub-species in our
collection. Table 2 presents a matrix comparison of A_β allleles in
group 4 with alleles in group 1 which are derived from separate Mus
sub-species.

Table 2. RF genotype comparisons of A_β alleles in separate sub-species of Mus.

Group	Mouse Strain	Mus Species	Group 4		Group 1		
			AZR2	MET4	MET1	BEL1	THON1
4	AZROU2	dom	-	.64	.27	.29	.27
	METKOVIC4	dom	14/22	-	.00	.10	.09
1	METKOVIC1	dom	6/20	0/22	-	.80	.64
	BELGRADE1	mus	6/19	2/21	16/20	-	.64
	THONBURI1	cas	6/20	2/23	14/22	14/22	-

METKOVIC1, BELGRADE1, and THONBURI1, which carry A_β alleles from evolutionary group 1, have H-2 haplotypes derived from domesticus, musculus, and castaneus, respectively. Comparisons of the RF genotypes of their A_β alleles yield values of .80, .64, and .64, indicating that the majority of the restriction fragments compared were identical. AZROU2 and METKOVIC4 have I-A alleles in evolutionary group 4 of Mus m. domesticus and have A_β alleles which are clearly much less related to that of METKOVIC4 than are the evolutionary group 1 A_β alleles derived from musculus and castaneus. These findings suggest that A_β evolutionary group 1, the most common group in domesticus, arose prior to the divergence of these Mus sub-species.

COMPARISONS OF I-A MOLECULES AND I-A RESTRICTION FRAGMENT GENOTYPES

Comparisons of the RF genotypes of I-A alleles provide information on DNA sequence variations throughout the interval of genomic DNA containing A_α and A_β, including sequences contained in exons, introns, and flanking regions. The size of the interval of genomic DNA analyzed with each probe can be estimated from the average size of the sum of all the restriction fragments detected with each restriction enzyme. For the 7 restriction enzymes used in this analysis, the A_β probe hybridized to an average of 9.4 kb of genomic DNA per restriction enzyme digest and the A_α probe hybridized to an average of 7.2 kb. This indicates that the polymorphic restriction enzyme sites assayed in this study are distributed over a large segment of genomic DNA. Since both A_α and A_β are each encoded by about 700 bp of DNA, the majority of the restriction enzyme sites detected reflect DNA sequence variations in non-coding regions. This observation suggests that evolutionary relationships detected by RFLP analysis may not be representative of polymorphisms occuring in the exons.

The evolutionary relationships of the exon portions of these I-A alleles are indirectly reflected by the structures of the A_α and A_β

subunits they encode. If the evolution of the exons is reflected in the evolutionary relationships detected by RFLP analysis, then the I-A molecules encoded by alleles in the same evolutionary group should be structurally more similar to each other than they are to I-A molecules encoded by alleles in different evolutionary groups. We have previously utilized high performance liquid chromatography (HPLC) tryptic peptide fingerprinting to compare the structures of A_α and A_β subunits encoded by I-A alleles (Wakeland and Klein 1983; Wakeland et al 1985). This technique can be used to quantitatively compare the structural variations which distinguish the subunits encoded by different I-A alleles. Table 3 presents a quantitative analysis of the structural variations distinguishing the A_β subunits encoded by alleles in 3 different A_β evolutionary groups.

Table 3. Structural comparisons of A_β subunits encoded by alleles in different evolutionary groups.

Group Strain	1			2			5	
	CAS2	R1ll	SM	M	WB	STC90	PL	BR
1 B10.CAS2	–	.63[a]	.59	.44	.47	.59	.53	.46
B10.R1ll	24/38[b]	–	.65	.61	.47	.63	.63	.57
B10.SM	20/34	22/34	–	.44	.47	.54	.53	.58
2 B10.M	16/36	22/36	14/32	–	.39	.63	.61	.61
B10.WB	18/38	18/38	16/34	14/36	–	.59	.47	.57
B10.STC90	22/37	26/37	18/33	22/35	22/37	–	.65	.83
5 B10.PL	20/38	24/38	18/34	22/36	18/38	24/37	–	.57
B10.BR	16/35	20/35	18/31	20/33	20/35	28/34	20/35	–

[a] Fraction of tryptic peptides which elute identically when these alleles are compared by HPLC tryptic peptide fingerprinting.

[b] Number of differences/total peptides scored.

The results in Table 3 indicate that the structural variations which distinguish these A_β subunits do not correlate well with the evolutionary groups defined by RFLP analysis. With the exception of B10.CAS2 and B10.SM of evolutionary group 1, every I-A allele compared encoded molecules which were more similar to I-A molecules encoded by alleles in another evolutionary group than they were to molecules in their own group. These results suggest that the structures of class II exons may be subject to selective pressures or evolutionary mechanisms which differ from those affecting non-coding regions and indicate that RF genotypes often will not accurately predict the structural relationships of allelic class II molecules. These observations suggest that attempts to correlate specific RFLPs of class II alleles with functional properties of the molecules they encode may not be successful.

The most intriguing data presented in Table 3 involves the structural variations which distinguish the I-A molecules encoded by B10.M, B10.WB, B10.BR, B10.PL, and B10.STC90. Table 4 presents a matrix comparison of the RF genotypes of the A_β alleles present in these 5 Mus m. domesticus-derived H-2 haplotypes.

Table 4. RFLP comparisons of Aβ alleles encoding Aβ subunits
which have been compared by tryptic peptide fingerprinting

Group	Mouse Strain	Group 2			Group 5	
		B10.M	B10.WB	B10.STC90	B10.BR	B10.PL
2	B10.M	–	.88	.57	.28	.10
	B10.WB	22/25	–	.54	.29	.13
	B10.STC90	12/21	13/24	–	.10	.0
5	B10.BR	6/21	7/24	2/21	–	.60
	B10.PL	2/20	3/23	0/19	12/20	–

The data in Table 4 demonstrate that the A$\underline{\beta}$ RF genotypes of B10.M
and B10.WB are very similar (F=0.88) while the A$\underline{\beta}$ RF genotypes of
B10.STC90 and B10.BR are very different (F=0.10). Figure 1 presents
the chromatograms of HPLC tryptic peptide fingerprint comparisons
of the A$_\beta$ subunits encoded by B10.M, B10.WB, B10.BR, and B10.STC90.

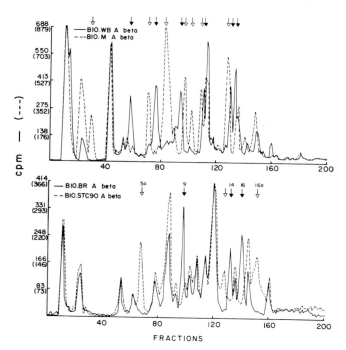

Figure 1. HPLC chromatography of A$_\beta$ tryptic peptides. A$_\beta$ tryptic
peptides from B10.WB are compared with B10.M in the upper panel and
A$_\beta$ tryptic peptides from B10.BR are compared with B10.STC90 in the
lower panel. The arrows at the top of the graphs identify peptides
which elute at different positions in the comparison.

We have previously demonstrated by radiochemical sequencing that the A_β subunits of B10.BR and B10.STC90 differ detectably by only 3 amino acid interchanges, all of which occur in the exon which encodes the amino terminal domain (Wakeland et al. 1985). Yet dispite the close structural similarity of these A_β subunits, they are clearly encoded by alleles in separate evolutionary groups (see Table 4) These observations suggest that exons with very similar sequences are present in A_β alleles with very dissimilar non-coding regions. The relationship of A_β from B10.WB and B10.M illustrates the reverse situation in which alleles with very similar non-coding regions encode A_β subunits with very dissimilar structures.

Taken together, these observations suggest that the exons of these A_β genes can be shifted between alleles with different intron and flanking region structures. Such an event might be mediated by genetic mechanisms such as gene conversion or a specialized type of intragenic recombination. In this regard, more than 90% of all wild mice tested have been shown to be heterozygous at $\underline{I}$ region loci (Duncan et al. 1979; Wakeland and Klein 1981). Thus, intragenic recombination could play a major role in the generation of diversity in the $\underline{I}$ region by utilizing mechanisms similar to the gene conversion mechanisms which are thought to mediate class I gene diversification. Further work in this area should be informative about the role of intragenic recombination in the genetic diversification of class II genes in wild mice.

REFERENCES

Choi EK, Mcintyre K, Germain RN, Seidman SG (1983) Murine I-A_β chain polymorphism: nucleotide sequences of three allelic I-A_β genes. Science 221:283

Cullen SE, Freed JH, Nathenson SG (1975) Structural and serological properties of murine Ia alloantigens. Tansplant Rev 30: 236

Duncan WR, Wakeland EK, Klein J (1979) Heterozygosity of H-2 loci in wild mice. Nature 281:322

Klein J (1975) Biology of the mouse histocompatibility-2 complex. Springer-Verlag, New York.

McConnell TJ, Darby B, Wakeland EK (to be published) Restriction fragment length polymorphisms of class II gene sequences in mice expressing minor structural variants of I-A^k and I-A^p. J Immunol

Nei M, Li WH (1979) Mathematical model for studying genetic variation in terms of restriction endonucleases. PNAS 76:5269

Sage RD (1981) Wild mice. In: Foster HL, Small JD, Fox JG (eds) The mouse in biomedical research, vol 1. Academic Press New York p 40

Steinmetz MK, Minard K, Horvath S, et al. (1982) A molecular map of the immune response region from the major histocompatibility complex of the mouse. Nature 300:35

Steinmetz M, Malissen M, Hood L, et al. (1984) Tracts of high or low sequence divergence in the mouse major histocompatibility complex. EMBO Journal 3:2995

Uhr J, Capra JD, Vitetta ES, Cook RG (1979) Organization of the immune response genes. Science 206:292

Wakeland EK, Klein J (1981) The polymorphism of $\underline{I}$ region encoded antigens among wild mice. In: Reisfeld RA, Ferrone S (eds) Current trends in histocompatibility, Plenum Press New York p322.

Wakeland EK, Klein J (1983) Evidence for minor structural variations of class II genes in wild and inbred mice. J Immunol 130:1280

Wakeland EK, Darby BR (1983) Recombination and mutation of class II histocompatibility genes in wild mice. J Immunol 131:3052

Wakeland EK, Darby BR, Coligan (1985) Localization of structural variations to the α_1 and β_1 domains. J Immunol 135:391

Gene-Specific Structures Within Class I Genes from *Mus musculus domesticus* are Conserved in Class I Genes from *Mus pahari*

M.J. Rogers, D.F. Siwarski, E. Jouvin-Marche, and S. Rudikoff

The class I genes from the Major Histocompatibility Complex (MHC) of Mus musculus domesticus are a highly polymorphic multigene family (Klein 1981). The members of the present day family are thought to have evolved from a single ancestral gene by a number of complex molecular mechanisms ultimately controlled by natural selection. These include gene duplication (Steinmetz 1982; Weiss 1984), mutation, recombination (Artzt 1985), and gene conversion (Weiss 1983; Schulze 1983; Miyada 1985). There is little doubt that the class I gene family expanded by gene duplication and that mutational and recombinational events are responsible for the variation in size and organization of this family seen among different strains of Mus musculus domesticus (Weiss 1984; Rogers 1985) and among different vertebrate species (Ploegh 1981). However, there is some controversy concerning the mechanisms that have generated the polymorphism seen in Mus musculus. A considerable body of evidence suggests that much of the polymorphism existed before speciation of the genus Mus. According to this view the alleles have evolved independently and polymorphism has been maintained by natural selection (Arden 1982). On the other hand there is compelling evidence that gene conversion events involving small (<50 base pairs) segments of DNA have occurred among the class I genes of Mus musculus domesticus. It has been suggested that such events could contribute to class I polymorphism and may be helping to maintain this polymorphism by spreading sequence differences within the family (Schulze 1983; Miyada 1985; Evans 1982).

We have been cloning and sequencing class I genes from a distantly related member of the genus Mus (Mus pahari from the subgenus Coelomys) in order to identify highly conserved, potentially functional non-coding sequences. In addition, we hoped to shed some light on the molecular events occurring during the evolution of this multigene family.

In order to make meaningful comparisons between class I genes from two different species, it is necessary to identify the same gene in both species. This is a formidable problem in Mus pahari which appears to have more class I genes than Mus musculus domesticus (Rogers 1985) and for which no inbred strains, congenic strains or well-characterized serological reagents exist.. In an attempt to overcome this problem, we adopted the following approach. While most class I genes have the same overall exon-intron structure, certain features seem to be gene or region specific. That is, specific DNA sequences and/or amino acid sequences seem to be uniquely associated with either a particular class I gene or all genes from the H-2K, H-2D, Qa or Tla regions of the MHC. Some of these features are summarized in Fig. 1. For example, a particular

NC2 region from the 3' end of a Qa gene will be associated with particular amino acid sequences in the transmembrane region. We reasoned that if a particular group of features found associated with Qa genes in Mus musculus domesticus were all associated with a particular gene from Mus pahari, it would be reasonable to conclude that that gene from Mus pahari is also from the Qa region. In this way, particular genes from Mus pahari could be compared with their counterparts from Mus musculus. Of course, if features from different Mus musculus genes were found associated on the same Mus pahari gene, meaningful evolutionary comparisons would not be possible. However, this would have important implications for the relationship of these structures to the functions of class I genes from different regions of the MHC.

VARIATIONS IN MURINE CLASS I GENE STRUCTURE

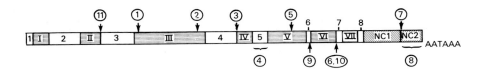

1   ~ 1200 extra bp containing ALU type repeats in Tla genes.
2   ~ 900 extra bp containing ALU type repeats in H2K, H2D and Qa genes.
3   Three additional 3' codons in exon 4 in H2D and Qa genes.
4   Some Qa genes contain mutations or deletions resulting in TRM in exon 5.
5   Intron V ~ 200 bp shorter in H2K, H2D, Qa than in Tla.
6   Three additional 5' codons in exon 7 of Tla genes.
7   Tla and H2D genes contain ALU repeats between NC1 and NC2.
8   NC2 region contains H2K or Qa specific sequenes.
9   Exon 6 is 2-3 times longer in Tla genes.
10 Mutations eliminating splice acceptor site for exon 7 in Qa genes.
11 Three extra codons at 5' end of exon 3 in Tla genes.

Fig. 1. At the top of the figure is a schematic diagram of a typical class I gene drawn approximately to scale including exons 1-8 (Arabic numerals), introns 1-7 (Roman numerals) and the 3' non-coding region up to the polyadenylation signal. The non-coding region has been divided into first and second segments (NC1 and NC2, respectively) on the basis of homology considerations pointed out by others (see Kress 1983; Xin 1982; and legend to Table 1). Arrows with circled numbers indicate the positions of unusual structural features which are thought to be region specific, i.e., associated with class I genes from the H-2K, H-2D, Qa or Tla regions of the MHC. These features are briefly described below the figure. References are as follows: 1,2,5,6 (Ronne 1985); 3 (Sher 1985; Steinmetz 1981); 4 (Steinmetz 1981; Cosman 1982); 7 (Obata 1985; Kress 1984); 8 (Xin 1982; Lalanne 1985; Kress 1983); 9,11 (Obata 1985; Fisher 1985); 10 (Steinmetz 1981; Mellor 1984).

From the point of view of evolution of class I genes, if particular features are associated in the same gene from both Mus pahari and Mus musculus domesticus, species that have been separated for approximately 10^7 years, it would strongly suggest that these associations predated the separation of these species. Moreover, the evolutionary stability of these associations would suggest that recombinational events involving these features have not occurred among class I genes or have not been selected for during the time that these species have been separated.

MATERIALS AND METHODS

Screening of the Mus pahari library

Between two and three genome equivalents of a Mus pahari library (Jouvin-Marche, this volume) were screened with the Q10 probe (Kress 1983) and pMHCI, a cDNA probe containing sequences from exons 2 and 3 of the H-2L^d gene (Evans 1982). Hybridizations were performed in 50% formamide, 5 X SSC and stringency washes were performed at 42°, 0.2 X SSC. Positive clones were plaque purified twice.

Sequencing

All sequencing was performed by the dideoxy method of Sanger (1980) using S^{35} labelled ATP.

Miscellaneous Procedures

Conditions for Southern blot hybridizations, preparation of DNA and restriction endonuclease digestions have been described (Rogers 1985).

RESULTS

Cloning of Class I Genes from a Mus pahari Library Using a Gene Specific Probe

In order to test whether the unusual structural features of particular class I genes remain associated during evolution, we attempted to clone the Q10 gene from Mus pahari. The Q10 gene is a Qa gene isolated from Mus musculus domesticus that encodes a secreted class I molecule (Cosman 1982; Mellor 1984). This gene was particularly well suited to our purposes because it contains several of the gene specific characteristics outlined in Fig. 1. In addition, precipitation with antiserum prepared against a specific peptide revealed that a very similar secreted protein was present in a large, representative sampling of species from the genus Mus, including Mus pahari (Siwarski 1985).

We performed a Southern blot hybridization with a Q10 specific
probe (Cosman 1982b) to DNA from a sampling of species representing
the entire genus Mus. This probe (a 146 base pair [bp] Pst I fragment composed of 43 bp from the NC1 region and 103 bp from the NC2
region) identified only one or two genes in all species tested
(Siwarski 1985). Using this low copy number probe we set out to
clone the class I gene(s) with the homologous NC2 sequence from a
Mus pahari library and then ask the question whether it also contained the other features associated with the Q10 gene.

We screened approximately 2-3 genome equivalents of a λJ1 library
from Mus pahari with both the Q10 probe and a coding region probe
from the H-2L^d gene that hybridized with most class I genes from
inbred Mus musculus domesticus (Evans 1982). From 175 phage clones
hybridizing to the class I coding region probe, only 12 hybridized
to the low copy number Q10 probe as well under conditions of high
stringency. Two of these, designated MPa5 and MPa51, were selected
for further study.

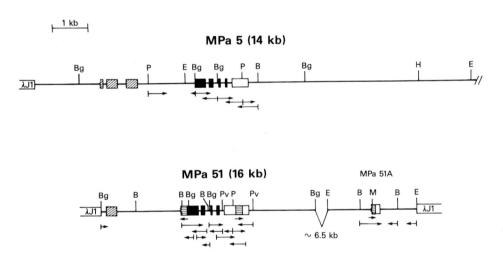

Fig. 2. Schematic diagrams of genomic clones containing class I
genes from Mus pahari. Closed, open or diagonally lined boxes
represent coding exons from class I genes. Open and closed exons
were determined by sequencing. Diagonally lined exons were inferred
by extensive restriction site mapping and hybridization to a variety
of class I probes from Mus musculus domesticus. Arrows with small
horizontal bars indicate sequencing strategy. The horizontally
lined boxes are B2 type repeat sequences and the arrows beneath them
indicate the 5'-- 3' orientation of the repeat. Restriction sites
are Bg, Bgl II; B, Bam HI; P, Pst I; Pv, Pvu II; E, Eco RI; M, Mbo I.
Open boxes labelled λJ1 indicate the limits of the genomic insert
and the beginning of vector sequences.

The restriction maps of these two clones are shown in Fig. 2. Clone
MPa5 contained a single, complete class I gene while clone MPa51
contained two partial genes. Gene MPa51A contained only a partial

B2 repeat, an NC2 region and 3' flanking region having homology to Mus musculus domesticus class I genes. Experiments are in progress to establish whether this is a cloning artifact or represents a partial gene generated by a mutational or recombinational event. Gene MPa51 contained exons 3-8 and 3' non-coding region but was interrupted in intron 2 by the cloning vector.

The sequence of exon 5 from genes MPa5 and MPa51 indicated that they would not encode secreted class I proteins similar to those from Mus musculus domesticus. Within this exon which encodes the transmembrane region, the Q10 gene contains a characteristic deletion and unique amino acid substitution (Cosman 1982). These were not present in exon 5 of gene MPa5 or gene MPa51.

The nucleotide sequences of the NC2 regions of the three Mus pahari genes are compared with the NC2 regions of representative class I genes from the 4 regions of the MHC of Mus musculus domesticus in Table 1. Gene MPa5 clearly falls into the H-2K,D class. The sequence of the NC1 region of gene MPa5 revealed that it hybridized to the Q10 probe by virtue of strong homology to the 43 bp of NCI region included in the probe (Cosman 1982b). The NC2 regions of genes MPa51 and MPa51A were more closely related to Q10 than to another Qa region gene, 27.1. Since, as mentioned above, neither gene could encode an secreted protein, these results and previous data (Siwarski 1985) suggest that several Q10 related genes exist in Mus pahari (see Discussion).

Table 1. Percent homologies[a] in the NC2 region of Mus pahari genes with class I genes from Mus musculus domesticus

| Gene or region of MHC[b] | Mus pahari gene | | |
	5	51	51A
K,D	82	66	64
Qa	76	71	76
Q10	66	80	83
Tla	59	71	61

[a] Nucleotide substitutions were counted directly. Sequence of Q10 probe was from Kress (1983). Deletions and insertions were counted as single events regardless of the number of bases involved. Inserted or deleted bases were not counted in the total when calculating percentages. Percent homology = 100 minus percent nucleotide substitutions.
[b] The genes used for comparison were: K,D, the H-2K gene from the b haplotype (Weiss 1983); Qa, the 27.1 gene from the d haplotype (Steinmetz 1981); Q10, the Q10 gene from the b haplotype (Mellor 1984); Tla, the T13 gene from the d haplotype (Fisher 1985).

These results indicate that the unique sequences of the NC2 region that are associated with distinguishable subgroups of class I genes in Mus musculus domesticus can be identified in the genes from Mus pahari. However, the data also show that the NC2 region is not better conserved than other non-coding regions within or near the gene. For example, when gene MPa5 is compared with the H-2K^b gene the percent homology is only 82% for the NC2 region, but 90% for the 3' flanking region, the NC1 region and the total introns (data not shown).

Structural Analysis of Mus pahari Class I Genes

The sequence of the NC2 region indicated that gene MPa5 was from the K or D region of the MHC and gene MPa51 was from the Qa region. Consequently we sequenced the 3' portions of these two genes beginning 100-200 bp 5' of exon 4 and continuing 100-200 bp 3' to the NC2 region (~1.7 kb, see Fig. 2). The sequences contained proper splice donor and acceptor sites, no stop codons within exons, and polyadenylation signals. Thus, both Mus pahari genes could be expressed provided that their 5' exons were intact. These sequences and the restriction maps in Fig. 2 were analyzed to see if other features of these genes also conformed to the classification indicated by the sequence of the NC2 region. Most of the features shown in Figure 1 were considered as well as certain specific amino acid sequences (Kimball, 1983) and overall nucleotide and amino acid sequence homology. The results are summarized in Table 2 and discussed below.

The sequences of Tla genes that have been obtained from Mus musculus domesticus are so unusual that they are immediately distinguishable from K, D or Qa genes (Obata 1985; Fisher 1985). It was clear from our sequence that neither gene MPa5 nor gene MPa51 was related to these Tla region genes. Therefore, further comparisons were made only with genes from the K, D and Qa regions. These genes were H-2K^b (Weiss, 1983), H-2L^d (Evans 1982; Moore 1982), the Qa region gene 27.1 (Steinmetz 1981), H-2K^d (Kvist 1983), Q10 (Mellor 1984, Kress 1983b), H-2D^d (Sher 1985), H-2D^b (Reyes 1982) and H-2K^q (Arnold 1985).

For most of the features analyzed, the Mus pahari genes could be clearly assigned to a particular region of the MHC based on identity or close similarity to the Mus musculus domesticus genes from that region. Where two regions are assigned in Table 2, it is not due to ambiguities in the Mus pahari gene, but because the Mus musculus domesticus genes from both regions share that feature.

We found that the nucleotide sequences of both Mus pahari genes were not strongly homologous to a particular gene from Mus musculus domesticus (Table 2, feature 3). The same was true for the predicted amino acid sequence of gene MPa51 (Table 2, feature 4). We attribute this to the fact that our sequences are not complete and do not include most of the introns from these genes. Ronne et al. (1985) have shown that the complete nucleotide sequences from introns reliably reflected evolutionary relationships among class I genes from various regions of the MHC, while sequences from exons did not.

Table 2. Features of genes MPa5 and MPa51 that are associated with
a particular region of the major histocompatibility complex
from Mus musculus domesticus[a]

Feature	MPa5	MPa51
1 Sequence of NC2 region	K,D	Qa
2 Length and structure of intron 3	K,D	Qa
3 Nucleotide sequence (exons 4-8, introns 4-7, 3' noncoding)	No decision possible	No decision possible
4 Amino acid composition (exons 4-8)	D	No decision possible
5 Amino acid residue 141	D,Qa	Not determined
6 Amino acids 296-299 (exon 5)	D,Qa	D,Qa
7 Amino acids 329-337 (exon 7)	D,Qa	D,Qa
8 Structure of exon 7	D,Qa	Qa
9 Repetitive sequence between NC1 and NC2	K,Qa	D

[a] Features are listed in the left column. K,D,Qa in the MPa5 or
MPa51 column indicates that with regard to that feature, the Mus
pahari genes are similar or identical to the Mus musculus domesticus genes of the H-2K, H-2D or Qa region, respectively. Where two
regions are indicated, the available data do not allow a distinction between the alternatives.

The sequence and the structure of exon 7 from the two Mus pahari
genes are unusual. Both of these genes have suffered a single base
deletion which eliminated the normal splice acceptor site at the
beginning of exon 7 found in most murine class I genes. A similar
alteration eliminating this splice acceptor is found in two Qa
region genes from Mus musculus domesticus that have been sequenced
(Steinmetz 1981; Mellor 1984). However, unlike the Qa genes, both
genes from Mus pahari contain an alternate splice acceptor 9 nucleotides upstream from the deletion. If these splice sites were used,
both gene MPa5 and MPa51 would encode a protein with 16 amino acids
in the second internal domain as opposed to 13 for the class I genes
from Mus musculus domesticus. On the basis of the characteristic
deletion in the splice acceptor site, we could assign both genes to
the Qa region (Table 3, feature 8). In addition, excluding the insertion of 9 extra nucleotides, the nucleotide sequence of exon 7
from gene MPa5 was 100% homologous to the H-2D[d] gene. Therefore,
we also assigned gene MPa5 to the D region on the basis of exon 7
sequence (Table 3, feature 8).

The summary in Table 2 illustrates that the Mus pahari genes are
remarkably similar to class I genes from Mus musculus domesticus
that bear the same NC2 regions. Gene MPa5 was most closely related
to D region genes from Mus musculus domesticus in 7 out of 8

features analyzed. Gene MPa51 was most closely related to Qa region
genes in 6 out of 7 features analyzed. The major discrepancy involved the presence or absence of a B2 interspersed repeat in the 3'
non-coding region.

DISCUSSION

While we have not yet succeeded in cloning the homologue of the Q10
gene from Mus pahari using the Q10 probe, our data support the contention that a probe from the NC2 region is capable of distinguishing
genes from different regions of the MHC. The data in Table 1 show
that the sequences of the NC2 regions of both Mus pahari genes were
clearly more homologous to Mus musculus domesticus class I genes
from a particular region. The summary in Table 2 indicates that
most features associated with a particular NC2 region in Mus
musculus domesticus genes were also associated with that NC2 region
in the genes from Mus pahari. The exceptions were the Qa-like deletion in the splice acceptor site for exon 7 in gene MPa5 (Table 2,
feature 8), the inappropriate B2 repeat present in the non-coding
region of MPa51, and the missing B2 repeat in the non-coding region
of MPa5 (Table 2, feature 9). Where two assignments were made, it
was not due to ambiguities in the structure of the Mus pahari gene,
but because that particular feature is shared by class I genes from
two regions of the MHC in Mus musculus domesticus.

Accumulating evidence suggests that the longer 48 nucleotide exon 7
in the Mus pahari genes is the ancestral form and that the shorter
39 nucleotide seventh exon seen in the H-2K and H-2D genes from Mus
musculus domesticus have been derived by a deletion mechanism (Marche
1985). Thus, the class I HLA genes from human and the RLA genes
from rabbit all contain an exon 7 that is 48 nucleotides in length
(Marche 1985; Sodoyer 1984). Moreover, some Tla region genes, which
appear to be the oldest genes in the MHC (Ronne 1985; Hood 1985),
the longer exon 7 (Obata 1985; Hood 1985), although it is not normally translated in many Tla genes. On the basis of these considerations, we conclude that the shorter exon 7 in the H-2K and H-2D
genes is restricted to Mus musculus domesticus and is not a general
feature of genes from this region.

If the structure of exon 7 is omitted as a distinguishing feature
on this basis, then the data are completely consistent with the
assignment of gene MPa5 to the H-2D region of the MHC with the
exception of the missing B2 repeat in the 3' non-coding region (Fig.
3). The data suggest, therefore, that the insertion of the B2 repeat
into the 3' non-coding portion of the H-2D region genes of Mus
musculus domesticus may have occurred after separation of this
species from Mus pahari. Alternatively, additional H-2D genes may
exist in the Mus pahari genomes that contain a B2 repeat in this
position.

Similarly, the data are completely consistent with the assignment of
gene MPa51 to the Qa region with the exception of the B2 repeat in
the 3' non-coding region. Our sequence comparisons suggested that
none of the Qa genes from Mus musculus domesticus that have been
sequenced represent the exact homologue of gene MPa51. Therefore,
it is conceivable that the true homologue of gene MPa51 may contain

a similar B2 repeat in the 3' non-coding region. Alternatively, this B2 repeat may also have been inserted subsequent to separation of the species.

Although, as mentioned above, none of the Mus pahari genes were equivalent to Q10, the data in Table 1 indicate that the NC2 regions of genes MPa51 and MPa51A are more homologous to Q10 than to another Qa gene. While other interpretations are possible, this suggests that genes MPa51 and MPa51A are part of a sub-group of Qa genes closely related to Q10 in Mus pahari. Moreover, one member of the group must be significantly more homologous to Q10 than either gene MPa51 or MPa51A, because the Q10 probe detected a different gene in Southern blots of genomic DNA from Mus pahari (Siwarski 1985).

These data are consistent with a model in which recombinational events involving large segments of genes from different regions of the MHC do not occur frequently, at least within the 3' region we have considered here. However, the data do not exclude the possibility of recombination between similar genes in the same region of the MHC or of gene conversion events involving short stretches of DNA. Sequences from the more polymorphic exons of the Mus pahari genes are needed to clarify this point. We are currently sequencing the 5' regions of these genes and preparing single copy probes from coding and flanking regions to determine whether the genes are expressed, and to locate them more precisely within particular regions of the MHC of Mus musculus domesticus. These studies should provide further insights into the evolution of class I genes.

REFERENCES

Arden B, Klein J (1982) Biochemical comparison of major histocompatibility complex molecules from different subspecies of Mus musculus: evidence for trans-specific evolution of alleles. Proc Natl Acad Sci USA 79:2342-2346

Arnold B, Burgert HG, Archibald AL, Kvist S (1985) Complete nucleotide sequence of the murine H-2K^b gene and comparison with three H-2K locus alleles. Nucleic Acids Res 12:9473-9482

Artzt K, Shin H, Bennett D, Dimeo-Talento A (1985) Analysis of major histocompatibility complex haplotypes of t-chromosomes reveals that the majority of diversity is generated by recombination. J Exp Med 162:93-104

Cosman D, Khoury G, Jay G (1982) Three classes of mouse H-2 mRNA distinguished by analysis of cDNA clones. Nature 295:73-76

Cosman D, Kress, M, Khoury G, Jay G (1982b) Tissue specific expression of an unusual H-2 (class I)-related gene. Proc Natl Acad Sci USA 79:4947-4951

Evans GA, Margulies DH, Camerini-Otero RD, Ozato K, Seidman JG, (1982) Structure and expression of a mouse major histocompatibility antigen, H-2L^d. Proc Natl Acad Sci USA 79:1994-1998

Fisher DA, Hunt SW, Hood L (1985) Structure of a gene encoding a murine thymus leukemia antigen and organization of the Tla gene in the BALB/c mouse. J Exp Med 162:528-545

Kimball ES, Coligan JE (1983) Structure of class I major compatibility antigens. In: Inman FP, Kindt TJ (eds) Contemporary topics in immunology, vol 9. Plenum Press, New York, p 1

Klein J, Figueroa F (1981) Polymorphism of the mouse H-2 loci. Immunological Rev 60:23-57

Kress M, Barra Y, Seidman JG, Khoury G, Jay G (1984) Functional insertion of an Alu type 2 (B2 SINE) repetitive sequence in murine class I genes. Science 226:974-977

Kress M, Glaros D, Khoury G, Jay G (1983b) Alternative splicing in the expression of the H-2K gene. Nature 306:602-604

Kress M, Liu WY, Jay E, Khoury G, Jay G (1983) Comparison of class I (H-2) gene sequences. Derivation of unique probes for numbers of this multigene family. J Biol Chem 258:13929-13936

Kvist S, Roberts L, Dobberstein B (1983) Mouse histocompatibility genes: structure and organization of a K^d gene. EMBO J 2:245-254

Lalanne JL, Transy C, Guerin S, Darche S, Meulien P, Kourilsky P (1985) Expression of clas I genes in the major histocompatibility complex: identification of eight distinct mRNAs in DBA/2 mouse liver. Cell 41:469-478

Marche PN, Tykocinski ML, Max EE, Kindt TJ (1985) Structure of a functional rabbit class I MHC gene: similarity to human class I genes. Immunogenetics 21:71-82

Mellor A, Weiss EH, Kress M, Jay G, Flavell RA (1984) A nonpolymorphic class I gene in the murine MHC. Cell 36:139-144

Miyada CG, Klofelt C, Reyes AA, McLaughlin-Taylor E, Wallace RB (1985) Evidence that polymorphism in the murine major histocompatibility complex may be generated by the assortment of subgene sequences. Proc Natl Acad Sci USA 82:2890-2894

Moore KW, Sher BT, Sun YH, Eakle KA, Hood L (1982) DNA sequence of a gene encoding a BALB/c mouse L^d transplantation antigen. Science 215:679-682

Obata Y, Chen Y, Stockert E, Old LJ (1985) Structural analysis of the TL genes of the mouse. Proc Natl Acad Sci USA 82:5475-5479

Ploegh HL, Orr HT, Strominger JL (1981) Major histocompatibility antigens: the human (HLA-A-B-C) and murine (H-2K, H-2D) class I molecules. Cell 24:287-299

Reyes AA, Schold M, Wallace RB (1982) The complete amino acid sequence of the $H-2D^b$ transplantation antigen as deduced by molecular cloning. Immunogenetics 16:1-9

Rogers MJ, Germain RN, Hare J, Long E, Singer DS (1985) Comparison of MHC genes among distantly related members of the genus Mus. J Immunol 134:630-636

Ronne H, Widmark E, Rask L, Peterson PA (1985) Intron sequences reveal evolutionary relationships among major histocompatibility complex class I genes. Proc Natl Acad Sci USA 82:5860-5864

Sanger F, Nicklen S, Coulson AR (1977) DNA sequencing with chain terminating inhibitors. Proc Natl Acad Sci USA 76:5463-5467

Schulze DH, Pease LR, Geier SS, Reyes AA, Sarmiento LA, Wallace RB, Nathenson SG (1983) Comparison of the cloned $H-2K^{bm1}$ variant gene with the $H-2K^b$ gene shows a cluster of seven nucleotide differences. Proc Natl Acad Sci USA 80:2007-2011

Siwarski DF, Barra Y, Jay G, Rogers MJ (1985) Occurrence of a unique MHC class I gene in distantly related members of the genus Mus. Immunogenetics 21:267-276

Sodoyer R, Dannotte M, Delovotch TL, Trucy J, Jordan BR, Strachan T (1984) Complete nucleotide sequence of a gene encoding a functional human class I histocompatibility antigen (HLA cw3). EMBO J 3:879-885

Sher BT, Nairn R, Coligan JE, Hood L (1985) DNA sequence of the mouse $H-2D^d$ transplantation antigen gene. Proc Natl Acad Sci 82:1175-1179

Steinmetz M, Moore KN, Frelinger JG, Sher BT, Shen FW, Boyse EA, Hood L (1981) Pseudogene homologous to mouse transplantation antigens: transplantation antigens are encoded by eight exons that correlate with protein domains. Cell 25:683-692
Steinmetz M, Winoto A, Minard K, Hood L (1982) Clusters of genes encoding transplantation antigens. Cell 28:489-498
Weiss EH, Golden L, Fahruer K, Mellor AL, Devlin JJ, Bullman H, Tiddens H, Bud H, Flavell RA (1984) Organization and evolution of the class I gene family in the major histocompatibility complex of the C57BL/10 mouse. Nature 310:650-655
Weiss E, Golden L, Zakut R, Mellor A, Fahrner K, Kvist S, Flavell RA (1983) The DNA sequence of the H-2K^b gene: evidence for gene conversion as a mechanism for the generation of polymorphism in histocompatibility antigens. EMBO J 2:453-462
Xin JH, Kvist S, Dobberstein B (1982) Identification of an H-2K^d gene using a specific cDNA probe. EMBO J 4:467-471

Genetic Variants of Histocompatibility Antigens from Wild Mice

K. Fischer Lindahl

INTRODUCTION

Had it not been for wild mice, the genetic analysis of Mta, a maternally transmitted histocompatibility antigen of mice, would have ended
five years ago. Testing 79 inbred strains of laboratory mice, we had
identified only two forms of Mta, positive (now known as Mta[α,a]) and
negative (Mta[β,a]), and shown that the difference was determined by a
maternally transmitted factor, Mtf (Fischer Lindahl et al. 1980;
Fischer Lindahl and Hausmann 1983). But then the plethora of genetic
variation in wild mice led to the identification of a chromosomal
gene, Hmt, involved in Mta expression (Fischer Lindahl et al. 1983),
yielded new alleles of Mtf, Hmt, and B2m (Robinson et al. 1984), gave
a clearer picture of the roles of Mtf and Hmt in expression of Mta
(Fischer Lindahl 1985a), and led to the discovery of new recombinational hot spots in the H-2 complex (Steinmetz et al., submitted).
This paper will briefly describe the new strains that are under inbreeding as a result of this work.

THE GENETICS OF Mta

Mta is a weak transplantation antigen, most easily detected by cytotoxic T cells and expressed on all nucleated cells. The antigenic
structure of Mta is determined jointly by the allelic forms of Mtf and
Hmt (Fischer Lindahl et al., submitted). Mtf is transmitted in the
egg and is strictly maternally inherited (Fischer Lindahl and Bürki
1982). Rare alleles of Mtf are correlated with unique mitochondrial
DNA restriction fragment patterns (Ferris et al. 1983; Fischer Lindahl
et al., in preparation). In somatic cell hybrids, the expression of a
particular Mta type is correlated with the presence of mitochondrial
DNA from the corresponding fusion partner (Smith et al. 1983; Huston
et al. 1985). Mtf is therefore thought to be a mitochondrial gene,
yet to be identified.

Monoclonal antibodies against β_2-microglobulin (β2m) block lysis by
Mta-specific killer cells (Fischer Lindahl et al. 1983), and variant
cell lines incapable of making β2m do not express Mta (Fischer Lindahl
and Langhorne 1981). The killer cells specific for Mta are not H-2-
restricted (Fischer Lindahl et al. 1980), and Hmt has been mapped to
the distal end of the H-2 complex, between Tla and Upg-1 (Fischer Lindahl et al. 1983). We have therefore proposed that Hmt codes for a
class I major histocompatibility antigen, expressed on the cell surface in association with β2m. The Mta target antigen is then formed
by the association of this class I molecule with a mitochondrially en-

Table 1. Mouse strains congenic for mitochondrial DNA

Strain	Donor	Background	N[a]
NZB.Mtf$^{\alpha}$ (ANN)[b]	A.CA/Ibm	NZB/Bom	20
B6.Mtf$^{\beta}$ (NMB)[b]	NMRI/Bom	C57BL/6JIbm	17
B6.Mtf$^{\gamma}$	WLA76	C57BL/6JIbm	11
D2.Mtf$^{\gamma}$	WLA76 (Toulouse/Guénet)[c]	DBA/2JIbm	9
B10.MilP	*M. m. domesticus* (Pavia/Winking)[c]	C57BL/10ScSn[d]	5
B6.Mtf$^{\delta}$	SUB-SHH	C57BL/6JIbm	6
BALB.Mtf$^{\delta}$	SUB-SHH (Shanghai/Moriwaki)[c]	BALB/cJIbm	4

[a] Number of generations of backcrossing as of October 1985.
[b] Older designation.
[c] Geographic origin and breeder.
[d] Strain is also congenic for H-2 (see Table 3).

coded protein (or a breakdown product thereof) that somehow reaches the cell surface (Fischer Lindahl 1985a; Hirama and Fischer Lindahl 1985).

THE Mtf ALLELES

We have isolated two new forms of Mtf from wild mice and shown that each of the four forms of Mtf determines a unique cell surface antigen together with a particular Hmt allele (Fischer Lindahl et al., in preparation). Because of the strict maternal inheritance (Fischer Lindahl 1985a), no typing is necessary to breed strains congenic for Mtf or mitochondrial DNA (Table 1).

Table 2. Strains carrying B2m alleles from wild mice

Strain	B2m donor	Source	Background	N[a]
B10.B2m^{w1}	*Mus spretus*	(Cadiz/Potter)	C57BL/10ScSn	6
B10.B2m^{w2}	*M. m. brevirostris*	(Azrou/Potter)	C57BL/10ScSn	5
BALB.B2m^{w3}	*M. m. bactrianus*	(Lahore/Moriwaki)	BALB/cJIbm	6
B.B.B2m^{w4}	*M. m. bactrianus*	(Lahore/Moriwaki)	BALB.B/OlaBii	6
B.B.B2m^{w5}	*M. m. domesticus*	(Isle of May/Triggs)	BALB.B/OlaBii	2

[a] Number of generations of backcrossing as of October 1985.

Table 3. Strains carrying H-2 haplotypes from wild mice with new
alleles of Hmt

Hmt	Strain[a]	H-2 donor (haplotype)	Source	N[b]
b	B6.CAS3	M. m. castaneus (cas3)	Thailand/Chapman	8
	B10.CAS3	M. m. castaneus (cas3)	Thailand/Chapman	6
	C3H.CAS3	M. m. castaneus (cas3)	Thailand/Chapman	8
	B10.CAS4	M. m. castaneus (cas4)	Thailand/Chapman	8
	C3H.CAS4	M. m. castaneus (cas4)	Thailand/Chapman	6
	B10.BAC2	M. m. bactrianus	Lahore/Moriwaki	6
	B10.MilII	M. m. domesticus	Milano/Winking	5
	B10.MilB	M. m. domesticus	Milano/Winking	6
	B10.MilP[c]	M. m. domesticus	Pavia/Winking	5
c	B10.SPA1	Mus spretus (sp1)	Cadiz/Potter	6
	B10.SPA2	Mus spretus (sp2)	Cadiz/Potter	5
	B10.SPE	SPE1 (sp3)	Granada/Guénet	2
d	B10.BAC1	M. m. bactrianus	Lahore/Moriwaki	9

a Background strains are B6 – C57BL/6JIbm, B10 – C57BL/10ScSn, and
C3H – C3H/HeJIbm.

b Number of backcross generations as of October 1985.

c Strain also congenic for Mtf$^\gamma$ (see Table 1).

THE B2m ALLELES

Only two forms of β2m have been detected in laboratory mice, the common β2m^a and the rare β2m^b (Michaelson 1983). β2m^a is characteristic
of Mus musculus domesticus and β2m^b of M. m. musculus, molossinus, and
castaneus, but our screening of wild mice also revealed several new
allelic forms that differ by their electrophoretic mobility, isoelectric point, and antigenic determinants (Robinson et al. 1984). These
new alleles are now being backcrossed to standard inbred strains for
further analysis (Table 2). None of them changes the antigenic specificity of Mta.

THE Hmt ALLELES

To date we have identified four alleles of Hmt. The a allele is by
far the most common, present in all subspecies of Mus musculus tested.
The c allele is characteristic of Mus spretus. The b allele was first
found among M. m. castaneus (Fischer Lindahl et al. 1983) and later
among wild mice from the Milano area (Fischer Lindahl et al., in preparation). The d allele came from a small stock of M. m. bactrianus
and its distribution is unknown (Fischer Lindahl et al., in preparation).

Table 4. Recombinant H-2 haplotypes from cas3 and cas4 backcrossing

Strain	H-2 donors	Background	K[a]	A	E	S	D	Q2	Tl	Ql	Hmt
R0	cas3/b (?)[b]	C57BL/10	c3'	b	b	b	b	b	b	b	b
R1	cas3/C3H	C57BL/10	c3	c3	c3	c3	c3	c3'	k	k	k
R2	cas4/C3H	C57BL/10	k '	c4	c4	c4	c4	c4	c4	c4	c4
R3	cas3/C3H	Extinct[c]	c3	c3	c3	c3'	k	k	k	k	k
R4	cas3/C3H	C3H.SW	k	k	k	k	k	k	k	k '	c3
R5	cas4/C3H	C3H.SW	k '	c4	c4	c4	c4	c4	c4	c4	c4
R6	cas4/C3H	Extinct[c]	k '	c4	c4	c4	c4	c4	c4	c4	c4
R7	cas3/B6	C57BL/6	c3	c3	c3	?	b	b	b	b	b
R8	cas3/R0	B10.BR	c3	c3	c3	?	b	b	b	b	b
R9	cas3/B6	C57BL/6	b	b	b	b	b	?	c3	c3	c3
R10	cas3/B6	C57BL/6	b	b	b	?	c3	c3	c3	c3	c3
R11	R3/C3H.SW	C3H/HeJ	b '	c3	c	c3	k	k	k	k	k
R12	R2/B10	C57BL/10	b	b	b	?	c4	c4	c4	c4	c4
R13	cas4/B10	C57BL/10	b	b	b	?	c4	c4	c4	c4	c4
R14	cas4/C3H	C3H.SW	c4	c4	c4	?	k	k	k	k	k
R16	cas3/B10	C57BL/10	b	b	b	b	b	?	c3	c3	c3
R18	R7/B6	C57BL/6	c3'	b	b	b	b	b	b	b	b
R22	R4/C3H.SW	Extinct[c]	k	?	?	?	b	b	b	b	b
R23	R8/B10.BR	C57BL/6	k '	c3	c3	?	b	b	b	b	b
R24	R0/B10.BR	C57BL/6	k	k	k	?	b	b	b	b	b
R25	R7/B6	C57BL/6	c3'	b	b	b	b	b	b	b	b
R28	cas4/B10	C57BL/10	c4	c4	c4	?	b	b	b	b	b
R29	cas4/B10	C57BL/10	b	b	b	?	c4	c4	c4	c4	c4
R30	R4/C3H.SW	C3H.SW	b	b '	k	k	k	k	k	k	c3

[a] Haplotype origin of the H-2 marker loci H-2K (K), I-A (A), E$_\alpha$ (E), Ss (S), H-2D (D), Qa-2 (Q2), Tla (T1), Qa-1 (Q1), and Hmt is indicated by lower case letters, not necessarily corresponding to standard allele designations. Position of most recent crossover is marked by ' or ?, when allele is still unknown.
[b] The R0 haplotype was found in the original M. m. castaneus stock and is presumed to be a recombinant.
[c] Haplotype lost in breeding.

In backcrossing the new alleles of Hmt onto inbred backgrounds (Table 3), I have taken advantage of the close linkage to H-2 by using the convenient serological assays for H-2, Ia and TL antigens (Fischer Lindahl, 1985b) rather than the cumbersome cytotoxic T cell assays for Hmt. I have therefore simultaneously isolated new alleles of various markers associated with the H-2 complex, including Tla and Qa-1, which await further characterization.

Table 5. Strains with H-2 alleles derived from the SUB-SHH stock

Strain	H-2 donor	K	A	E$_\alpha$	D	Tla	N[a]
B10.SHH1	SUB-SHH	sl	sl	sl	sl	sl	3
B10.SH1(R17)	SHH1/C57BL/10	sl	sl	sl	b	b	4
B10.SH1(R20)	SHH1/C57BL/10	sl	sl	sl	b	b	5
B10.SH1(R21)	SHH1/B10.CAS2	sl	sl	sl	wl7	wl7	4
B10.SH1(R27)	SHH1/C57BL/10	b	b	b	?	sl	5
B10.SHH2	SUB-SHH	s2	s2	s2	s2	s2	2
B10.SH2(R19)	SHH2/B10.CAS2	s2	s2	?	wl7	wl7	4

[a] Number of generations of backcrossing as of October 1985.

RECOMBINATIONAL HOT SPOTS

Obviously the tight linkage of Hmt to H-2 is also a disadvantage, as the stronger H-2 antigens will interfere with any immunological characterization of new forms of the Hmt gene product. So far, only the Hmt[b] allele of the cas3 haplotype has been isolated from H-2 by recombination (Table 4). The breeding of the castaneus H-2 haplotypes has made it clear that recombinational events are not randomly distributed. For instance, we have four recombinants between H-2D and Hmt of the cas3 haplotype, but none with cas4, despite a larger number of mice typed.

The most striking recombinational hot spots were found in the chromosomal interval from the H-2K to the A$_\beta$ gene. Typing of some 9,000 laboratory mice yielded only two recombinants in that interval (Klein 1975); typing of 900 cas3 and cas4 backcross progeny yielded eight (Table 4). Not only is the recombination frequency for the interval increased forty-fold, but all the crossovers are clustered within two small chromosomal regions, one for the cas3 and one for the cas4 haplotype (Steinmetz et al., submitted; see also Steinmetz, this volume). A similar phenomenon has been reported for a molossinus H-2 haplotype (Shiroishi et al. 1982), and a weaker recombinational hot spot was identified in the E$_\beta$ gene of common laboratory haplotypes a, b, d, k, and s (Steinmetz et al. 1982).

Once the E$_\alpha$ gene has been linked to the H-2D locus at the molecular level, it will be possible to test whether the many recombinants in that interval are also clustered around hot spots. In addition to the castaneus haplotypes, I have found at least one H-2 haplotype in a stock from Shanghai that may have a hot spot in this interval. Among 130 backcross progeny typed were four recombinants (Table 5).

CONCLUSIONS

Wild mice represent a valuable source of genetic variation, and it is clearly faster to screen representative stocks of different species and subspecies than to induce mutations in the desired gene in laboratory mice, even with the most effective technique available (Peters

1985). Even the drudgery that follows, if the new allele must be extracted for study on a standard inbred background, may have its re-
wards in the form of interesting recombinants. <u>Mus spretus</u> is the
most distant species that will still breed with laboratory mice, and,
not unexpectedly, we found species-specific new alleles of both <u>B2m</u>
and <u>Hmt</u> from <u>spretus</u>. However, evolutionary distance does not guaran-
tee new alleles. Thus we were surprised that the <u>Mtf</u> of <u>spretus</u> and
laboratory mice are indistinguishable despite a 10% divergence in the
nucleotide sequence of their mitochondrial DNA (Fischer Lindahl et
al., submitted). Other new alleles of histocompatibility antigens
were found only in a single area, stressing the need to test wild mice
from many different places all over the world.

ACKNOWLEDGEMENTS

I wish to thank especially Dr. Peter Hjorth, Århus University, Denmark, who provided my first samples of wild mice, and to express my
gratitude to all those mouse fanciers who have since generously shared
their stocks. Typing for β2m was done in collaboration with Dr. Peter
Robinson, German Cancer Research Center, Heidelberg. The Basel Institute for Immunology was founded and is supported by F. Hoffmann-
La Roche and Co., Ltd., Basel, Switzerland.

REFERENCES

Ferris SD, Ritte U, Fischer Lindahl K, Prager EM, Wilson AC (1983)
   Unusual type of mitochondrial DNA in mice lacking a maternally
   transmitted antigen. Nucleic Acids Res 11:2917-2926
Fischer Lindahl K (1985a) Mitochondrial inheritance in mice. Trends
   Genet 1:135-139
Fischer Lindahl K (1985b) Tissue typing using biosynthetically la-
   beled monoclonal antibodies. In: Lefkovits I, Pernis B (eds) Im-
   munological methods, vol 3. Academic Press, New York, p 187
Fischer Lindahl K, Bürki K (1982) Mta, a maternally inherited cell
   surface antigen of the mouse, is transmitted in the egg. Proc Natl
   Acad Sci USA 79:5362-5366
Fischer Lindahl K, Hausmann B (1983) Cytoplasmic inheritance of a
   cell surface antigen in the mouse. Genetics 103:483-494
Fischer Lindahl K, Langhorne J (1981) Medial histocompatibility anti-
   gens. Scand J Immunol 14:643-654
Fischer Lindahl K, Bocchieri M, Riblet R (1980) Maternally trans-
   mitted target antigen for unrestricted killing by NZB T lymphocytes.
   J Exp Med 152:1583-1595
Fischer Lindahl K, Hausmann B, Chapman VM (1983) A new H-2-linked
   class I gene whose expression depends on a maternally inherited factor. Nature 306:383-385
Fischer Lindahl K, Hausmann B, Robinson PJ, Guénet JL, Wharton DC,
   Winking H (submitted) Mta, the maternally transmitted antigen, is
   determined jointly by the chromosomal <u>Hmt</u> and the extrachromosomal
   <u>Mtf</u> genes.
Hirama M, Fischer Lindahl K (1985) Mouse mitochondria and the cell
   surface. In: Quagliariello E, Slater EC, Palmieri F, Saccone C,
   Kroon AM (eds) Achievements and perspectives of mitochondrial research, vol 2: Biogenesis. Elsevier, Amsterdam, in press

278

Huston MM, Smith III R, Hull R, Huston DP, Rich RR (1985) Mitochondrial modulation of maternally transmitted antigen: analysis of cell hybrids. Proc Natl Acad Sci USA 82:3286-3290

Klein J (1975) Biology of the mouse histocompatibility-2 complex. Springer, Berlin Heidelberg New York

Michaelson J (1983) Genetics of beta-2-microglobulin in the mouse. Immunogenetics 17:219-259

Peters J (1985) Ethylnitrosourea as a mouse mutagen. Trends Genet 1:5-6

Robinson PJ, Steinmetz M, Moriwaki M, Fischer Lindahl K (1984) Beta-2-microglobulin types in mice of wild origin. Immunogenetics 20:655-665

Shiroishi T, Sagai T, Moriwaki K (1982) A new wild-derived H-2 haplotype enhancing K-IA recombination. Nature 300:370-372

Smith III R, Huston MM, Jenkins RN, Huston DP, Rich RR (1983) Mitochondria control expression of a murine cell surface antigen. Nature 306:599-601

Steinmetz M, Minard K, Horvath S, McNicholas J, Frelinger J, Wake C, Long E, Mach B, Hood L (1982) A molecular map of the immune response region from the major histocompatibility complex of the mouse. Nature 300:35-42

Steinmetz M, Stephan D, Fischer Lindahl K (submitted) Gene organisation and recombinational hot spots in the proximal portion of the murine major histocompatibility complex.

Polymorphism and Recombinational Hot Spots in the Murine MHC

M. Steinmetz

GENE ORGANIZATION

Over the past five years enormous progress has been made in the elucidation of the molecular biology of the murine major histocompatibility complex (MHC) (for reviews see Klein et al, 1983; Mengle-Gaw and McDevitt 1985; Steinmetz 1985). Forty-six genes have been cloned and identified from the MHC of the BALB/c mouse and ordered into six gene clusters encompassing more than 1600 kb of DNA (Fig. 1). The largest cluster spans 600 kb of DNA and links the 2 class I genes located in the K region to the 7 class II genes in the I region. A gap of unknown size separates this cluster from a 250 kb cluster located entirely in the S region containing 6 genes unrelated to class I and class II genes. These genes code for the complement components C2, Bf and C4, for the C4-related Slp molecule and for 21-hydroxylase, an enzyme involved in steroid biosynthesis. The second largest cluster, 500 kb in size, links the D to the Qa region and contains 13 class I genes. Finally, 18 class I genes have been mapped into 3 gene clusters, 160, 80 and 40 kb in size, all located in the Tla region.

The function for only 3 of the 33 class I genes and 4 of the 7 class II genes is known. The K, D and L genes code for the α chains of the corresponding class I, and the A_α, A_β, E_α and E_β genes code for α and β chains of the I-A and I-E class II molecules. These class I and class II molecules are involved in the presentation of foreign antigens to cytotoxic and helper T cells (for a review, see Schwartz 1985). The function of the remaining class I and class II genes is unknown.

RECOMBINATIONAL HOT SPOTS

Three recombinational hot spots, defined as sites where crossing-over events occur repeatedly at high frequencies, have been identified in the 600 kb gene cluster spanning the K and I regions of the MHC (Steinmetz et al. 1982; Kobori et al. 1984; Steinmetz, Stephan and Fischer Lindahl, submitted; see also Fischer Lindahl, this volume) (Fig. 2). Two hot spots have been found between the K and A_β genes, one in the cas3 haplotype and one in the cas4 haplotype of M.m. castaneus. Eight independent recombination events have occured at these hot spots at a frequency of 0.6-1.5%. In contrast, recombinants which have been found at a comparatively low frequency of 0.02% in genetic crosses of different laboratory mouse strains have undergone crossing-over at distinct locations (Fig. 2). This indicates that recombinational hot spots do not occur in laboratory strains of mice between the K and A_β genes. On the other hand it appears that the wild-derived MHC haplotype of the B10.MOL-SGR mouse strain, which

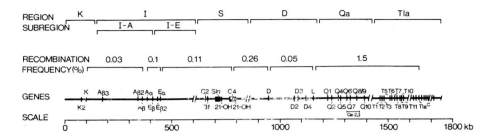

Fig. 1   Molecular map of the major histocompatibility complex of the BALB/c mouse. The 6 gene clusters have been correlated with the genetic map of the MHC, divided into six regions and two subregions. Recombination frequencies between marker loci of laboratory mouse strains are indicated. The map is based on published and unpublished results (Fisher et al. 1985; Mellor et al. 1985; Steinmetz et al. 1982 and manuscripts in preparation).

shows 2% recombination frequency between the K and I region marker loci, also contains a recombinational hot spot in this portion of the MHC (Shiroishi et al. 1982).

A third recombinational hot spot has been mapped to the large intervening sequence in the Eβ gene, between the two exons coding for the β1 and β2 external domains of the β chain (Steinmetz et al. 1982; Kobori et al. 1984). Nine independent recombination events have occurred at this position (Fig. 2) at a frequency of 0.1%. Part of the intron has been sequenced (Saito et al. 1983) and a search for an unusual structure that could form the molecular basis of the recombinational hot spot revealed a CAGG tetramer, repeated in tandem about 20 times (Steinmetz, Stephan and Fischer Lindahl, submitted). This sequence bears a low homology (62%) to the Chi sequence, known to be a hot spot in phage λ. More significantly, it also contains 21 intermingled copies with 50-80% homology to the human hypervariable minisatellite core sequence (Jeffreys et al. 1985), believed to be a recombinational hot spot.

Finding a similar repeat sequence at the two other recombinational hot spots discussed above would substantially strengthen the idea that the repeat constitutes the hot spot. Alternatively, chromatin organization might suppress recombination over extended regions of DNA except for small stretches which are accessible to the recombination machinery and are therefore scored as hot spots. However, it has been shown that site specific recombination in the human β globin locus is not reduced in cells which do not express the gene as compared to those showing active transcription (Smithies et al. 1985). Furthermore, recombination suppression in t haplotypes when crossed with wild-type chromosomes appears to be due to a chromosomal inversion rather than a different chromatin organization (Artzt et al. 1982). Thus the hypothesis that a special DNA sequence forms the basis for recombination hot spots is presently favored.

The genetic length of the mouse genome is about 1600 centiMorgans and its physical size 3 x 10^9 bp. If recombination frequency and physical length would be proportional, 1 centiMorgan should correspond to about 2000 kb of DNA. Clearly, such a proportionality does not exist. For instance, in laboratory mouse strains, a ratio of 0.1 centiMorgan per 1000 kb is observed between K and Aβ and 1.8 cen-

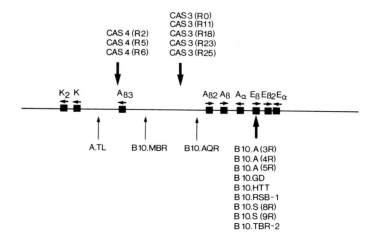

Fig. 2   Location of 20 independent recombination events in the proximal part of the MHC.   Genes are indicated by boxes.   Horizontal arrows show 5' to 3' orientation.   Recombinational hot spots are indicated by heavy vertical arrows.   Recombinants obtained from crosses between M.m. castaneus and laboratory mouse strains are listed on the top, those obtained from crosses between different laboratory strains on the bottom.   Laboratory strains appear to lack a hot spot between K and A_β.   For a more detailed discussion see Steinmetz, Stephan and Fischer Lindahl (submitted).

tiMorgan per 1000 kb between A_α and E_α.   Thus, recombination frequencies are lower than the average (0.5 centiMorgan/1000 kb) in regions where recombinational hot spots are absent (between K and A_β), but higher where hot spots are present (between A_α and E_α).   The activity of a recombinational hot spot might also vary.   For instance, the recombinational hot spots which are found between the K and A_β genes and between the A_α and E_α genes enhance recombination by a factor of 10 and 3, respectively, as compared to the average.   The calculation is based on the reasonable assumption that the physical distance between the K and A_β genes is not drastically different in BALB/c and M.m. castaneus mouse strains.

POLYMORPHISM

DNA sequence information for several class I and class II alleles has confirmed the extreme polymorphism of certain MHC genes in the mouse. Thus the K, D, A_α, A_β and E_β genes vary extensively between different strains (e.g. 16% of the amino acid residues are different between the K^b and K^d molecules) while for instance the Q10, $E_{\beta2}$ and E_α genes are more conserved.   The variability observed in the highly polymorphic MHC molecules is primarily confined to 3 or 4 hypervariable regions in the $\alpha1$ and $\alpha2$ domains of class I and the $\alpha1$ and $\beta1$ domains of class II molecules.   The functional significance of this extreme polymorphism is unclear. It might be important for covering "holes" in the T cell repertoire that arise in individual members of a spe-

282

cies due to self tolerization. Since T cells show specificity for both the foreign antigen and the MHC allomorph, the polymorphic residues must be involved in antigen recognition. Crystallographic analyses will be needed to understand the precise molecular interactions between T cell receptor, antigen and MHC molecule.

At least 3 recombinational mechanisms operate on MHC genes to generate and maintain polymorphism: homologous equal and unequal crossing-over and gene conversion. First, gene expansion and contraction events by unequal crossing-over alter the number of MHC genes and occasionally generate new hybrid genes. Variation in gene number between strains of mice has been found for genes located in the S, D, Qa and Tla regions (Weiss et al. 1984; Lévi-Strauss et al. 1985; Steinmetz unpubl. results). Hybrid genes, apparently generated by unequal crossing over, have been identified in the B10.D2-H-2^{dml} mouse strain (a D/L hybrid gene, Sun et al. 1985) and in BALB/c mice (a Q8/Q9 hybrid gene and an additional Q6/Q7 hybrid gene in the BALB/cBy substrain, Weiss et al. 1984; Mellor et al. 1985). Presumably the unequal crossing-over events in the distal portion of the MHC are favored by the large number of closely-spaced class I genes, most of which appear to have the same 5' to 3' orientation and high sequence homology.

Second, gene conversion-like events introduce mutations into class I and class II genes. Evidence that important functional alterations are generated this way has been obtained in the C57BL/6 mouse (Pease et al. 1983). Most, if not all, of the spontaneous mutations, which have occured in the K^b gene at an unusually high rate (2.2 x 10^{-4} per locus per gamete) and led to the rejection of skin grafted from the mutant to the parent, appear to result from the transfer of a block of sequence (perhaps up to 50 bp in length) from one of several potential donor genes to the K^b acceptor gene (Mellor et al. 1983, Nathenson et al. 1985). Furthermore, the Aβ^{bml2} mutant gene appears to have been generated by a sequence transfer from the Eβ^b to the Aβ^b gene (McIntyre and Seidman, 1984). Thus, gene conversion-like events appear to occur at a high rate in C57BL/6 mice, presumably in coding and non-coding sequences. From the pool of mutated sequences those MHC genes that contain biologically useful variations in their coding sequences will be selected and established in the population.

Third, homologous recombination, preferentially occurring at recombinational hot spots, shuffles alleles between different haplotypes thus generating individuals with new sets of MHC molecules. Recombinant haplotypes will be subject to positive and negative selective forces, which might favor variability in the population for some segments of the MHC but not for others. In this regard it is interesting to note that in the mouse the highly polymorphic class II alleles, A$_\alpha$, A$_\beta$ and E$_\beta$, are clustered and that recombinational hot spots are found to the left and right of the polymorphic sequences but not in between (Fig. 2). If the E$_\alpha$ gene or a gene closely linked to it is under tight selectional constraint while variability in the A$_\alpha$, A$_\beta$ and E$_\beta$ genes is favored, then placing the E$_\alpha$ gene away from the other class II genes onto a different chromosome might be useful - unless linkage is required for other reasons, e.g. to coregulate the genes or to promote gene conversion-like events. Under such circumstances, the placement of a recombinational hot spot between these genes might reflect the optimal solution. Evidence that the recombinational hot spot in the E$_\beta$ gene constitutes a boundary between a polymorphic and a more conserved tract of DNA has indeed been obtained (Steinmetz et al. 1984).

SUMMARY AND CONCLUSIONS

It is likely that most of the DNA from the MHC of the BALB/c mouse
has now been cloned. Forty-six genes spread over 1600 kb of DNA have
been identified. It remains to be seen whether additional genes are
present on the clones already isolated or will be found once the
remaining gaps have been closed by chromosome walking experiments.
One of many surprising findings made during the molecular exploration
of the MHC is the discovery of recombinational hot spots. It is likely
that selective forces have established recombinational hot spots in the
MHC to promote the generation and maintenance of polymorphism. Thus
at least 3 recombinational mechanisms, homologous equal and unequal
crossing-over and gene conversion-like events, contribute to the unusual variability observed for MHC molecules between individual members of a species.

ACKNOWLEDGEMENTS

I thank Kirsten Fischer Lindahl for comments on the manuscript. The
Basel Institute for Immunology was founded and is supported by
F. Hoffmann-La Roche, Limited Company, Basel, Switzerland.

REFERENCES

Artzt K, Shin H-S, Bennett D (1982) Gene mapping within the T/t
complex of the mouse. II. Anomalous position of the H-2 complex in
t haplotypes. Cell 28:471-476
Fisher DA, Hunt III SW, Hood LE (1985) Structure of a gene encoding
a murine thymus leukemia antigen and organization of Tla genes in
the BALB/c mouse. J Exp Med 162:528-545
Jeffreys AJ, Wilson V, Thein SL (1985) Hypervariable minisatellite
regions in human DNA. Nature 314:67-73
Klein J, Figueroa F, Nagy ZA (1983) Genetics of the major histocompatibility complex: The final act. Ann Rev Immunol 1:119-142
Kobori JA, Winoto A, McNicholas J, Hood L (1984) Molecular characterization of the recombination region of six murine major histocompatibility complex (MHC) I-region recombinants. J Mol Cell Immunol 1:125-131
Lévi-Strauss M, Tosi M, Steinmetz M, Klein J, Meo T (1985) Multiple
duplications of complement C4 gene correlate with the H-2
controlled testosterone independent expression of its sex-limited
isoform. Proc Natl Acad Sci USA 82:1746-1750
McIntyre KR, Seidman JG (1984) Nucleotide sequence of mutant
I-Aβbm12 gene is evidence for genetic exchange between mouse
immune response genes. Nature 308:551-553
Mellor AL, Weiss EH, Ramachandran K, Flavell RA (1983) A potential
donor gene for the bml gene conversion event in the C57BL mouse.
Nature 306:792-795
Mellor AL, Antoniou J, Robinson PJ (1985) Structure and expression
of genes encoding murine Qa-2 class I antigens. Proc Natl Acad Sci
USA: in press
Mengle-Gaw L, McDevitt HO (1985) Genetics and expression of murine
Ia antigens. Ann Rev Immunol 3:367-396
Nathenson SG, Geliebter J, Geier SS, Mashimo H, Hemmi S, Kumar A,
McGovern D, Nakagawa M, Pfaffenbach G, Pontarotti P, Zeff R (1985)
The study of H-2 major histocompatibility complex mutants reveals
structure-function relationships and mechanisms of generation of
diversity and polymorphism. In: Streilein et al. (eds) Advances in

gene technology: molecular biology of the immune system. Cambridge
University Press, Cambridge p37-40

Pease LR, Schulze DH, Pfaffenbach GM, Nathenson SG (1983) Spontaneous H-2 mutants provide evidence that a copy mechanism analogous to gene conversion generates polymorphism in the major histocompatibility complex. Proc Natl Acad Sci USA 80:242-246

Saito H, Maki RA, Clayton LK, Tonegawa S (1983) Complete primary
structures of the Eβ chain and gene of the mouse major histocompatibility complex. Proc Natl Acad Sci USA 80:5520-5524

Schwartz RH (1985) T-lymphocyte recognition of antigen in association with gene products of the major histocompatibility complex.
Ann Rev Immunol 3:237-261

Shiroishi T, Sagai T, Moriwaki K (1982) A new wild-derived H-2
haplotype enhancing K-IA recombination. Nature 300:370-372

Smithies O, Gregg RG, Boggs SS, Koralewski MA, Kucherlapati RS (1985)
Insertion of DNA sequences into the human chromosomal β-globin
locus by homologous recombination. Nature 317:230-234

Steinmetz M, Minard K, Horvath S, McNicholas J, Frelinger J, Wake C,
Long E, Mach B, Hood L (1982) A molecular map of the immune
response region from the major histocompatibility complex of the
mouse. Nature 300:35-42

Steinmetz M, Malissen M, Hood L, Örn A, Maki RA, Dastornikoo GR,
Stephan D, Gibb E, Romaniuk R (1984) Tracts of high or low
sequence divergence in the mouse major histocompatibility complex.
EMBO J 3:2995-3003

Steinmetz M (1985) Genes of the immune system. In: Rigby PWJ (ed)
Genetic engineering, vol 5 Academic Press, London, in press

Sun H, Goodenow RS, Hood L (1985) Molecular basis of the dml mutation in the major histocompatibility complex of the mouse: A D/L
hybrid gene. J Exp Med: in press

The *t*-Complex and Ovarian Teratocarcinogenesis

J.H. Nadeau and D. Varnum

INTRODUCTION

Two of the many unanswered questions about the t-complex are the nature of the lethal effects controlled by recessive genes within the t-complex and whether recombination is suppressed between the t-complex and the centromere. Ovarian teratomas, which occur frequently in LT/Sv females (Stevens and Varnum 1974) and females of related strains, can be used to study both problems. Because ovarian teratomas originate from oocytes that have completed the first but not the second meiotic division (Eppig et al 1977), the vast majority of teratomas in heterozygous females are homozygous, unless recombination occurred between the centromere and a marker locus in which case the teratoma would be heterozygous. A number of congenic strains are being produced in which a t-complex is being transferred to the LT/Sv inbred strain or to the closely related LT.MA-$Glo-1^b$ congenic strain. During construction of the LT.MA- + $Glo-1^b$.TT6- t^6 $Glo-1^c$ congenic strain, which is hereafter designated LT-t^6/+ and which is now at the 14th generation of back-crossing, it became apparent that heterozygosity for the t^6-haplotype affected the frequency of ovarian teratomas. The purpose of this note is to document this effect and to present results of experiments whose purpose was to identify factors contributing to the reduced frequency.

The frequency of spontaneous ovarian teratomas in LT-t^6/+ females

Both t^6/+ and +/+ segregants of LT-t^6/+ females were autopsied at about three months of age (+/- 10 days) and the presence of macroscopically detectable teratomas was scored. Since the frequency of teratomas did not vary significantly either between generations N4 to N14 or between reciprocal crosses, data were pooled. The frequency of teratomas in LT-t^6/+ (t^6/+) females was about 4-fold less than the frequency in both their +/+ sisters and in LT.MA-$Glo-1^b$ females (Table 1) and about 10-fold less than the frequency in LT/Sv females (Stevens and Varnum 1974). Experiments were undertaken to determine which step in the process leading to teratomas was affected in these LT-t^6/+ congenic females.

The incidence of parthenogenetically activated oocytes

One hypothesis to account for the reduced frequency of teratomas is that the t^6-haplotype reduced the frequency of parthenogenetically activated oocytes. Histological analysis of ovaries from LT-t^6/+ females that were approximately 3-months old showed that the frequencies of activated oocytes in LT-t^6/+ (t^6/+) females and their +/+ sisters were significantly different (Table 1). However, the 1.4-fold reduction in the frequency of activated oocytes was insufficient to account for the 4-fold reduction in the frequency of macroscopic teratomas. In addition, the products of induced ovulation in LT-t^6/+ (t^6/+) females, their +/+ sisters, and LT.MA-$Glo-1^b$ females were examined for parthenogenetically activated oocytes, but no significant differences were found (Table 1).

The size of ovarian teratomas in LT-t^6/+ females

It could be hypothesized that activated oocytes in females heterozygous for the t^6-haplotype were less likely to become teratomas or, alternatively, once they become teratomas their stem cells were less likely to proliferate. Ovaries from 3-month old females were histologically examined and the frequency of microscopic teratomas was estimated. The frequencies of microscopic teratomas in LT-t^6/+ (t^6/+) females and their +/+ sisters were not significantly different (Table 1). This result suggests that the reduced frequency of macroscopic teratomas in LT-t^6/+ (t^6/+) females results from a failure of stem cells in small teratomas to proliferate.

Homozygous teratomas in heterozygous females

Another hypothesis to account for the reduced frequency of macroscopic teratomas is that teratomas homozygous for the t^6-haplotype are inviable; the t^6-haplotype has a recessive gene that results in embryonic lethality at about the egg cylinder stage (Glucksohn-Schoenheimer 1940). This explanation does not account for the magnitude of the reduction, however, because less than 50% of spontaneous teratomas are expected to be homozygous for the t^6-haplotype. Lethality would at most produce a 2-fold reduction.

Table 1. Characteristics of (LT.MA-Glo-1^b × LT-t^6/+) F_1 and LT.MA-Glo-1^b females.

	Strain	Frequency	N	χ^2	P
Frequency of	LT.MA-Glo-1^b	0.23	53	-	-
macroscopic	LT-t^6/+ +/+	0.22	68		
teratomas	t^6/+	0.05	186	17.40	< 0.001
Frequency of	LT-t^6/+ +/+	0.84	38		
ovaries with	t^6/+	0.62	71	5.79	< 0.05
activated oocytes					
Frequency of	LT.MA-Glo-1^b	0.23	354	-	-
activated oocytes	LT-t^6/+ +/+	0.21	109		
among products of	t^6/+	0.29	79	1.62	NS
induced ovulation					
Frequency of	LT-t^6/+ +/+	0.29	38		
microscopic	t^6/+	0.23	71	0.56	NS
teratomas					

Another explanation is that teratomas that are homozygous for H-2, i.e. t^6/t^6 or +/+, are rejected in H-2 heterozygous (t^6/+) females (cf Cudkowitz and Stimpfling 1964). This hypothesis was tested by determining the Glo-1 genotype of spontaneous macroscopic teratomas in LT-t^6/+ (t^6 H-2^{w30} Glo-1^c/+ H-2^d Glo-1^b) heterozygous females. Of the five teratomas from LT-t^6/+ (t^6/+) heterozygous females that were typed, two were (t^6 Glo-1^c/t^6 Glo-1^c), two were (+ Glo-1^b/+ Glo-1^b), and one was (t^6 Glo-1^c/+ Glo-1^b). The occurrence of homozygous t^6/t^6 and +/+ teratomas, even in this limited sample, suggests that resistance to H-2 homozygous teratomas in H-2 heterozygous females does not account for the reduced frequency of teratomas. These results also suggest that teratomas homozygous for the t^6-haplotype were viable and that recombination occurred between the t^6-haplotype and the centromere.

The composition of teratomas

Histological analysis revealed that teratomas in LT-t^6/+ (t^6/+) females were composed almost exclusively of trophoblastic giant cells, yolk sac and Reichert's membrane, all of which are extra-embryonic derivatives. Occassionally, immature neuroepithelium and brain cells were observed. Noteably absent were muscle, cartilage, bone, and endodermal derivatives, while only 1 of 16 teratomas had undifferentiated cells. All of these are common in ovarian teratomas from LT/Sv females (Stevens and Varnum 1974). The composition of teratomas in LT-t^6/+ (+/+) females has not been fully characterized because too few +/+ teratomas were available for histological examination.

SUMMARY

There was a dramatic reduction both in the frequency of large teratomas and in the frequency of teratomas with tissues such as muscle, cartilage, and bone. By contrast, neither the frequency of parthenogenesis nor of small teratomas appear to be affected. We hypothesize that one or more loci within the t^6-haplotype, and perhaps its wild-type homologue, restrict the differentiation or proliferation of some, but not all, homozygous teratoma cells arising in t^6/+ heterozygous females.

ACKNOWLEDGEMENTS

This work was supported by NSF grant PCM8215004 to JHN

REFERENCES

Cudkowicz G, Stimpfling JH (1964) Hybrid resistance to parental bone marrow grafts: Association with the K region of H-2. Science 144:1339-1340

Eppig JJ, Kozak LP, Eicher EM, Stevens LC (1977) Ovarian teratomas in mice are derived from oocytes that have completed the first meiotic division. Nature 269: 517-518

Gluecksohn-Schoenheimer S (1940) The effect of an early lethal (t^0) in the house mouse. Genetics 25:391-400

Stevens LC, Varnum D (1974) The development of teratomas from parthenogenetically activated ovarian mouse eggs. Devel Biol 37:369-380

T-Cell Receptor

The Context of T Cell Receptor β Chain Genes Among Wild and Inbred Mouse Species

K. Huppi, L. A. D'Hoostelaere, and E. Jouvin-Marche

INTRODUCTION

The organization of the mouse T cell receptor (TCR) genes has been extensively reviewed (Hood 1985). The structure of the TCR alpha (α), beta (β) and gamma (γ) genes is analogous to the immunoglobulin (Ig) gene organization in the mouse. This homology probably reflects similar requirements for diversity in binding antigen. The major source of diversity for Ig genes comes from (1) multiple germline variable (V_K, $V\lambda$ and V_H) regions, diversity (D_H) regions and joining (J_K, $J\lambda$ and J_H) elements; (2) combinatorial joining of V, D and J; (3) somatic mutation and (4) multiple alleles present in inbred and wild mice (Tonegawa 1983). Preliminary findings among the TCRα and β chains of the mouse inbred strains indicate fewer germline variable ($V_{T\alpha}$, $V_{T\beta}$) genes are available (30-40 each) (Becker 1985; Barth 1985; Behlke 1985a) than V_K and V_H genes (100-300 each) (Valbuena 1978; Cory 1981; Brodeur and Riblet 1984). Furthermore, studies indicate that the frequency of somatic mutation in TCRα and TCRβ chain genes although present is as much as 10% or less than that of Ig genes (Augustin and Sim 1984; Ikuta 1985). The apparent lack of extensive $V_{T\alpha}$ or $V_{T\beta}$ germline gene repertoire or somatic mutation places more emphasis on the alternative sources of TCR diversification such as is found in recombination events and larger allelic gene pools. The J_T region genes in the mouse genome are located 5' to each of two constant beta genes ($C_{T\beta}1$, $C_{T\beta}2$), one constant alpha gene ($C_{T\alpha}$) and three constant gamma genes ($C_{T\gamma}7.5$, $C_{T\gamma}10.5$ and $C_{T\gamma}13.4$).

Although only two major haplotypes have been determined for $C_{T\beta}$ in the mouse (Epstein 1985; Sim 1985; Cazenave, this volume), it is possible that significantly diverse alleles may be found among the wild mouse population. A recent report (Kotzin 1985) has found a deletion of the entire $C_{T\beta}1$ gene and $J_{T\beta}2$ region genes in the inbred mouse NZW. This raises questions as to whether deletions of this sort result in impaired T cell function. Alternatively, absence of particular $C_{T\beta}$ or $J_{T\beta}$ genes may be a common feature among wild mouse populations.

We have examined the content and context of the TCR $V_{T\beta}1$, $J_{T\beta}$ and $C_{T\beta}$ genes among inbred and wild mouse species by Southern hybridization analysis. In a survey of this kind individuals from the wild mouse population have been chosen to represent at best a broad phylogenetic spectrum of mouse species. Southern hybridization analysis of restriction fragment length polymorphism (RFLP) is only useful when particular restriction sites differ among samples. In the absence of RFLPs there can be no conclusion that every base pair of the DNA sequence is identical between individuals. Therefore, our

Southern hybridization survey permits us to examine whether a single $V_{T\beta 1}$ gene and two $C_{T\beta}$ genes are consistently found among commensal and feral mice. We can also determine to some degree the extent of allelic polymorphism of the TCR_β genes among the wild mouse population.

Source of DNA Probes and Mice

The inbred mice used in this study were obtained largely from The Jackson Laboratory, Bar Harbor, ME. All of the wild mouse species and the following inbred mouse strains are maintained at Hazelton Laboratories under contract no. NO1-CB-25584: AKR/N, AL/N, BALB/cAnPt, BALB/cJ, C57BL/Ka, C57BL/6J, DBA/2N, STS/A, SJL/JLwPt. Livers were harvested from individual mice and DNA was extracted as described (Huppi 1985). The stringency of wash conditions for all hybridizations performed in this study is 15 mM sodium chloride, 1.5 mM sodium citrate at 65°C.

The $C_{T\beta}$ specific probe was isolated from the $86T_5$ cDNA clone and includes $J_{T\beta 1}$ and $C_{T\beta 1}$ regions (Hedrick 1984). The $V_{T\beta 1}$ probe is derived from the $86T_1$ cDNA clone (Hedrick 1984) and reflects the nomenclature for $V_{T\beta}$ genes adopted (Barth 1985; Behlke 1985). The $J_{T\beta 1}$ specific probe was isolated from the genomic phage clone WSB1.1.1 which contains the $C_{T\beta 1}$ region of M. m. domesticus (WSB). The $J_{T\beta 1}$ probe represents the $3'$ side of the $J_{T\beta 1}$ cluster including at least $J_{T\beta 5}$ and $J_{T\beta 6}$ (manuscript submitted).

Two $C_{T\beta}$ Regions are Found Among Mouse Species

Hybridization of $C_{T\beta}$ to a panel of DNA from inbred or rat strains and wild mouse species indicates that three restriction fragment (RF) bands are consistently observed (Fig. 1). In BALB/c, $C_{T\beta}$ hybridizes to 5.0 kilobase (kb) 5.5 kb and 10.0 kb BamHI RF bands corresponding to 5' $J_{T\beta 1}$, $C_{T\beta 2}$ and $J_{T\beta 1}$-$C_{T\beta 1}$-$J_{T\beta 2}$ regions, respectively. Although many of the inbred mouse strains exhibit the same $C_{T\beta}$ BamHI RF patterns as BALB/c, there is a distinct RFLP in the SJL/J strain (D'Hoostelaere 1985; Epstein 1985 and Fig. 1). The SJL BamHI RF band for $C_{T\beta 1}$ is 6.7 kb rather than 10 kb as found in BALB/c. The wild mouse species M. m. domesticus (WSB and CLA), M. m. brevirostris and Mus spretus display $C_{T\beta}$ Bam RF patterns similar to SJL/J. In the case of WSB and CLA, the $C_{T\beta}$ RF pattern is identical, however, subsequent restriction digestions with Hind III or EcoRI (manuscript in preparation) show the $C_{T\beta}$ haplotypes for WSB, CLA and SJL/J are not identical. M. m. brevirostris contains a combination of RF bands similar in size to BALB/c and SJL/J with $C_{T\beta}$. This individual mouse has previously been documented to be heterozygous for a locus closely associatd with TCR_β on mouse chromosome 6, Ig-K (Huppi 1985). Therefore, it is not unexpected that the individual mouse may also be heterozygous for $C_{T\beta}$ carrying both the SJL/J and BALB/c Bam HI RF patterns. Mus spretus contains the same $C_{T\beta}$ BamHI RF pattern as SJL/J with the exception of a 6.5 kb band which corresponds to the 5.0 kb region 5' of $J_{T\beta 1}$ in BALB/c (unpublished data). Therefore, M. spretus contains the SJL/J $C_{T\beta}$ BamHI RF pattern with the exception of the $J_{T\beta 1}$ region. Other musculus subspecies such as M. m. musculus (Czech II) and M. m. castaneus carry the $C_{T\beta}$ BamHI RF pattern of BALB/c. There is an exception to the RF pattern in M. m. castaneus, however, in that the BamHI RF band corresponding to the 5' side of $J_{T\beta 1}$ is polymorphic with

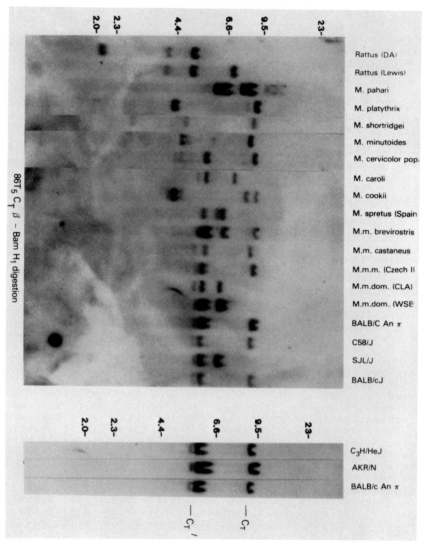

Fig. 1. BamHI Southern hybridization analysis of $C_T\beta$ among mouse species. BamHI digested liver DNAs from mice representing the four subgenera of the Mus lineage were hybridized to $C_T\beta$. The $C_T\beta$ probe is a 1.35 kb EcoRI fragment derived from the $86T_5$ cDNA clone (Hedrick 1984) and encodes $J_T\beta$ and $C_T\beta$ regions. The size markers (λ HindIII) are noted in kilobases on the left. C_T' and C_T refer to the expected 5.5 kb $C_T\beta_2$ and 10.0 kb $C_T\beta_1$ BamHI RF bands.

respect to BALB/c. Thus, the M. m. castaneus and Mus spretus individuals both have the $C_{T\beta}$ RF context of a haplotype of BALB/c or SJL
but differ in their $J_{T\beta 1}$ regions. More detailed examination of
$J_{T\beta}$ region sequences (see below) will resolve whether $J_{T\beta}$ regions
may be more diverse than their $C_{T\beta}$ counterparts.

Other mouse species such as Mus cookii, Mus caroli, Mus cervicolor
popaeus, Mus minutoides, Mus shortridgei, Mus platythrix and Mus
pahari as well as the genus Rattus display very polymorphic $C_{T\beta}$
BamHI banding patterns. However, in each case, two intense $C_{T\beta}$ RF
bands and one faint $J_{T\beta 1}$ RF band are consistently found. ($J_{T\beta 2}$
region has insufficient homology to cross hybridize with many of the
$J_{T\beta 1}$ regions including those used in this survey.) We conclude
that two $C_{T\beta}$ regions are maintained throughout the wide spectrum
of mouse species and they exhibit a considerable amount of RF polymorphism. More detailed studies are required to accurately assess
the extent of polymorphism of $C_{T\beta}$ in these mice.

$V_{T\beta 1}$ is found as a single nonpolymorphic gene.

Reports have demonstrated that $V_{T\beta}$ gene families, as defined by
Southern hybridization, consist of only 1-3 members among inbred
strains (Behlke 1985; Barth 1985). Since about 18-20 distinct
$V_{T\beta}$ groups have been defined, only 20-60 $V_{T\beta}$ genes are predicted in
the inbred mouse genome. Some strains of mice such as SJL, SWR/J,
C57BR and C57L/J have lost approximately 50% of their $V_{T\beta}$ repertoire
(Behlke 1985; Augustin 1985). These mouse strains were originally
derived from different sources, therefore one questions whether
$V_{T\beta}$ gene deletion is a result of inbreeding or whether wild mouse
populations contain greatly varying numbers of $V_{T\beta}$ gene families.
We have begun a systematic hybridization survey of the $V_{T\beta}$ gene
families to determine the content of $V_{T\beta}$ genes among wild mice. We
hybridized $V_{T\beta 1}$ ($86T_1$) to the same panel of BamHl digested DNA
of individuals (Fig. 2). A single $V_{T\beta 1}$ BamHl RF band is found
in all inbred strains surveyed to date including the strains SJL/J,
C57L/J, SWR/J and C57BR. However, a BamHl $V_{T\beta 1}$ RFLP is observed
with SJL/J as a 12 kb BamHl band rather than the 9.8 kb RF band
found for BALB/c. The 12 kb $V_{T\beta 1}$ RF band is also found in M. m.
domesticus (CLA), M. m. brevirostris and Mus minutoides. Consistent
with the results of $C_{T\beta 1}$, M. m. brevirostris appears with a
heterozygous pattern for $V_{T\beta 1}$ with two RF bands of 11 kb and 12
kb. The 12 kb RF band is SJL in context and the 11 kb is found
among many of the wild mouse species such as M. m. domesticus (WSB),
M. m. musculus (Czech II), M. m. castaneus, Mus spretus, Mus
cookii, Mus cervicolor popaeus and Mus shortridgei. Surprisingly,
although the $V_{T\beta 1}$ BamHl RF band of 11 kb is found predominantly
among wild mouse species, none of the inbred mouse strains surveyed
contain this RF band. Likewise none of the wild mice contain the
9.8 kb BALB/c RF pattern. In conclusion it is evident that only one
$V_{T\beta 1}$ gene is found among the wild mouse species surveyed. Furthermore, the $V_{T\beta 1}$ gene does not appear to be polymorphic. The results
presented here have been confirmed by further restriction analysis
with EcoRl and HindIII (manuscript submitted).

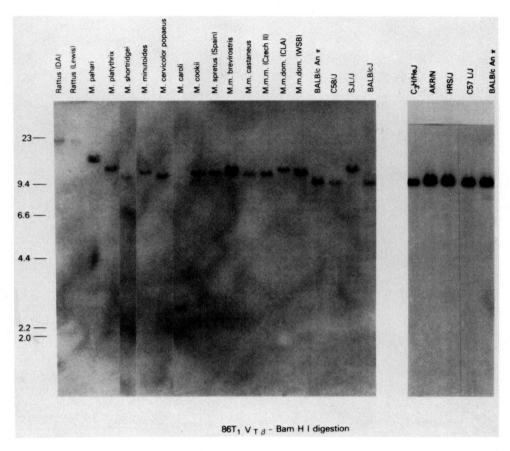

Fig. 2. BamHI Southern hybridization analysis of $V_T{}^o{}_1$ among mouse species. The   HindIII size markers are denoted in kilobases on the left.

$J_T\beta_1$ displays two major haplotypes among inbred strains.

In view of the apparent lack of diversity of $V_T\beta$ and $C_T\beta$ genes, we have turned our focus to the context of $J_T\beta$ among the inbred mouse strains. A survey of mouse inbred strains and wild mouse species with a $J_T\beta_1$ specific probe (Fig. 3 and Table 1) establishes that two major haplotypes of $J_T\beta$ can be observed. Among most mouse inbred strains, a 9.5 kb EcoRl RF band is found. The strains SJL and SWR/J contain a polymorphic 7.0 kb EcoRl RF band. Several wild mouse species from the subgenus Mus such as M. m. domesticus (CLA,

296

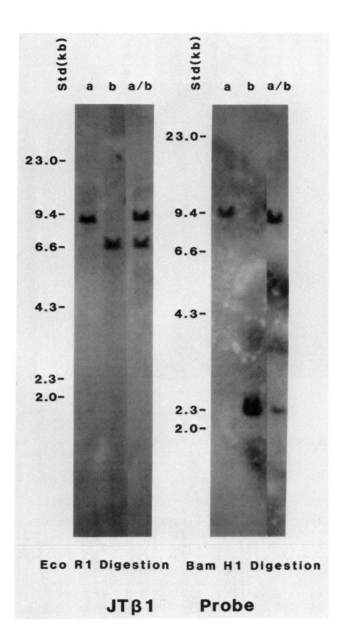

Fig. 3. BamHI or EcoRI Southern hybridization with the JTβ1 specific probe to representatives of the two major JTβ1 haplotypes. The designations "a" and "b" refer to JTβ1 haplotypes. The size marker (λ HindIII) is on the left hand sides of each respective blot.

Table 1. $J_T\beta_1$ haplotypes[a]

Haplotype designation	EcoRl RF Size	Strain or Species
$J_T\beta_1{}^a$	9.5 kb	A/J, AL/N, BALB/cAnPt, BALB/cJ, BDP, BSVS, C3H/HeJ, C57BL/6J, C57BL/Ka, C57L/J C58/J, CBA/J, CE/J, DBA/2n, HRS/J, I, MA/MyJ, MRL, NH, NZB, NZW, PL/J, RF/J, STS/A, ST/bJ, YBR, 129/J, <u>M. m. musculus</u>, <u>M. m. brevirostris</u>[b]
$J_T\beta_1{}^b$	7.0 kb	<u>M. m. domesticus</u> (WSB or CLA), <u>M. m. castaneus</u>, <u>M. m. poschiavinius</u>, <u>M. abbotti</u>, <u>M. m. praetextus</u>, <u>M. m. brevirostris</u>[b]

[a] Other <u>Mus</u> species tested which have widely varying EcoRl RF patterns and are not categorized are: <u>Mus spretus</u>, <u>Mus cookii</u>, <u>Mus caroli</u>, <u>Mus cerv. popaeus</u>, <u>Mus minutoides</u>, <u>Mus shortridgei</u>, <u>Mus platythrix</u>, <u>Mus pahari</u>.

[b] <u>M. m. brevirostris</u> carries both alleles of $J_T\beta_1{}^a$ and $J_T\beta_1{}^b$ as tested and as a heterozygote, falls into both categories.

WSB) <u>M. m. castaneus</u>, <u>M. m. poschiavinus</u>, <u>Mus abbotti</u>, <u>M. m. domesticus praetextus</u>, and <u>M. m. domesticus brevirostris</u> also display this 7.0 kb $J_T\beta_1$ EcoRl RF band. Other wild species used in this report contain diverse and unrelated RF patterns for $J_T\beta_1$. As expected, <u>M. m. brevirostris</u> carries both alleles of $J_T\beta_1$ which we have designated $J_T\beta_1{}^a$ (BALB/c, A/J, etc.) and $J_T\beta_1{}^b$ (SJL/J, SWR/J, etc.).

The segregation of inbred strains and wild mouse species for $J_T\beta_1$ is consistent with the finding of $C_T\beta$ polymorphism for mouse inbred strains (Epstein 1985) and wild mouse species (also see Cazenave, this volume). Although the $J_T\beta_1{}^a$ haplotype is the predominant allele among mouse inbred strains there is no evidence of this allele among the wild mouse species. This result corresponds precisely to the observations for $V_T\beta_1$ in that the most common inbred haplotype is not found in our survey of wild mouse species. Furthermore, the $V_T\beta_1$ and $J_T\beta_1{}^b$ haplotypes associated with SJL/J are indeed found among several wild species.

298

DISCUSSION

We conclude from our survey of wild mouse species that one $V_{T\beta 1}$ and two $C_{T\beta}$ genes are maintained throughout the genus <u>Mus</u>. In addition, very few polymorphisms of $V_{T\beta 1}$ are found in <u>the</u> genus <u>Mus</u>. $V_{T\beta 1}$ is conserved as a single gene which implies that the $V_{T\beta}$ repertoire, as reported for BALB/c or SJL/J is restricted. The fact that $J_{T\beta}$ and $C_{T\beta}$ RF patterns appear to be much more polymorphic than $V_{T\beta 1}$ among wild species suggests that J_T and C_T regions may be more important in the diversification of the mouse TCR. That the $V_{T\beta}$ regions are not as important as their Ig counterparts in diversification is further supported by the absence of 50% of the $V_{T\beta}$ repertoire in SJL/J, SWR/J, C57BR, and C57L/J (Behlke 1985; Sims 1985). SJL/J, SWR/J, C57BR and C57L/J are considered to be immunologically competent. Therefore, DNA sequence comparison of the $V_{T\beta}$ and $J_{T\beta}$ regions among the wild mouse population, particularly those of the $J_{T\beta 1}{}^b$ haplotype will be important in studies of TCR diversity.

ACKNOWLEDGEMENTS

We appreciate the generous gift of 86T1 and 86T5 cDNA clones from Dr. Mark M. Davis. We also wish to thank Mary Millison and Victoria Rogers for their expert assistance in preparing this manuscript.

REFERENCES

Arden B, Klotz JL, Siu G, Hood L (1985) Diversity and structure of genes of the α family of mouse T-cell antigen receptor. Nature 316: 783-787

Augustin A, Sim GK (1984) T-cell receptors generated via mutations are specific for various major histocompatibility antigens. Cell 39:5-12

Barth RK, Kim BS, Lon NC, Hunkapiller T, Sobieck N, Winoto A, Gershenfeld H, Hansburg D, Weissman I, Hood L (1985) The murine T-cell receptor uses a limited repertoire of expressed Vβ gene segments. Nature 316:517-522

Becker DM, Patten P, Chien Y-h, Yokota T, Eshhar Z, Giedlin M, Gascoigne NR, Goodnow L, Wolf R, Arai K, Davis MM (1985) Variability and repertoire size of T-cell receptor Vα gene segments. Nature 317:430-434

Behlke MA, Spinella DE, Chou HS, Sha W, Hartl DL, Loh DY (1985) T-cell receptor β-chain expression: dependence on relatively few variable region genes. Science 229:566-570

Behlke, MA, Chou HS, Huppi K, Loh DY, Murine T-cell receptor V β deletion mutants. Proc Natl Acad Sci (USA) in press

Brodeur PH, Riblet R (1984) The immunoglobulin heavy chain variable region (Igh-V) locus in the mouse. I. One hundred Igh-V genes comprise seven families of homologous genes. Eur J Immunol 14: 922-926.

Cazenave PA, Bonhomme F, Guenet J-L, Kindt TJ (1985) Correlation of
  C$_T$β phenotype with origins of laboratory mouse strains (this
  edition)
Cory S, Tyler BM, Adams JM (1981) Sets of immunoglobulin V genes
  homologous to ten cloned V sequences: implications for the numbers
  of germline V genes. J Mol Appl Genet 1:103-116
D'Hoostelaere LA, Jouvin-Marche E, Huppi K (1985) Localization of
  C$_T$β and Cκ on mouse chromosome 6. Immunogenetics 22:277-283
Epstein R, Roehm N, Marrack P, Kappler J, Davis MM, Hedrick S, Cohn
  M (1985) Genetic markers of the antigen-specific T cell receptor
  locus. J Exp Med 161:1219-1224
Hedrick SM, Nielsen EA, Kavaler J, Cohen DI, Davis MM (1984) Sequence
  relationships between putative T-cell receptor polypeptides and
  immunogloublins. Nature 308:153-158
Hood L, Kronenberg M, Hunkapiller T (1985) T cell antigen receptors
  and the immunoglobulin super gene family. Cell 40:225-229
Huppi K, Jouvin-Marche E, Scott C, Potter M, Weigert M (1985) Genetic
  polymorphism at the κ chain locus in mice: comparisons of restriction
  enzyme hybridization fragments of variable and constant region genes.
  Immunogenetics 21:445-457
Huppi K, Jouvin-Marche E, D'Hoostelaere LA, Mushinski JF, Rudikoff S
  (1985) T cell receptor α and β gene diversity among mouse species
  (Submitted)
Ikuta K, Ogura T, Shimizu A, Honjo T (1985) Low frequency of somatic
  mutation in β chain variable region genes of human T-cell recep-
  tors. Proc Natl Acad Sci (USA) 82:7701-7705
Kotzin BL, Barr VL, Palmer E (1985) A large deletion within the
  T-cell receptor beta-chain gene complex in New Zealand white mice.
  Science 229:167-170
Sim GK, Augustin AA (1985) Vβ gene polymorphism and a major poly-
  clonal T cell receptor idiotype. Cell 42:89-92
Tonegawa S (1983) Somatic generation of antibody diversity. Nature
  302:575-581
Valbuena O, Marcu KB, Weigert M, Perry RP (1978) Multiplicity of
  germline genes specifying a group of related mouse κ chains with
  implications for the generation of immunoglobulin diversity.
  Nature 276:780-784

Correlation of $C_T\beta$ Phenotype with Origins of Laboratory Mouse Strains

P.-A. Cazenave, F. Bonhomme, J. L. Guénet, and T.J. Kindt

INTRODUCTION

The majority of laboratory mouse strains have been derived from relatively limited pools from the Mus musculus species. The original breeders, with a few exceptions, originated from European and North American pet dealers and Japanese mice fanciers. The primary source of these pet dealers probably trace back to wild mice caught in restricted areas like England and eastern North America (domesticus) and Japanese animals related to the musculus group through the Japanese fancy tradition, resulting in a genetic melting pot for classical inbred strains that are more or less all related to each other. Besides these, a few lines were independently derived from wild stocks. Among the exceptions are the SJL and certain related strains which are derived from the so called "Swiss" stock. SJL mice have been shown to contain genes for lambda L chains (Lieberman 1977; Arp 1982) and certain kappa L chain V regions (Huppi 1985) that are different from other laboratory mice. More recently, many wild derived inbred and partially inbred strains of known geographical origin and systematical status make it possible to assess the precise origin of variation found in laboratory stocks (Bonhomme 1984).

The locus encoding the beta chain of the T cell receptor in mouse, man and rabbit has been shown to contain two constant genes in close proximity (Gascoigne 1984; Malissen 1984; Sims 1984). Only limited polymorphism of the $C_T\beta$ genes has been observed by molecular studies for man (Robinson and Kindt 1985) and rabbit (Mage, personal communication; Marche, Wetterskog and Kindt, unpublished). Restriction fragment length polymorphisms (RFLP) that distinguish $C_T\beta$ genes in BALB/c and SJL strains have been reported (Epstein 1985; D'Hoostelaere 1985).

The present study concerns the distribution of RFLP for $C_T\beta$ in various mouse strains classified according to the criteria proposed by Bonhomme (1984). It was found with few exceptions that strains of the Mus2 type carried the BALB/c $C_T\beta$ allele (C) whereas nearly all Mus1 strains were of the SJL (S) type. In addition, other Swiss mice from several sources were heterozygous with respect to the $C_T\beta$ genes.

Source of Wild Mouse Strains

The origins of strains used in this study are given in Table I . The classifications are according to the biochemical criteria of Bonhomme (1984). The designation I for inbred is given those strains with more than 20 generations of brother-sister crosses. These strains are maintained in the Institut des Sciences del'Evolution in Montpellier and the Departement d'Immunologie of the Institut Pasteur in Paris. DNA samples were isolated from mouse livers as described (Kindt 1985).

Table 1. Inbred (I) and partially inbred (P) wild-derived strains used in this study

Biochemical group	Strains	Geographical origin	I or P
Mus 1	ULA	Palaiseau, France	P
	WLA	Issus, France	I
	WBG	Bois-Guillaume, France	P
	DGD	Doirani, Greece	P
	DBP	Pomorie, Bulgaria	P
	DFL	Larzac, France	P
	DOT	Tahiti	P
	DFA	Annemasse, France	P
	BNC	Cairo, Egypt	P
	BEP	Palma de Mallorca, Spain	P
	BFM/2	Montpellier, France	I
	BZO	Oran, Algeria	P
	BIB/a	Sede Boger, Israel	P
	BIB/b	Sede Boger, Israel	P
	BIK/g	Kefar Galim, Israel	P
	24BI	Binasco, Italy	P
	DFC	Corse	P
	DIO	Italy	P
	38CH	Chiarello, Italy	P
	WMP	Monastir, Tunisia	P
	WAS	Athens, Greece	P
	BIA/b	Afula, Israel	P
	BEM	Minorque, Spain	P
	WGQ	France	P
	DBV	Vlas, Bulgaria	P
Mus 2A	PWK	Prague Zoo, Czechoslovakia	I
	MBT	General Toshevo, Bulgaria	I
	MBV	Vrania, Bulgaria	P
	MAI	Illmitz, Austria	I
	MYL	Lubljana, Yugoslavia	P
	MPW	Varsovia, Poland	P
	MBK	Kranero, Bulgaria	P
	MBB	Bania, Bulgaria	P
	MBS	Bulgaria	P
Mus 2B	MOL	Japan	I
Mus 2C	CAS	Thailand and Indonesia	P

RFLP in Wild Derived Mouse Strains

High molecular weight DNA samples were digested with BamHI and subjected to Southern blot analysis using a $C_T\beta$ probe derived from the clone 86T1 (Hedrick 1984). Only two patterns were observed in the inbred or partially inbred strains tested here. At the high stringency conditions used (65°C 0.1 x SSC), all samples contained a band at 6.6 Kb whereas the second band was variable appearing at 8 Kb in the SJL sample and at 12 Kb in BALB/c. These RFLP were designated S and C types. The thirteen Mus1 derived samples were all identical and were all of the S type (Fig. 1). The Mus2 samples with the exception of MYL were of the C type. Analysis of additional strains confirmed observed preponderance of S type in Mus1 strains and C type in Mus2 (see Table 2).

302

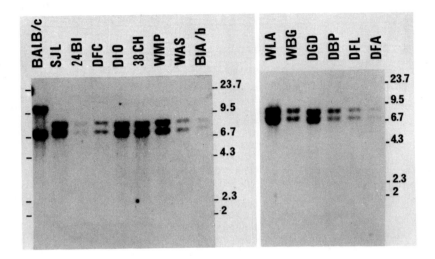

Fig. 1. Southern blot analysis of BamHI digested DNA samples from livers of BALB/c, SJL and Mus1 strains. The probe used was a 615 bp BamHI/EcoRI fragment from the clone 86TI (a kind gift of Mark Davis). The filters were washed at a final temperature of 65°C in 15 mM NaCl/1.5 mM sodium citrate and exposed to Kodak X-omat AR film at -70°C using Dupont lightning plus screens.

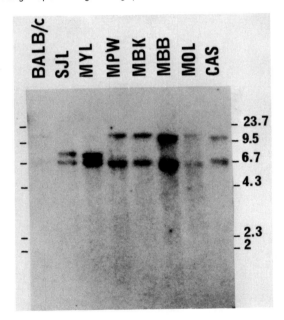

Fig. 2. Southern blot analysis of BamHI digested DNA samples from BALB/c, SJL and various Mus2 strains. Conditions as in Fig. 1.

An exception to the association of type C with Mus2 is found in the MYL strain. This strain originates from a region in Yugoslavia near the boundary between areas in which Mus1 and Mus2 animals predominate (Bonhomme 1983). The area is close enough to the hybrid zone that some introgression cannot be ruled out. An exception of Mus1 association with the S type is found in the DBV strain which is heterozygous C/S. This strain originates from a region in Bulgaria near this same boundary.

Table 2. $C_{T}\beta$ typing of Mus1 and Mus2 mouse strains

Mus1

  C type[a]: DBV

  S type : ULA, WLA, WBG, DGD, DBP, DFL, DOT, DFA, BNC, BEP, BFM/2, BZO, BIB/a, BIB/b, BIK/g, 24BI, DFC, DIO, 38CH, WMP, WAS, BIA/b, BEM, WGQ

Mus2

  C type : PWK, MBT, MBV, MAI, MPW, MBK, MBB, MBS, MOL, CAS

  S type : MYL

[a] The C and S types are defined by RFLP detected in BamHI digests hybridized with a $C_{T}\beta$ probe. The C type has fragments of 6.6 and 11 Kb, the S type has fragments of 6.6 and 8.0 Kb.

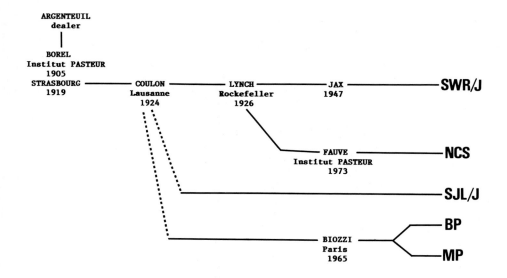

Fig. 3. Origin of SJL/J and other related inbred mouse strains. Adapted from Potter and Klein (1979) with additional information from the Archives of the Institut Pasteur, Paris, courtesy of Dr. Robert Fauve and Guido Biozzi.

304

C$_T$β Types of Swiss Derived Mice

Because SJL is one of strains derived from stock given the designation "Swiss" it
was of interest to type other strains of this origin. As diagrammed in Fig. 3 the
Swiss stock originated from mice bred at the Institut Pasteur by Amedee Borel in the
beginning of this century. The mice were from a dealer in Argenteuil a suburb of
Paris. Additional mice of Swiss derivation were obtained from the Charles River
Corporation. These are designated CD1, CF1 and CFW in Figure 4.

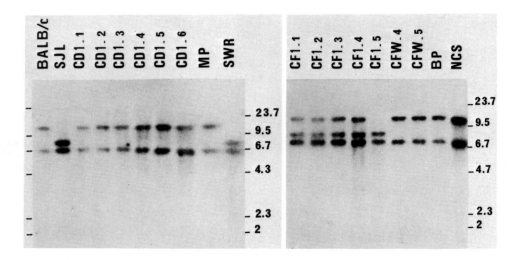

Fig. 4. Southern blot analyses of BamHI digested DNA samples from livers of BALB/c,
SJL and inbred (SWR, NCS, BP and MP) strains and outbred (CF1, CD1 and CFW) strains
all derived from "Swiss" stock.

The S haplotype was found for the SWR inbred strain and the C haplotype was found
for the NCS, BP and MP inbred strains. This observation suggests that both C and S
types were present in the original population. The results with outbred animals
verify this supposition in that heterozygotes as well as homozygotes of both types
are found. The observation of homozygotes of both S (CF1.5) and C (CFW and CD1)
types in the outbred Swiss mice argues against the occurrence of a duplication of C$_T$β
genes in this line.

DISCUSSION

Geographical and biosystematical evidence is presented for the separate origins of
the C$_T$β genes in BALB/c and SJL mouse strains. The RFLP described for C$_T$β of BALB/c
(C) is found in each of the strains classified as Mus2 (except MYL) whereas Mus1
strains carried exclusively the S type for which the prototype is SJL (except for
DBV). The origins of the SJL from so called Swiss mice can be traced to a French

dealer by records available from the Institut Pasteur. The Swiss derived mice apparently carried both $C_T\beta$ types. Of the inbred strains derived from this lineage and tested here, SJL and SWR carry the S/S type.

Appreciation of the functional significance of the $C_T\beta$ polymorphism awaits further investigation. It must be determined whether $V_T\beta$ gene families linked to the S and C types are different and whether these differences are reflected in immune responsiveness. It is known that SJL mice are prone to autoimmune disease and it is not unreasonable to suspect a linkage of this trait with Tβ genes.

The polymorphism observed with BamHI is most likely located to the 5' side of the $C_T\beta1$ gene. The fragment of 6.6 Kb that remains constant includes the $C_T\beta2$ gene which does not vary in BamHI sites. When samples of Mus1 and Mus2 DNA were digested with EcoRI a similar distribution of RFLP was seen (data not shown). Studies of mice falling into the biochemically determined group 3 and 4 showed conservation of the SJL pattern with some small variation in fragment size; no patterns were similar to the C type. The presence of a Mus2 gene widely represented in laboratory stock is compatible with what we know from the study of other markers concerning the admixture of Musculus-like and domesticus genomes in classical inbred strains (Bishop 1985; Bonhomme and Guenet in preparation).

ACKNOWLEDGEMENTS

The authors thank Dr. Mark Davis for providing the $C_T\beta$ probe used here. The expert technical assistance of Carine Gris and Viviane James and the secretarial help of Michelle Berson and Virginia Shaw is gratefully acknowledged. The valuable information provided by Drs. Fauve and Biozzi was critical to this study.

REFERENCES

Arp B, McMullan MD, Storb U (1982) Sequences of immunoglobulin λ1 genes in a λ1 defective mouse strain. Nature 298:184-186

Bishop CE, Boursot P, Baron B, Bonhomme F, Hatat D (1985) Most classical Mus musculus domesticus laboratory mouse strains carry a Mus musculus musculus Y chromosome. Nature 325:70-72

Bonhomme F, Catalan J, Gerasinov S, Orsini Ph, Thaler L (1983) Le complexe d'especes du genre Mus en Europe centrale et orientale. I. Genetique. Z. f Saugetierkunde 1:312-317

Bonhomme F, Catalan J, Britton-Davidian J, Chapman VM, Moriwaki D, Nevo E, Thaler L (1984) Biochemical diversity and evolution in the genus Mus. Biochem Genet 22:275-303

D'Hoostelaere LA, Jouvin-Marche E, Huppi K (1985) Localization of $C_T\beta$ and C_κ on mouse chromosome 6. Immunogenetics 22:277-283.

Epstein R, Roehm N, Marrack P, Kappler J, Davis M, Hedrick S and Cohn M (1985) Genetic markers of the antigen-specific T cell receptor locus. J. Exp Med. 161:1219-1224

Gascoigne NRJ, Chien Y-h, Becker DM, Kavaler J, Davis MM (1984) Genomic organization and sequence of T-cell receptor beta-chain constant- and joining-region genes Nature 310:387-391

Hedrick SM, Cohen DI, Nielsen EA, David MM (1984) Isolation of cDNA clones encoding T cell-specific membrane-associated proteins. Nature 308:149-152

Huppi K, Jouvin-Marche E, Scott C, Potter M, Weigert M (1985) Genetic polymorphism of the kappa chain locus in mice: Comparisons of restriction enzyme hybridization fragments of variable and constant region genes. Immunogenetics 21:448-474

Kindt TJ, Gris C, Guenet JL, Bonhomme F, Cazenave PA (1985) Lambda light chain
    constant and variable gene complements in wild-derived inbred mouse strains.
    Eur J Immunol 15:535-540

Lieberman R, Humphrey W, Chien CC (1977) Identification and genetics of λ1 light
    chain allotype in the mouse. Immunogenetics 5:515

Malissen M, Minard K, Mjolsness S, Kronenberg M, Goverman J, Hunkapiller T,
    Prystowsky MB, Yoshikai Y, Fitch F, Mak TW, Hood L (1984) Mouse T cell antigen
    receptor: structure and organization of constant and joining gene segments
    encoding the beta polypeptide. Cell 37:1101-1110

Potter M, Klein J, (1979) Contributors: Genealogy of the more commonly used inbred
    mouse strains. In: Altman PL, Katz DD (eds) Inbred and Genetically Defined
    Strains of Laboratory Animals. Federation of American Societies for Experimental
    Biology, p 16-17

Robinson MA, Kindt TJ (1985) Segregation of polymorphic T-cell receptor genes in
    human families. Proc Natl Acad Sci USA 82:3804-3808

Sims JE, Tunnacliffe A, Smith WJ and Rabbitts TH (1984) Complexity of human T-cell
    antigen receptor beta-chain constant- and variable-region genes. Nature
    312:541-545

Genes Determining Resistance and Susceptibility to Infections

Susceptibility of *Mus musculus musculus* (Czech I) Mice to *Salmonella typhimurium* Infection

A. D. O'Brien, D. L. Weinstein, L. A. D'Hoostelaere, and M. Potter

INTRODUCTION

When inbred or outbred mice are challenged with Salmonella typhimurium, they develop a disease which is similar in its pathogenesis to typhoid fever in man. Whether the animals ultimately survive the infection depends on the virulence of the bacterial strain, the route of challenge, and the genetic constitution of the mice. Although mice of some inbred strains and many outbred strains survive parenteral inoculation with up to 10,000 virulent salmonellae, mice of other inbred strains invariably succumb to low-dose (< 10 bacteria) challenge. Several distinct host genes have been identified which regulate this differential susceptibility to murine typhoid. Some of these genes act early in the course of the disease (Ity, Lps, and the C3HeB/FeJ gene), and mice that express the susceptibility allele at any one of these loci (e.g., Ity^s or Lps^d) usually die by day 10 of infection with a virulent strain of S. typhimurium (Plant and Glynn 1976; Hormaeche 1979; O'Brien et al. 1980, O'Brien and Rosenstreich 1983). Other salmonella-response genes confer a salmonella-susceptible phenotype (xid, nu or the C57L/DBA/2 gene), and mice homozygous for any one of these genes tend to die between the second and third week of infection with a virulent strain of S. typhimurium (O'Brien et al. 1979; O'Brien and Metcalf 1982; O'Brien et al. 1984). Recently, Hoermache et al. (1985) reported that genes within the major histocompatibility complex of mice are responsible for the ultimate clearance of salmonellae from the reticuloendothelial cell system of Ity^s mice challenged with an S. typhimurium strain of intermediate virulence. The purpose of this study was to determine whether salmonella susceptibility is a characteristic of domesticated mice or whether wild mice can also exhibit genetically-controlled susceptibility to murine tyhpoid.

SCREENING WILD MICE FOR SUSCEPTIBILITY TO S. typhimurium

Wild mice of different geographic origin were tested for suscep-
tibility to S. typhimurium strain TML by monitoring the size of the bacterial population in their spleens 10 days after subcutaneous infection with approximately 1,000 organisms. Mice were trapped in Czechoslovakia [Mus musculus musculus (Czech I)], Japan (Mus musculus molossinus), or the Eastern Shore of Maryland [Mus musculus domesticus (Watkins Star), and Mus musculus domesticus (Starlight)]. Among these groups of wild mice, only Czech I mice were susceptible to S. typhimurium (Table 1). Inbred Ity^r (C57L/J) and Ity^s (C57BL/6J) mice were included in the experiment as controls.

310

Table 1. Susceptibility of Mice to _Salmonella typhimurium_
          strain TML

Mice	Number Tested	Log_{10} geometric mean number of TML per spleen[a]	Phenotype[b]
M. m. musculus (Czech I)	4	7.9	S
M. m. molossinus	3	3.2	R
M. m. domesticus (Watkins Star)	5	3.1	R
M. m. domesticus (Starlight)	3	2.7	R
C57L/J	5	3.1	R($\underline{\text{Ity}}^r$)
C57BL/6J	5	6.3	S($\underline{\text{Ity}}^s$)

[a] Mice that died before day 10 of infection were considered to have 10^8 organisms per spleen. Because of the small sample size of some groups, standard errors were not calculated.

[b] R mice, log_{10} geometric mean number of TML per spleen ≤ 4.9.

ANALYSIS OF THE GENETIC BASIS FOR CZECH I SUSCEPTIBILITY TO S. typhimurium

Expression of any one of the early-phase salmonella response genes could account for the susceptibility of Czech I mice to S. typhimurium. To examine the possibility that Czech I mice are $\underline{\text{Ity}}^s$, the animals were crossed with inbred BALB/c ($\underline{\text{Ity}}^s$) mice, and the F_1 hybrids tested for sensitivity to S. typhimurium. We reasoned that hybrids would be susceptible to murine typhoid if the Czech I parents were $\underline{\text{Ity}}^s$ and resistant if the Czech I parents were $\underline{\text{Ity}}^r$ because $\underline{\text{Ity}}^s$-mediated susceptibility is a recessive trait. As shown in Table 2, the progeny of Czech I and BALB/cⅡ matings were salmonella resistant. Both male and female F_1 mice were tested from crosses in which the Czech I animals were the mothers (not shown); all such progeny were resistant to S. typhimurium. Thus, Czech I mice are not homozygous for $\underline{\text{Ity}}^s$ and do not appear to carry a sex-linked recessive gene. As anticipated, matings between Czech I and $\underline{\text{Ity}}^r$ mice [C.D2($\underline{\text{Ity}}^r$)congenic mice, or CE/J mice, or A/J mice], also produced salmonella resistant progeny(Table 2). The Czech I mice have not as yet been successfully mated with inbred mice that carry other early-phase salmonella response genes, such as $\underline{\text{Lps}}^d$ or the C3HeB/FeJ gene. However, the strong response of Czech I spleen cells to the mitogenic stimulus of protein-free lipopolysaccharide (data not shown) suggests that the animals are not endotoxin hyporesponsive, i.e., of the $\underline{\text{Lps}}^d$ genotype.

Table 2. Susceptibility of parental and F_1 mice to Salmonella
typhimurium strain TML

Mice	Ity phenotype	Number tested	Log_{10} TML per spleen $\pm$ 2SE
Czech I	?	38	6.8 ± 0.4
BALB/cⅡ	S	27	6.7 ± 0.7
C.D2(Ity^r)	R	5	4.0 ± 0.5
CE/J	R	9	3.8 ± 1.4
(Czech I x BALB/cⅡ)F_1	?/S	10	3.2 ± 0.3
(BALB/cⅡ x CzechI)F_1	S/?	12	3.5 ± 0.3
(Czech I x C.D2)F_1	?/R	12	2.7 ± 0.4
(Czech I x CE/J)F_1	?/R	8	2.8 ± 0.4
(CE/J x CzechI)F_1	R/?	6	2.9 ± 0.3
(Czech I x A/J)F_1	?/R	7	2.2 ± 0.2

SUMMARY

Mus musculus musculus (Czech I) were observed to be highly susceptible to infection with the mouse-virulent S. typhimurium strain
TML. Genetic analyses indicated that this susceptibility was not
due to expression of Ity^s or an X-linked susceptibility gene.
Furthermore, Czech I mice do not appear to be Lps^d. Taken together,
the findings suggest that Czech I mice either express the C3HeB/FeJ
salmonella susceptibility gene or an as yet undefined gene(s) that
confers a salmonella susceptible phenotype.

REFERENCES

Hormaeche CE (1979) Natural resistance to Salmonella typhimurium
   in different inbred mouse strains. Immunology 37:311-318
Hormaeche CE, Harrington KA, Joysey HS (1985) Natural resistance
   to salmonellae in mice: control by genes within the major
   histocompatibility complex. J Infect Dis 152:1050-1056
O'Brien AD, Scher I, Cambell GH, MacDermott RP, Formal SB (1979)
   Susceptibility of CBA/N mice to infection with Salmonella
   typhimurium: influence of the X-linked gene controlling B
   lymphocyte function. J Immunol 123:720-724
O'Brien AD, Metcalf ES (1982) Control of early Salmonella
   typhimurium growth in innately salmonella-resistant mice does
   not require functional T lymphocytes. J. Immunol 129:1349-1351
O'Brien AD, Taylor BA, Rosenstreich DL (1984) Genetic control
   of natural resistance to Salmonella typhimurium in mice during
   the late phase of infection. J Immunol 133:3313-3318

Plant J, Glynn AA (1976) Genetics of resistance to infection with <u>Salmonella</u> <u>typhimurium</u> in mice. J Infect Dis 133:72-78

Genetically Controlled Resistance to Flaviviruses Within the House Mouse Complex of Species

M. Y. Sangster and G. R. Shellam

INTRODUCTION

One of the consequences of the interaction of an infectious microorganism and its normal host is the selection of individuals with a genetic constitution which confers a survival advantage. In man the greater resistance to yellow fever in areas of Africa where the virus is endemic has been regarded as an example of this phenomenon (Sabin, 1954), although direct evidence is lacking. Experimental studies in mice have also established the occurrence of genetically determined resistance to infection with a number of infectious agents. The first observation of resistance to yellow fever virus in mice dates back over fifty years (Sawyer and Lloyd, 1931) and resistance was shown to be due to an inherited factor (Lynch and Hughes, 1936). Sabin (1952) working with mice of the PRI strain showed that an autosomal dominant gene conferred resistance, not only to yellow fever virus, but also to a number of other arthropod-borne viruses. These viruses are now known to be flaviviruses, and the genetically-determined resistance appears to be flavivirus specific (Sabin, 1952a; Hanson and Koprowski, 1969). Interestingly however this resistance has only been described in the Det (Lynch and Hughes, 1936), BRVR and BSVR (Webster, 1937) and PRI (Sabin, 1952) strains of mice and not in the commonly used strains of inbred mice (Darnell, Koprowski, and Lagerspetz, 1974; Sangster and Shellam, unpublished observations). The resistance gene *RV* carried by PRI mice has been introduced into the C3H/He strain to create congenic resistant C3H.RV mice (Groschel and Koprowski, 1965), thus greatly facilitating the study of its mode of action. However the unusual distribution of resistance in laboratory mice may not reflect the prevalence of resistance in wild populations.

In order to determine how widely the *RV* and possibly other flavivirus resistance genes are distributed in nature, we have studied resistance to these viruses in the house mouse complex of species. Since we planned to study wild mice trapped in Australia we chose an Australian flavivirus, Murray Valley Encephalitis virus (MVE) as the challenge agent. An *RV*-like gene has been described in wild mice in the United States (Darnell *et al.*, 1974), and we have therefore compared resistance in wild mice to the known effects of the *RV* gene.

We have found evidence of resistance to MVE in populations of wild mice from several parts of Australia and in inbred strains of mice derived from Asian species of *Mus*. In some cases the resistance closely resembles the known effect of the *RV* gene.

RESULTS

1. THE EFFECT OF THE *RV* GENE ON THE GROWTH OF AUSTRALIAN FLAVIVIRUSES IN MICE.

Because we wished to study resistance to flaviviruses in populations of wild mice, including mice trapped in Australia, it was necessary to establish that a resistance gene (*RV*) which was known to control the replication of a number of flaviviruses could influence the growth of flaviviruses with a predominantly Australian distribution. Accordingly the growth of the Australian flavivirus Murray Valley encephalitis virus (MVE) was compared in C3H.RV and C3H/HeJ (susceptible) mice. Adult males were inoculated intracerebrally (i.c.) with 10^4 $TCID_{50}$ of MVE (equivalent to 300 i.c. LD_{50} in C3H mice), and brains were removed 3 or 6 days later for the estimation of viral content. Ten percent homogenates were prepared using a Ten Broek homogeniser and were stored at $-70^{\circ}C$ until titration. Viral titers were determined using PS-EK cells in 96-well microtiter trays with serial ten-fold dilutions of homogenate in a volume of 0.1 ml per well. Twenty replicates of each dilution were used and the cytopathic effect was scored 7 days later. The $TCID_{50}$ was calculated using the Kaerber method.

Table 1. The effect of the *RV* gene on Murray Valley encephalitis virus (MVE)

Brain titer*
(days post infection)

Mouse strain	MVE		SFV	
	3 days	6 days	2 days	4 days
C3H/HeJ	6.27 ± 0.13	7.55 ± 0.02	6.45 ± 0.09	8.15 ± 0.33
C3H.RV	3.30 ± 0.21	4.95 ± 0.21	5.98 ± 0.32	7.43 ± 0.23

*$\log_{10}$ $TCID_{50}$/0.1g brain tissue after i.c. inoculation of 10^4 $TCID_{50}$ of MVE.

The *RV* gene was clearly very effective in controlling the growth of MVE (Table 1) and a reduction in titer of 300 to 1000-fold in C3H.RV compared with C3H/HeJ has been observed consistently. This effect is essentially the same as that reported for West Nile

virus and other flaviviruses. In addition we have observed a
marked reduction in the growth of the other predominantly
Australian flaviviruses, Alfuy, Kunjin and Kokobera, in the brains
of C3H.RV mice (unpublished observation). As a specificity control
the alphavirus Semliki Forest virus (SFV) was used. As can be seen
(Table 1) the *RV* gene did not restrict the growth of SFV, and this
is consistent with experience with other non-flaviviruses (Sabin,
1952a; Hanson and Koprowski, 1969). Accordingly MVE was chosen for
the study of resistance genes in populations of wild mice. This
appears to be the first report of the effect of the *RV* gene on
these particular flaviviruses.

2. THE STUDY OF RESISTANCE TO MVE IN AUSTRALIAN WILD MICE

Feral mice were trapped in three widely separated regions of Australia, Dubbo (New South Wales), Geraldton (Western Australia) and
the southwest of Western Australia. The mice from Geraldton were
shown by Dr P. Baverstock of the South Australian Museum to be *Mus
domesticus* by isozyme electrophoresis. None of 100 mice from Geraldton or Dubbo areas were found to have serum antibodies to MVE.

Adult mice of both sexes were challenged i.c. with a dose of MVE
which was uniformly lethal to C3H/HeJ mice, and the mice were
observed for four weeks. The results (Table 2) indicate that a
proportion (18-25%) of wild mice survived this challenge which was
lethal to 100% of C3H/HeJ mice. In addition wild male mice which
survived the challenge were mated with C3H and their progeny were
challenged at 8-10 weeks of age with MVE. Clearly, a significant
proportion survived an otherwise lethal challenge (Table 2),
strongly suggesting the inheritance of a resistance factor.

Table 2. Resistance of adult mice to i.c. challenge with MVE

LOCATION	% SURVIVAL		
	WILD	(C3H X WILD)F$_1$	C3H/HeJ*
Dubbo (NSW)	18 (3/17)	49 (23/47)	2 (1/44)
Geraldton (WA)	20 (20/102)	50 (9/18)	0 (0/25)
South West (WA)	25 (5/20)	35 (8/23)	0 (0/25)

* C3H/HeJ and (C3H X WILD) F$_1$ were challenged simultaneously

Given that about 50% of the F_1 mice originating from matings involving mice from Dubbo or Geraldton were resistant, the data suggests that resistant mice from these regions were heterozygous for a dominant resistance gene. This possibility is currently being studied further in F_2 and backcross breedings. No sex differences were observed in the mortality of F_1 mice, and no sex differences have been reported in the resistance to flaviviruses of PRI mice (Sabin, 1952). The data therefore suggest the operation of an autosomal gene. In addition to studies of mortality, virus titers were determined in the brains of [C3H x Wild (Dubbo)] F_1 and C3H/HeJ mice six days after i.c.infection with MVE. The titers in the F_1 fell into two distinct groups; 60% had a titer essentially identical to that of susceptible C3H, and 40% had a titer which was 1.7 $\log_{10}$ units lower than that of C3H. The state of health of the mice at the time of sampling corresponded to their brain titers.

In order to determine whether these resistance genes are the same as the *RV* gene, the complementation of gene action is being studied in the progeny of *RV* and resistant wild mice. These studies are in progress.

3.   RESISTANCE TO MVE IN INBRED STRAINS DERIVED FROM WILD MICE.

As an alternative to the study of resistance factors in feral mice, evidence for genetic control of resistance was sought in inbred strains which have been recently derived from wild mice,since the existence of these strains offers the opportunity to study resistance factors in genetically homogeneous populations. Accordingly, adult CASA/Rk mice which were derived from *Mus castaneus* and MOLD/Rk which were derived from *Mus molossinus* were challenged i.c. with 10^4 $TCID_{50}$ units of MVE, and brain titers were measured (Table 3). These mice were the kind gift of Professor Ian McKenzie and were obtained from the Jackson Laboratories.

Table 3. Resistance to MVE in inbred wild-derived strains

Strain	Brain titer* (days post infection)			
	2 days	3 days	4 days	6 days
C3H/HeJ	4.51 ± 0.31	6.30 ± 0.09	7.65 ± 0.15	7.53 ± 0.06
MOLD/RK	3.67 ± 0.40		5.97 ± 0.18	6.95 ± 0.07
CASA/RK		4.37 ± 0.17		5.20 ± 0.32

* $\log_{10}$ $TCID_{50}$/0.1g brain tissue

Clearly both strains exhibited resistance to the growth of MVE compared with C3H/HeJ mice. The resistance in CASA/RK was very similar in magnitude to the effect of the *RV* gene (Table 1) and the reduction in titer in the CASA/Rk strain was highly significant (p< 0.001 at day 3, p< 0.01 at day 6). The resistance in MOLD mice was less marked but was statistically significant on days 4 (p< 0.001) and 6 (p< 0.01).

The nature of the resistance in CASA/Rk mice was studied further in (CASA x C3H)F_1 (Table 4). The F_1 were more resistant than C3H. Their brain titers were significantly lower at 4 days (p< 0.05) and 7 days (p< 0.01) after infection. The F_1 mice also exhibited lower mortality than C3H. Thus, although further work needs to be done to establish the nature of this effect, resistance to infection with MVE is clearly genetically controlled in the CASA/Rk strain.

Table 4. Resistance to MVE in (C3H x CASA)F_1 mice

	Brain titer* (days post infection)		% Mortality**
	4 days	7 days	
C3H/HeJ	4.5±0.3	6.7±0.1	100
(C3HxCASA)F_1	3.3±0.1	5.2±0.2	29

*$\log_{10}$ TCID$_{50}$/0.1g brain tissue

**Mice were observed for 28 days

DISCUSSION

We have identified genetically-controlled resistance to MVE in wild mice from several different Australian regions. This resistance resembles the *RV* gene in its degree of effect. In addition to *Mus domesticus*, we have obtained evidence for flavivirus resistance in two other members of the house mouse complex of species, CASA/Rk (derived from *Mus castaneus*) and MOLD/Rk (derived from *Mus molossinus*). The resistance of MOLD/Rk mice is significant but relatively weak compared with the effect of the *RV* gene. We have also suggestive evidence for the existence of such modest protective effects in populations of Australian feral mice (M. Sangster, unpublished observation). In contrast, resistance in CASA/Rk mice was more pronounced and closely resembled the magnitude of effect exerted by the *RV* gene. However the relationship between the *RV* gene and the genetic factors controlling resistance in CASA/Rk mice remains to be determined. The existence of a powerful resistance gene(s) in an inbred strain (CASA/Rk) will greatly facilitate these investigations.

318

It has been suggested that the *RV* gene may protect wild mice in the United States against natural flavivirus infection (Darnell *et al.*, 1974). Indeed our observation of the retention of apparently similar resistance genes in diverse members of the house mouse complex of species supports the notion of a useful role for such resistance factors. However, there is no direct evidence that mice are other than occasional hosts for mosquito-borne flavivirus infections, although tick-borne viruses may have been a selective force in the past. Alternatively, the effect of the *RV* gene on flavivirus replication may be entirely coincidental rather than its primary function.

Our future studies are aimed at identifying resistance genes in other members of the house mouse complex of species and elucidating their mechanism of action.

REFERENCES

Darnell, MB, Koprowski, H, Lagerspetz, K (1974). Genetically determined resistance to infection with group B arboviruses I. Distribution of the resistance gene among various mouse populations and characteristics of gene expression *in vivo*. J. Infect. Dis. 129: 240-256.
Groschel, D, Koprowski, H (1965). Development of a virus-resistant inbred mouse strain for the study of innate resistance to arbo B viruses. Arch ges Virus forsch. 17: 379-391.
Lynch, CJ, Hughes, TP (1936). The inheritance of susceptibility to yellow fever encephalitis in mice. Genetics 21: 104-112.
Sabin, A (1952). Nature of inherited resistance to viruses affecting the nervous system. Proc Nat Acad Sci (USA) 38: 540-546
Sabin, A (1952a). Genetic, hormonal and age factors in natural resistance to certain viruses. Ann NY Acad Sci 54: 936-944.
Sabin, A (1954). Genetic factors affecting susceptibility and resistance to virus diseases of the nervous system. In: Proceedings of the Association for Research in Nervous and Mental Disease, vol 33 p 64.
Sawyer, WA, Lloyd, W (1931). The use of mice in tests of immunity against yellow fever. J Exp Med 54: 533-555.
Webster, LT (1937). Inheritance of resistance of mice to enteric bacterial and neurotropic virus infections. J Exp Med 65: 261-286.

Variable Resistance to Ectromelia (Mousepox) Virus Among Genera of *Mus*

R. M. L. Buller, M. Potter, and G. D. Wallace

INTRODUCTION

Ectromelia virus, an orthopoxvirus, is a member of the poxvirus family. It replicates in the cytoplasm of infected cells producing progeny virions which are "brick-shaped" with dimensions of approximately 200 by 300 nm, and contain a double-stranded DNA genome of $130\text{-}140\times10^6$ daltons MW. (Mackett and Archard 1979). The virus naturally infects M. m. domesticus in animal colonies causing a severe disease (mousepox) in certain strains (A/J, DBA/2J, BALB/cByJ), and a subclinical infection in others (AKR/J, C57BL/6J, C57BL) (Schell 1960; Wallace and Buller 1985). Much speculation has centered on the question of a potential wildlife host for ectromelia virus. Fenner examined 150 wild mice from the area of Melbourne, Australia without finding evidence for prior exposure to this virus (Fenner 1949). Kaplan et al. (1980) have presented serologic evidence suggesting that field mice (Apodemus) and voles (Microtus and Clethrionomys) can be infected with an orthopoxvirus, but no direct evidence that these species are natural reservoirs for ectromelia virus is available. Thus it was of interest to study closer relatives of M. m. domesticus for susceptibility to ectromelia virus.

RESULTS

Resistance of Various Mus Genera to Mousepox

In the last several years, representatives of four genera of Mus have been introduced into the laboratory. These mice are currently maintained in a conventional breeding colony housed at Litton Bionetics, Rockville, Maryland under an NCI contract No 1CB 25584.

Mice were transferred from this colony to a BL4 isolation facility at NIH, and inoculated with ectromelia virus into the rear footpad (approximates the natural route of infection). The number of deaths and the mean day of death for both male and female mice in each group is given in Table 1. Mus platythrix (genus Pyromys) and M. pahari (genus Coelomys) had no deaths and showed no signs of mousepox. Furthermore, the expected severe swelling of the footpad due to the inflammatory response to virus replication at the site of the inoculation (Fenner 1947; Wallace and Buller 1985), and a primary lesion were not observed in both of these populations. Mus minutoides, a representative of the genus Nannomys developed ectromelia virus infections some of which were lethal. The mean day of death was 6.3 ± 0.5 and the disease course resembled the responses seen in some genus mus species (M. cookii, M. caroli, and M. cervicolor popaeus). Thus M. minutoides mice appear to be heterogenous in their response to ectromelia virus, some develop lethal infections with no lesions, others recovered from disease and developed a local lesion.

Table 1.   Mortality in various Mus genera following footpad inoculation of ectromelia virus (Strain NIH 79)[a]

Genus	Species	Males		Females		Totals	
		Deaths	Mean Death-Day	Deaths	Mean Death-Day	Deaths	Mean Death-Day
Pyromys	platythrix[c]	0/7(0)	NM[b]	0/23(0)	NM	0/30(0)	NM
Coelomys	pahari[d]	0/12(0)	NM	0/9(0)	NM	0/21(0)	NM
Nannomys	minutoides[e]	3/13(23)	6.3±0.6	4/16(25)	6.3±0.5	7/29(24)	6.3±0.5
Mus	caroli[f]	12/12(100)	6.2±0.4	14/14(100)	6.5±0.9	26/26(100)	6.3±0.5
Mus	cookii[g]	13/13(100)	5.9±0.5	15/15(100)	5.9±0.6	28/28(100)	5.9±0.6
Mus	cervicolor popaeus[h]	21/21(100)	6.4±0.8	13/13(100)	6.8±1.1	34/34(100)	6.6±0.9
Mus	musculus musculus (Czech I)[i]	9/15(60)	12.5±2.8	8/25(32)	11.9±1.1	17/40(43)	12.2±2.1
Mus	musculus domesticus (eastern shore)[j]	5/16(31)	12.4±2.7	2/16(13)	12.0±2.8	7/32(22)	12.3±2.5
Mus	spretus (Spain)[k]	8/12(67)	8.4±1.7	13/21(62)	8.1±1.8	21/33(64)	8.2±1.7
Mus	spretus (Morocco)[l]	4/13(31)	9.5±3.0	4/10(40)	8.0±0.8	8/23(35)	8.8±2.2

[a] Mice were inoculated by the footpad (fp) route with 0.05 ml of a suspension containing 50-200 plaque forming units (pfu) of mouse-passed ectromelia virus (strain NIH 79). Deaths between the 2nd and 21st day (numerator) were expressed as a fraction of the total number of mice injected (denominator). The bracketed value is the percentage mortality. When assayed on BS-C-1 cells (Wallace and Buller 1985), spleens from dead animals contained greater than 10^7 pfu of ectromelia virus per gram of tissue

[b] NM = no mortality.

[c] M. platythrix (Mysore, India) was obtained from T.H. Yosida via R. Callahan NCI.

[d] M. pahari (Dr. J.T. Marshall, Tak Province, Thailand).

[e] M. minutoides (Mr. Issa Aggundey, National Museum of Kenya, in a field near Kenyatta University in 1981.)

[f] M. caroli (Dr. J.T. Marshall, Chonburi Province, Thailand).

[g] M. cookii (Dr. J.T. Marshall, Loei, Tak Province, Thailand).

[h] M. cervicolor popaeus (Dr. J.T. Marshall, Chonburi Province, Thailand).

[i] M. m. musculus (Studenec, Morovia, Czechoslovakia).

[j] M. m. domesticus (Centreville, Queen Anne's Co., Maryland)

[k] M. spretus (Dr. R. Sage, Puerto Real Cadiz, Spain and Azrou, Morocco.)

Seven species in the genus mus were studied. Two types of responses were observed. Mus cookii, caroli, cervicolor popaeus , uniformly developed fulminating systemic infections with no local lesions and died between 5.9 ± 0.6 and 6.8 ± 1.1 days post-inoculation. The M. m. musculus, M. m. domesticus and the two M. spretus populations from Spain and Morocco developed local lesions associated with recovery or lethal infections, and resembled M. minutoides in this respect although the observed mean day of death was greater.

Subclincial Infection of M. platythrix and M. pahari by Ectromelia Virus

Although Table 1 suggests that M. platythrix and M. pahari are resistant to mousepox it does not rule out a subclinical infection as is the case of an ectromelia virus infection of C57BL6/J mice by the footpad route (Wallace and

Buller 1985). Consequently, M. platythrix, M. pahari and C57BL/6J mice were inoculated with large doses of ectromelia virus (10,000-fold more virus than used in experiments described in Table 1) by the footpad and intraperitoneal routes. Mortality rates, infectivity titers at the site of inoculation, and neutralizing antibody titers in survivors are presented in Table 2.

Table 2. Responses of M. platythrix, M. pahari and C57BL6/J mice following inoculation of ectromelia virus (strain NIH 79) by the footpad or intraperitoneal route[a]

Species/strain	Route of Inoculation	Mortality	pfu per foot	Reciprocal of neutralizing antibody titre
M. pahari	Fp	0/4	2.2×10⁶ ×÷ 2.1	799 ×÷ 1.3[b] (522-1684)
M. pahari	Ip	0/4	NA[c]	371 ×÷ 1.1[b] (300-436)
M. pahari	Mock	0/4	NA	< 160
M. platythrix	Fp	0/4	1.3×10⁶ ×÷ 7.1	2359 ×÷ 1.5[b] (756-5052)
M. platythrix	Ip	0/4	NA	1739 ×÷ 1.3[b] (1040-2286)
M. platythrix	Mock	0/4	NA	< 160
C57BL/6J	Fp	0/6	3.8×10⁹ ×÷ 1.2	6570 ×÷ 1.1[b] (6128-7044)
C57BL/6J	Ip	6/6	NA	NA
C57BL/6J	Mock	0/4	NA	< 160

[a] Mus pahari, M. platythrix and C57BL6/J mice were inoculated either by the footpad or the intraperitoneal route with 5×10⁵ pfu of ectromelia virus (NIH 79). At 7 days post-inoculation, 3 mice from each group inoculated by the footpad route were sacrificed and spleen, liver, and foot tissue (where appropriate) were collected. Virus infectivity in the tissues was measured using standard procedures (Wallace and Buller 1985). At 21 days post-inoculation, the surviving mice were bled from the orbital sinus. Plasma was heat-inactivated at 56°C for 30 min, and virus neutralization assays were carried out by standard methods (Lennette and Schmidt 1979). The highest dilution of plasma that produced a 50% reduction in the number of virus plaques (intracellular band-purified WT virus) was chosen as the assay end-point. The geometric mean and relative standard error was calculated from 2 to 4 neutralizing titers obtained for each inoculation series. The bracketed values indicate the titer range.
[b] Significantly different from mock infected control values (P<0.05), student's t-test.
[c] NA = Not available.

No deaths were observed by either route except in the group of C57BL/6J mice that received virus by the ip route. Similar results have been noted by Schell (1960). The virus infectivity detected in the inoculated foot of M. pahari and M. platythrix mice was of the same order of magnitude as the input inoculum (ie. 5×10⁵ pfu), which would suggest that only very limited virus replication had taken place. Significantly this quantity of virus was 1000-fold lower than the level detected in the feet of similarly infected C57BL/6J mice. Furthermore, no virus could be detected in the spleens and livers from the M. pahari and M. platythrix mice at 7 days post inoculation, whereas in C57BL/6J mice 6.7×10⁴ ×÷ 1.3 and 1.3×10³ ×÷ 1.8 pfu/g were detected in the spleen and liver, respectively. Spleens and livers from similarly inoculated susceptible inbred strains A/J or BALB/cByJ or outbred Mus strains M. caroli, M. cookii and M. cervicolor popaeus yielded virus titers greater than 10⁷ pfu/g. of spleen or liver tissue (R.M.L. Buller, unpublished results). Ectromelia virus neutralizing antibody was detected in survivors in all groups. The antibody titers were lowest from M. pahari mice followed by M. platythrix and C57BL/6J mice. The mechanism of resistance to ectromelia virus infection in M. pahari and M. platythrix mice appears to be very different from the mechanism operative in the C57BL6/J mouse.

DISCUSSION

The pattern of resistance to ectromelia virus infection observed in the outbred mouse populations tested suggested that genera Pyromys (M. platythrix) and Coelomys (M. pahari) are unlikely to transmit or maintain ectromelia virus in the wild since ectromelia virus replicated only to a limited extent at the site of inoculation, and no primary lesion was observed. Similarly, only limited replication was noted in ectromelia virus infection of members of genus Rattus (Burnet and Lush 1936; Mooser 1943). Mus caroli, M. cervicolor popaeus and M. cookii are also poor candidates as the animal reservoir for ectromelia virus as the severity of the disease could potentially eliminate the natural population. These Mus species (i.e. M. caroli, M. cookii and M. cervicolor popaeus) are considered to have evolved before M. musculus and thus susceptibility to ectromelia virus (or lack of resistance) is a very ancient trait. This may also suggest that ectromelia virus was not endemic to the areas of Southeast Asia where these mice are indigenous. The appearance of resistance to ectromelia virus in populations of M. minutoides (genus Nannomys) and Mus genus species: M. m. domesticus and musculus and M. spretus (Morocco and Spain), could point to a common ancestor of genera Mus and Nannomys which was first to experience a mousepox-like disease. The Nannomys and Mus genera have been separated since the Pliocene period when a tropical land bridge that linked Asia with Africa became arid thus isolating the two groups (Missone 1969). These results also suggest that at least in Europe, populations of mice exist which could maintain ectromelia virus in the wild.

ACKNOWLEDGEMENTS

We are grateful to the Jackson Laboratory for furnishing (without cost) the mice used, and the following National Institutes of Health (NIH) intramural research programs, and divisions, for support: National Cancer Institute; National Heart, Lung, and Blood Institute; National Institute of Arthritis, Diabetes and Digestive and Kidney Diseases; National Eye Institute; National Institute of Mental Health; Clinical Center; National Center for Drugs and Biologics; and the Division of Research Services. The support of the Division of Safety, Office of Director, NIH was essential to the operation of the laboratory. We also would like to thank Dr. D. Alling for expert statistical advice and Dr. H.C. Morse III for a critical review of the manuscript.

REFERENCES

Burnet FM, Lush D (1936) Inapparent (subclinical) infection of the rat with the
  virus of infectious ectromelia of mice.   J Path Bacterol 43:469-476
Fenner F (1947) Studies in infectious ectromelia of mice. I. Immunization of mice
  against ectromelia with living vaccinia virus. Aust J Exp Biol Med Sci 25:257-274
Fenner F (1949) Mousepox (infectious ectromelia of mice): A review. J Immunol 63:341-37?
Kaplan C, Healing TD, Evans N, Healing L, Prin A (1980) Evidence of infection by
  viruses in small British field rodents. J Hyg 84:285-294.
Lennette EH, Schmidt NJ (1979) Diagnostic Procedures for viral, rickettsial and
  chlamydial infectious (American Public Health Association Inc. 1979) p 291
Mackett M, Archard LC (1979) Conservation and variation in orthopoxvirus genome
  structure. J Gen Virol 45:683-701
Missone X (1969) African and Australia Murida Evolutionary Trends.
  Belgique Annales Serie in 80 Sciences Zoologiques No 172, 1-213
Mooser IT (1943) Uber die Mischinfektion der weissen Maus mit einem Stamm Klassichen
  Fleckfiebers und dem virus der infectiosen Ektromelie. Z Path Bakteriol 6:463-472
Schell K (1960) Studies on the innate resistance of mice to infection with
  mousepox. II. Route of inoculation and resistance; and some observations
  on the inheritance of resistance. Aust J Exp Biol Med Sci 38:289-300
Wallace GD, Buller RML (1985) Kinetics of ectromelia virus (mousepox) transmission
  and clinical response in C57BL/6J, BALB/cByJ and AKR/J mice. Lab Animal Sci 35:41-46

Expression of the Natural Resistance Gene *(Lsh)* in Wild Mice Infected Experimentally with *Leishmania donovani* or *Salmonella typhimurium*

J.M. Blackwell and J.E. Plant

INTRODUCTION

Leishmania species are obligate intracellular protozoan parasites of the host's mononuclear phagocyte system. The particular tissue tropism of the parasite (cutaneous versus visceral) is determined largely by the species of leishmanial parasite but, within each species, a broad spectrum of disease profiles results from variations in the host's ability either to control growth of the parasite population early in infection (Bradley 1979; Crocker, Blackwell & Bradley 1984a) and/or to mount an effective cell mediated immune response as the disease progresses (Skov & Twohy 1974; Rezai, Farrell & Soulsby 1980). In inbred mouse strains ability to control early proliferation of L. donovani in the viscera is determined by a single gene, Lsh, which segregates for dominant resistant and recessive susceptible alleles (Bradley 1974 & 1977) and maps to a position between Idh-1 and ln on mouse chromosome 1 (Bradley, Taylor, Blackwell, Evans & Freeman 1979). This gene is indistinguishable by traditional genetic analysis from the separately described genes, Ity and Bcg, which control early resistance and susceptibility to Salmonella typhimurium (Plant, Blackwell, O'Brien, Bradley & Glynn 1982) and Mycobacterium bovis (Skamene, Gros, Forget, Kongshavn, St. Charles & Taylor 1982). Functional studies also suggest that the genes are identical. Studies with all three pathogens have shown that expression of resistance does not require a functional T cell population (Bradley & Kirkley 1972; O'Brien & Metcalfe 1982; Gros, Skamene & Forget 1983), can be transferred with the donor haematopoietic system in reciprocal radiation bone marrow chimaeras (Hormaeche 1979; Gros et al. 1983; Crocker, Blackwell & Bradley 1984b), and correlates with a reduction in rate of proliferation of each microorganism in liver or spleen in vivo (Bradley 1979; Hormaeche 1980; Crocker et al. 1984a) or in peritoneal macrophages in vitro (Stach, Gros, Forget & Skamene 1984). It is now generally agreed that the gene is expressed at the macrophage level, various reports having claimed that it is expressed in vitro in resident peritoneal macrophages for S. typhimurium (Lissner, Swanson & O'Brien 1983) and M. bovis (Stach et al. 1984), in splenic macrophage populations for S. typhimurium (Lissner et al., 1983), and in resident liver macrophages isolated from congenic B10 and B10.L-Lsh^r mice for L. donovani (Crocker et al. 1984a; Blackwell, Crocker & Channon 1985). The molecular basis for the action of the gene remains unknown.

Distribution of resistant and susceptible alleles for Lsh amongst inbred mouse strains

Figure 1 shows the distribution of resistant and susceptible alleles for **Lsh** among different inbred mouse strains. It is not possible to

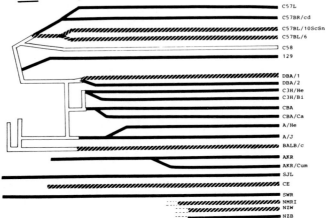

Fig. 1. Distribution of susceptible (///////) and resistant (▬▬▬▬) alleles for **Lsh** among different inbred mouse strains. Origin of strains modified from Potter & Lieberman (1967).

trace all inbred strains back to one origin but, from the information presented, it seems unlikely that either allele arose as a single mutational event. Various attempts (Table 1), although by no means exhaustive, have failed to isolate leishmanial parasites from wild caught **Mus musculus** so we cannot be sure whether or not they act as potential reservoirs for the disease. It seems plausible, nevertheless, that functional polymorphism for resistant and susceptible alleles at **Lsh** might be maintained in wild mice in response to fluctuations in natural infection with any one of the intracellular macrophage pathogens. We therefore set out to determine whether both resistant and susceptible alleles were present in wild **Mus musculus** populations.

Table 1. Unsuccessful attempts to isolate **Leishmania** spp. from wild caught **Mus musculus**.

Reference	Methods	Locality	Number of mice examined
Pringle 1956	? Organ smears	Iraq	35
Hoogstraal & Heyneman 1966	Inoculation into hamsters	Sudan	7
Lopez et al. 1966	?	Mexico	?
Bray & Dabbagh 1968	Spleen smears & promastigote culture	Iraq	6

325

Experimental L. donovani infection in wild caught Mus musculus

A total of 253 wild caught <u>Mus musculus</u> were infected experimentally with a standard inoculation of 10^7 <u>L. donovani</u> LV9 amastigotes and examined for liver parasite load 15 days later. Details of collection of mice appear elsewhere (Blackwell 1983). British and Peru-Coppock mice were all <u>Mus musculus domesticus</u>. The subspecies of mice from Iraq was not determined. Earlier studies in Iraq (Pringle 1956) quote <u>Mus musculus bactriana</u> as the subspecies caught in Baghdad city. All of the mice had liver parasite loads (e.g. Fig. 2) which fell within the range of counts obtained for control <u>Lsh</u> resistant inbred mice. There was no evidence for increased resistance in wild mice which might result from complementation between many loci or from cross-immunity acquired through other infections experienced in the wild.

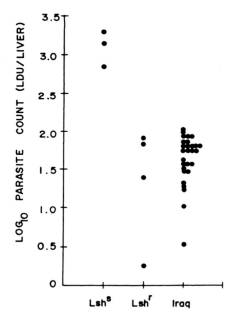

Fig. 2. Individual liver parasite counts (LDU) for some of the wild caught <u>Mus musculus</u> compared with counts for control inbred <u>Lsh</u> susceptible and resistant mice from the same infection experiments.

Mendelian inheritance of resistance and susceptibility in F2 and backcross generations from inbred x wild matings.

In order to determine more precisely the genetical basis for the early resistant phenotype observed in wild caught <u>Mus musculus</u>, crosses were performed between inbred C57BL/10ScSn (B10; <u>Lsh</u> susceptible) females and wild caught males from Long Sutton in Somerset, England, and between inbred NMRI (<u>Lsh</u> susceptible) females and males from the Peru-Coppock colony. Mice from the F1, the F2 and the backcross to susceptible inbred mice were again infected experimentally with <u>L. donovani</u> and liver parasite loads determined at day 15. The bimodality of the log LDU scores obtained in F2 and backcross mice (e.g. Fig. 3) and the close fit to Mendelian ratios (Table 2) for

326

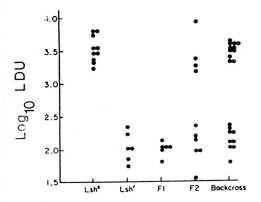

Fig. 3. Individual liver parasite counts (LDU) for some of the F1, F2 and backcross to B10 progeny bred from the original B10 x Long Sutton crosses (see Table 2). Counts are compared against control inbred Lsh susceptible and resistant mice from the same infection experiment.

Table 2. Numbers of resistant (R) and susceptible (S) progeny obtained from (A) five F1, nine F2 and five backcross to B10 families reared after initially crossing five male mice from Long Sutton to five homozygous Lsh susceptible B10 females; and (B) two F1, three F2 and three backcross to NMRI families reared from crossing two male mice from the Peru-Coppock colony to two homozygous Lsh susceptible NMRI female mice. Observed ratios do not differ significantly from expected Mendelian ratios for single gene control: F1 all R; F2 3R:1S; backcross 1R:1S.

Cross	F1		F2		Backcross	
	R	S	R	S	R	S
A	20	0	39	13	21	19
B	27	0	19	8	13	17

resistant and susceptible phenotypes in the progeny were consistent with single gene control and suggest that wild mouse populations are monomorphic for the Lsh resistant allele. If the resistant phenotype observed in wild mice had been due to other loci masking expression of the Lsh susceptible allele, it would be unlikely that the susceptible phenotype would be so clearly expressed on the mixed wild and inbred genetic backgrounds of F2 and backcross mice. In every experiment at least of 0.5 log LDU difference between the highest resistant and lowest susceptible counts was observed while within each phenotype the distributions of counts were similar to those observed in the parental susceptible and resistant mice.

Experimental S. typhimurium infection in wild caught Mus musculus

While our observation of monomorphism for the Lsh resistant allele leaves us with no clear solution to the question of the origin of

the susceptible allele in inbred mouse strains, it tempts speculation
as to the selective pressures which might maintain the resistant allele
at high frequency in wild populations of <u>Mus musculus</u>. Since the
<u>Lsh</u>/<u>Ity</u> susceptible allele is lethal even to very low inoculations of
<u>S. typhimurium</u> we wondered whether natural infections of this pathogen
in the wild might favour survival of mice carrying the resistant
allele. Again, when we infected wild caught mice experimentally with
<u>S. typhimurium</u> C5, 10 day viable counts in the spleen (Fig. 4) and
liver (data not shown) fell within the range normally observed in
<u>Lsh</u>/<u>Ity</u> resistant inbred mice. Faecal pellets taken from the mice
before experimental infection failed to produce any viable <u>Salmonella</u>
colonies (Table 3). Similarly, previous attempts to isolate <u>Salmonella</u>
from wild caught mice in Britain (Table 4) have proved unsuccessful.
Wild mouse populations don't appear to constitute a reservoir for
infection of domestic animals or man. In Iran the situation is
different. Various salmonellae have been isolated from the faeces of
wild mice (Table 4) leading workers there (Shimi, Keyhani & Hedayati
1979) to postulate that the house mouse might be an important reservoir

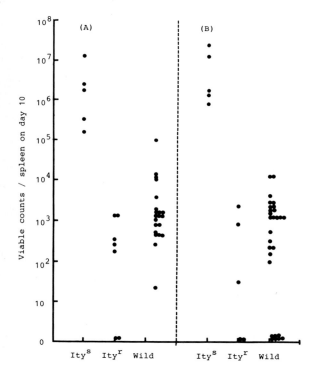

<u>Fig. 4</u>. Individual viable bacterial counts in the spleens of wild
caught <u>Mus musculus</u> from Somerton, England infected experimentally with
(A) 4.5×10^3 or (B) 1.1×10^3 viable <u>S. typhimurium</u> C5.

Table 3. Viable bacteria in pooled faecal pellets from the two samples of wild caught Mus musculus used in the experimental S. typhimurium infection experiment (Fig. 4).

Bacteria	Total viable colonies	
	Sample 1	Sample 2
Escherichia coli	1.0×10^5	1.6×10^4
Stretococcus sp.	5.5×10^4	6.2×10^4
Bacillus sp.	3.0×10^3	6.0×10^2
Coliforms	2.0×10^4	-
Staphlococcus epidermidis	2.0×10^4	1.2×10^5

Table 4. Attempts to isolate Salmonella spp. from wild caught Mus musculus

Reference	No. mice examined	Locality	Result	
Brown & Parker, 1957	73	Manchester (ships)	1 (1.4%)	S. typhimurium
			1 (1.4%)	S. stanley
			71	-ve
Brown & Parker, 1957	35	Manchester (docks)	35	-ve
Brown & Parker, 1957	256	Manchester (city)	1 (0.4%)	S. enteritidis (from rodenticide)
			255	-ve
Jones & Twigg, 1976	364	Berkshire (ships)	1 (0.3%)	S. typhimurium
			7 (2.6%)	S. dublin (from cattle)
			356	-ve
Shimi et al, 1979	170	Iran	17 (10%)	Salmonella spp.
			153	-ve

of human and animal salmonellosis. Whether the currently observed uniform resistance of wild mice has resulted from direct selection pressure from Salmonella infection, past or present, remains unre-solved. The broad spectrum of pathogens coming under Lsh gene control (Brown, Glynn & Plant 1982, Plant et al. 1982, Skamene et al. 1982, Goto, Nakamura, Takahashi & Tokunaga 1984, Skamene, Gros, Forget, Patel & Nesbitt 1984) raises other intrigueing possibilities, although it is interesting that for other loci (e.g. the H-2 complex) continual selection pressure from a large range of pathogens is thought to maintain high levels of polymorphism in wild mouse populations (Klein, Gotze, Nadeau & Wakeland 1981). In some systems too resistant hosts have been shown to have lower reproductive performance than uninfected susceptible hosts (Macdonald 1976; Minchella & Loverde 1983). In wild mice nothing is known about the reproductive cost of maintaining the resistant allele for Lsh/Ity/Bcg at high frequency. Presumably resistance confers an overall selective advantage. Further studies on the interactions between this gene and natural pathogens in wild Mus musculus populations, as well as in experimental mouse colonies where the susceptible allele and a pathogen of choice could be introduced, may provide important new insight into the genetical processes which govern the regulation of host populations.

Acknowledgements

Research reported here was supported by ·the Medical Research Council and the Wellcome Trust. J. Blackwell is a Wellcome Trust Senior Lecturer.

REFERENCES

Blackwell JM (1983) Regulation of Leishmania populations within the host. V. Resistance to L. donovani in wild mice. J Trop Med Hyg 86:17-22

Blackwell JM, Crocker PR, Channon JY (1985) The role of the macrophage in genetically controlled resistance and susceptibility to leishmaniasis. In: Mononuclear phagocytes. Characteristics, physiology, and function (ed. R van Furth), Martinus Nijhoff Publishers, Boston, Dordrecht, Lancaster, pp 677-683

Bradley DJ (1974) Genetic control of natural resistance to Leishmania donovani. Nature 250:353-354

Bradley DJ (1977) Regulation of Leishmania populations within the host. II. Genetic control of acute susceptibility of mice to Leishmania donovani infection. Clin Exp Immunol 30:130-140

Bradley DJ (1979) Regulation of Leishmania populations within the host. IV. Parasite and host cell kinetics studied by radioisotope labelling. Acta Tropica 36:171-179

Bradley DJ, Kirkley J (1972) Variation in susceptibility of mouse strains to Leishmania donovani infection. Trans Roy Soc Trop Med Hyg 66:527-528

Bradley DJ, Taylor BA, Blackwell JM, Evans EP, Freeman J (1979) Regulation of Leishmania populations within the host. III. Mapping of the locus controlling susceptibility to visceral leishmaniasis in the mouse. Clin Exp Immunol 37:7-14

Bray RS, Dabbagh MA (1968) Investigations into the epidemiology of leishmaniasis. Unsuccessful search for the reservoir host of kala-azar in Baghdad. J Trop Med Hyg 71:46-47

Brown CM, Parker MT (1957) Salmonella infections in rodents in Manchester. Lancet 273,1277-1279

Brown IN, Glynn AA, Plant J (1982) Inbred mouse strain resistance to Mycobacterium lepraemurium follows the Ity/Lsh pattern. Immunology 47:149-156

Crocker PR, Blackwell JM , Bradley DJ (1984a) Expression of the natural resistance gene Lsh in resident liver macrophages. Infect Immun 43: 1033-1040

Crocker PR, Blackwell JM, Bradley DJ (1984b) Transfer of innate resistance and susceptibility to Leishmania donovani infection in mouse radiation bone marrow chimaeras. Immunology 52:417-422

Goto Y, Nakamura RM, Takahashi H, Tokunaga T (1984) Genetic control of resistance to Mycobacterium intracellulare infection in mice. Infect Immun 46:135-140

Gros P, Skamene E, Forget A (1983) Cellular mechanisms of genetically controlled host resistance to Mycobacterium bovis (BCG). J Immunol 131:1966-1972

Hoogstraal H, Heyneman D (1969) Leishmaniasis in the Sudan Republic. 30. Final epidemiologic report. Amer J Trop Med Hyg 18:1091-1210

Hormaeche CE (1979) The natural resistance of radiation chimaeras to S. typhimurium. Immunology 37:329-332

Hormaeche CE (1980) The in vivo division and death rates of Salmonella typhimurium in the spleen of naturally resistant and susceptible mice measured by the super-infecting phage technique of Meyell. Immunology 41:973-979

Jones PW, Twigg GI (1976) Salmonellosis in wild mammals. J Hyg, Camb 77:51-54

Klein J, Gotze D, Nadeau JH, Wakeland EK (1981) Population immunogenetics of murine H-2 and t systems. Symp Zool Soc Lond 47:439-453

Lissner CR, Swanson RN, O'Brien AD (1983) Genetic control of innate resistance of mice to Salmonella typhimurium: expression of the Ity gene in peritoneal and splenic macrophages isolated in vitro. J Immunol 131:3006-3013

Lopez MR, Martinez GA, Molinari JL, Biagi FF (1966) Kala-azar en Mexico. Primeras observaciones sobre posibles reservorios. Rev de Fac de Med (Mexico) 8:533-538

Macdonald WW (1976) Mosquito genetics in relation to filarial infection. Symp Brit Soc Parasitol 14:1-24

Minchella DJ, Loverde PT (1983) Laboratory comparison of the relative success of Biomphalaria glabrata stocks which are susceptible and insusceptible to infection with Schistosoma mansoni. Parasitology 86:335-344

O'Brien AD, Metcalf ES (1982) Control of early Salmonella typhimurium growth in innately Salmonella-resistant mice does not require functional T lymphocytes. J Immunol 129:1349-1351

Plant JE, Blackwell JM, O'Brien AD, Bradley DJ, Glynn AA (1982) Are the disease resistance genes Lsh and Ity at one locus on mouse chromosome 1. Nature 297:510-511

Potter M, Lieberman R (1967) Genetics of immunoglobulins in the mouse. Adv Immunol 7:91-145

Pringle G (1956) Kala azar in Iraq: preliminary epidemiological considerations. Bull End Dis 1:275-293

Rezai HR, Farrell J, Soulsby EL (1980) Immunological responses of Leishmania donovani infection in mice and significance of T cell resistance to experimental leishmaniasis. Clin Exp Immunol 40:508-514

Shimi A, Keyhani M, Hedayati K (1979) Studies on salmonellosis in the house mouse, Mus musculus. Lab Anim 13:33-34

Skamene E, Gros P, Forget A, Kongshavn PAL, St Charles C, Taylor BA (1982) Genetic regulation of resistance to intracellular pathogens. Nature 297:506-509

Skamene E, Gros P, Forget A, Patel PJ, Nesbitt MN (1984) Regulation of resistance to leprosy by chromosome 1 locus in the mouse. Immunogenetics 19:117-124

Skov CB, Twohy DW (1974) Cellular immunity to Leishmania donovani. 1. the effect of T cell depletion on resistance to L. donovani in mice. J Immunol 113:2004-2011

Stach J-L, Gros P, Forget A, Skamene E (1984) Phenotypic expression of genetically-controlled natural resistance to Mycobacterium bovis (BCG). J Immunol 132:888-892

Genetic Resistance to Influenza Virus in Wild Mice

O. Haller, M. Acklin, and P. Staeheli

INTRODUCTION

Resistance of mice to influenza viruses is governed by the Mx gene locus on chromosome 16 (Lindenmann 1964; Haller 1981; Staeheli et al. 1986). Mice of the inbred laboratory strain A2G carry the resistance allele Mx^+ and are highly resistant to most influenza A viruses examined, including neurotropic (Lindenmann 1964), pneumotropic (Haller et al. 1979) and hepatotropic strains (Haller et al. 1976). In contrast, all other laboratory mouse strains tested so far are Mx^- (lacking the influenza virus resistance allele) and are uniformely susceptible to influenza viruses (Haller 1981). Resistance of Mx^+ mice selectively affects influenza viruses; susceptibility to other viruses is not influenced by the Mx gene (Haller et al. 1980). The expression of the resistance phenotype requires the action of interferon (IFN) (Haller et al. 1979, 1980). Murine IFN alpha or beta (but not IFN gamma) induces in Mx^+ cells the synthesis of a 75,000 dalton protein, termed Mx protein (Horisberger et al. 1983; Staeheli et al. 1984). The Mx protein accumulates in the cell nucleus (Dreiding et al. 1985) and inhibits influenza virus replication presumably by affecting influenza viral mRNA synthesis (Krug et al. 1985). IFN- responsive cells from influenza virus susceptible Mx^- mice are unable to synthesize the Mx protein and do not develop a comparable antiviral state towards influenza viruses.

Recently, a cDNA encoding the Mx protein has been cloned and sequenced (Staeheli et al. 1986). Southern analysis of chromosomal DNA has revealed that Mx^- mice carry deletions at the Mx locus (Staeheli et al 1986). These data indicate that despite the high frequency of Mx^- alleles in laboratory mice, the wild allele is Mx^+. The A2G strain is thought to have originated from an illegitimate mating between strain A (known to be Mx^-) and an unknown mouse (Staats 1980). We report here that the Mx^+ allele is present in a second inbred mouse strain and also in some wild mice.

RESISTANCE TO INFLUENZA VIRUS IS RARE IN LABORATORY MICE

A number of mouse strains have been tested over the years in our laboratory for their ability to survive lethal infection with influenza viruses. Table 1 lists all mouse strains found to be susceptible. We did not find another example of resistance in contemporary mouse strains. Where did the Mx^+ allele of A2G mice originate from? The unknown mouse that contaminated strain A at Glaxo Laboratories and presumably carried the wild type Mx^+ allele was either a laboratory or a wild mouse. As discussed by Lindenmann and Klein (1966), it is unlikely that the Mx^+ allele was distributed to any large extent in early European stocks of mice. In those days,

laboratory mice were frequently used for influenza virus titrations, and investigators were struck by the regularity with
which death would follow virus inoculation (Andrewes et al.
1934). We therefore started to investigate the situation in
wild mice.

Table 1

List of mouse strains susceptible to influenza virus

A/BrA	CBA/BrA	DD/He	P/J	WLL/BrA
A/BrAf	CBA/J	DBA/LiA	PL/J	129/J
A/He/Cum	CE/J	DBA/LiAf	PRI	129/MA
A/J	C3H/Exm	DBA/1J	RF/J	129/SVSL
A/JHan	C3H/HeA	DBA/2J	RIII/J	
AKR/FuA	C3H/HeAf	E/Gw	RIII/SeA	
AKR/J	C3H/HeDiSnAf	GRS/A	SEA/GnJ	
AL/Ks	C3H/HeJ	LG/Mi	SEC/1ReJ	
AU/J	C57BL/ImrHeA	LG/J	S/Gw	
BaB/Gw	C57BL/KsJ	LMH	SJL/Ola	
BALB/cCdA	C57BL/LiA	LP/J	SM/J	
BALB/cCrgl	C57BL/6J	MA/J	ST/aFibBom	
BALB/cJ	C57BL/10ScSnA	MA/MyJ	ST/bJ	
BDP/J	C57L/J	NFS/NA	STS/A	
BUA/Le	C58/JA	NZB/NBom	SWR/J	

GENETIC RESISTANCE TO INFLUENZA VIRUS IN WILD MICE

Laboratory-reared offspring of Mus musculus originally trapped
near Lake Casitas in Southwestern Ventura County, California,
were kindly provided by Murray B. Gardner (1978). The animals
were infected with 500 LD_{50} of TURH virus. This hepatotropic
avian influenza A virus causes acute liver failure and death
within 2-3 days in susceptible Mx^- mice (Haller 1975). Resistant
Mx^+ mice easily survive up to 10,000 LD_{50} (Haller et al. 1976).
Only 7 out of 21 infected wild mice died within the time period
expected for susceptible animals (Table 2, group 1). Two surviving males were then mated with Mx^- females and their offspring
were again tested for influenza virus resistance. Approximately
50% of the F1 animals survived infection (Table 2, group 2).
Resistant F1 males were then backcrossed to females of the
parental inbred strain; the ratio of susceptible to resistant
backcross mice was approximately 1:1 (Table 2, group 3). The
simplest explanation is that the wild mouse parents carried an
autosomal, dominant resistance allele in heterozygous form.

Table 2

Inheritance of resistance to influenza A virus in wild mice

Group	Mouse strain and crosses	Sex	No. tested	No. susceptible	No. resistant
1	WILD MICE (W)	f	7	2	5
		m	14	5	9
		total	21	7	14
2	F1,				
	(BALB/c x W1)	f	11	6	5
		m	13	3	10
		total	24	9	15
	(BALB/c x W2)	f	15	9	6
		m	5	2	3
		total	20	11	9
3	BC-1,				
	(BALB/c x F1)	f	3	2	1
		m	10	5	5
		total	13	7	6

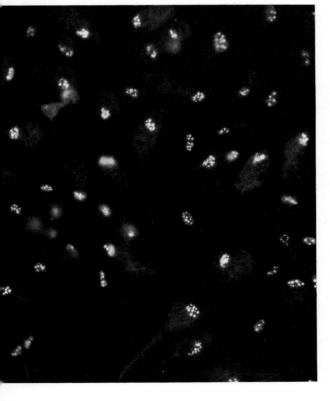

Fig. 1. Detection of Mx protein in macrophages from a resistant wild mouse. Peritoneal macrophages were analyzed for the presence of IFN- induced Mx protein by immunofluorescence with mo- noclonal antibody 2C12 as described (Dreiding et al. 1985). Mx protein accumu- lates in the nuclei.

RESISTANCE OF WILD MICE IS DUE TO A FUNCTIONAL Mx LOCUS

If the resistance locus of wild mice were similar or identical to
Mx, it would be expected to code for an IFN-induced protein cross-
reacting with antibodies to protein Mx in immunofluorescence assays.
Fig. 1 illustrates that this was the case. The wild mouse protein
had the same apparent molecular weight as Mx protein of A2G mice and
was induced by mouse IFN alpha or beta but not by IFN gamma (not
shown).

INBRED STRAIN SL/NiA IS HOMOZYGOUS FOR THE RESISTANCE ALLELE Mx^+

We have since analyzed more wild mice from various locations in
Europe and California. Mx^+ alleles seemed to be quite common among
these populations. We then started to look for additional Mx^+ car-
riers among some rare inbred mouse strains. SL/NiA mice established
and kept in Japan (Hiai et al. 1982) had the same degree of resistance as A2G mice. Again, IFN induced the synthesis of a karyophilic
protein that crossreacted with monoclonal antibodies to protein Mx.
The results in table 3 show that SL/NiA mice are homozygous for a
dominant resistance allele which is either closely linked to or
within the Mx locus of A2G mice (if not, group 5 would have 35
susceptible backcross mice (25%) instead of only one).

Table 3

Inheritance of resistance to influenza virus in SL/NiA mice

Group	Mouse strain and crosses	Sex	No. tested	No. susceptible	No. resistant
1	SL/NiA	f	7	0	7
		m	8	0	8
		total	15	0	15
2	F1, (BALB/c x SL/NiA)		14	0	14
	(SL/NiA x BALB/c)		9	0	9
3	BC-1, (BALB/c x F1*)	f	25	10	15
		m	30	14	16
		total	55	24	31
4	F1, (A2G x SL/NiA)		23	0	23
5	BC-1, (BALB/c x F1+)	f	68	1	67
		m	74	0	74
		total	142	1	141

F1* were (BALB/c x SL/NiA)F1 resistant males. F1+ were (A2G x
SL/NiA)F1 male offspring.

SOUTHERN ANALYSIS OF THE Mx GENE

We compared the Eco RI restriction pattern of eight different mouse strains. As shown before (Staeheli et al. 1986), the Mx⁻ genes of the 5 virus susceptible strains analyzed fell into two classes (which differed from the Mx⁺ pattern). However, the restriction patterns of the influenza virus resistant SL/NiA strain and of strain (T9 x CBA)FLU₊(carrying the Mx gene of a wild mouse) were identical to the Mx⁺ pattern of congenic strain BALB.A2G-Mx.

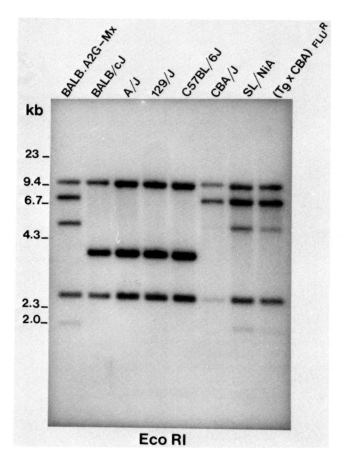

Fig. 2. Southern transfer analysis of murine genomic sequences related to Mx cDNA. Eco RI digested liver DNAs from the different mouse strains indicated were probed with the radiolabeled 1.65 kb Bam HI fragment of pMx41 as described by Staeheli et al. (1986). BALB/c and congenic BALB.A2G-Mx mice differ at alleles at the Mx locus. (T9 x CBA)FLUR mice represent the influenza virus resistant fifth backcross generation of a resistant wild male and a susceptible CBA/J female.

SUMMARY

Most inbred strains of laboratory mice carry deletions at the influenza virus resistance locus $\underline{Mx}$ on chromosome 16. The wild type
allele is present, as far as we can tell, only in two inbred
strains, A2G and SL/NiA, but is widespread in wild mice. Mice carrying the wild type allele ($\underline{Mx}^+$) are much more resistant towards
infections with influenza virus than mice with deletions ($\underline{Mx}^-$). The
$\underline{Mx}^+$ allele codes for an interferon- induced protein, called Mx
protein, that accumulates in the cell nucleus and is inhibitory to
orthomyxoviruses. It is not clear whether the prevalence of the $\underline{Mx}^-$
alleles in laboratory strains is due to a founder effect or to
selection.

ACKNOWLEDGEMENTS

We thank Murray B. Gardner and Joe Hilgers for gifts of mice and
Jean Lindenmann and Charles Weissmann for helpful discussions. This
study was supported by the Swiss National Science Foundation, Grant
3.507-083.

REFERENCES

Andrewes CH, Laidlaw PP, Smith W (1934) The susceptibility of
    mice to the viruses of human and swine influenza. Lancet II:
    859-862
Dreiding P, Staeheli P, Haller, O (1985) Interferon-induced
    protein Mx accumulates in nuclei of mouse cells expressing
    resistance to influenza viruses. Virology 140:192-196
Gardner MB (1978) Type C viruses of wild mice: Characterization
    and natural history of amphotropic, ecotropic, and xenotropic
    MuLV. Curr Top Microbiol Immunol 79:112-259
Haller O (1975) A mouse hepatotropic variant of influenza virus.
    Arch Virol 49:99-116
Haller O (1981) Inborn resistance of mice to orthomyxoviruses.
    Curr Topics Microbiol Immunol 92:25-52
Haller O, Arnheiter H, Gresser I, Lindenmann J (1979) Geneti-
    cally determined, interferon-dependent resistance to influenza
    virus in mice. J Exp Med 149:601-612
Haller O, Arnheiter H, Lindenmann J (1976) Genetically deter-
    mined resistance to infection by hepatotropic influenza A
    virus in mice: Effect of immunosuppression. Infect Immun 13:
    844-854
Haller O, Arnheiter H, Lindenmann J, Gresser I (1980) Host gene
    influences sensitivity to interferon action selectively for
    influenza virus. Nature 283:660-662
Hiai H, Ikeda H, Kaneshima H, Odaka T, Nishizuka Y (1982)
    Slvr-1: A new epistatic host gene restricting expression of
    endogenous ecotropic virus in SL/Ni mice is distinct from
    Fv-4. Proc Jap Cancer Assoc 41:335
Horisberger MA, Staeheli P, Haller O (1983) Interferon induces a
    unique protein in mouse cells bearing a gene for resistance to
    influenza virus. Proc Natl Acad Sci USA 80:1910-1914

Krug RM, Shaw M, Broni B, Shapiro G, Haller O (1985) Inhibition
   of influenza viral messenger RNA synthesis in cells expressing
   the interferon-induced Mx gene product. J Virol 56:201-206
Lindenmann J (1964) Inheritance of resistance to influenza in
   mice. Proc Soc Exp Biol Med 116:505-509
Lindenmann J, Klein, PA (1966) Further studies on the resistance
   of mice to myxoviruses. Arch ges Virusforsch 19:1-12
Staats J (1980) Standardized nomenclature for inbred strains of
   mice, seventh listing. Cancer Res 40:2083-2128
Staeheli P, Haller O, Boll W, Lindenmann J, Weissmann C (1986)
   Mx protein: Constitutive expression in 3T3 cells transformed
   with cloned Mx cDNA confers selective resistance to influenza
   virus. Cell 44:147-158
Staeheli P, Horisberger MA, Haller O (1984) Mx-dependent resistance to influenza virus is induced by mouse interferons alpha
   and beta but not gamma. Virology 132:456-461

Molecular Mechanism of an Ecotropic MuLV Restriction Gene Akvr-1/FV-4 in California Wild Mice

M. Gardner, S. Dandekar, and R. Cardiff

The Akvr-1 restriction gene was discovered as a dominant allele segregating in a feral population of mice (M. domesticus) at a squab farm near Lake Casitas (LC) in Southern California (Gardner et al. 1980). This gene prevented viremia of AKR endogenous retrovirus and virus-mediated lymphoma in LC (Akvr-1^{RR} x AKR) F1 hybrids. This effect was not due to the Fv-1 gene, which prevents AKR viremia and associated lymphoma in lab mice (Pincus et al. 1977), because LC viruses are N-tropic and LC mice appear to be monomorphic for Fv-1^N (Gardner 1978). The Akvr-1^R gene conferred a strong resistance to in vivo and in vitro infection of various ecotropic murine leukemia viruses (MuLV) (N-tropic, B-tropic or NB tropic) but did not restrict infection with wild mouse amphotropic MuLV strains (Rasheed and Gardner 1983). In these properties, Akvr-1^R closely resembled the Fv-4^R allele previously identified on chromosome 12 in certain Japanese inbred (FRG strain) and feral mice (M. molossinus) (Odaka et al. 1980; Odaka et al. 1981). Genetic crosses between LC (Akvr-1^{RR}) and FRG (Fv-4^{RR}) mice showed that these resistance loci were allelic (O'Brien et al 1983). Both Akvr-1^R and Fv-4^R alleles have now been molecularly cloned and characterized and their identicality confirmed. We summarize here the evidence showing that Akvr-1^R and Fv-4^R are the same gene and that this locus represents an evolutionarily conserved defective endogenous MuLV provirus which encodes an ecotropic envelope protein apparently interfering at the cell surface with entry of exogenous ecotropic MuLV.

To determine the cellular level at which ecotropic MuLV was restricted, we analyzed Hirt supernatents of cultured fibroblasts from resistant and susceptible mice for unintegrated proviral DNA following acute infection with ecotropic virus at high input. All of these cell lines were free of infectious MuLV and no retrovirus was induced from the wild mouse cells following treatment with 5 iododeoxyuridine (Rasheed and Gardner 1983). No viral DNA was found in the resistant cells indicating that the cellular block to infection occurred early, either before or during reverse transcription (Fig. 1). By contrast, the same cells that were resistant to ecotropic MuLV were fully susceptible to infection with amphotropic MuLV. We then found by Western blot analysis that this resistance was correlated with the presence on the cell surface of an ecotropic MuLV related envelope glycoprotein (gp70) in the absence of other viral proteins or replicating virus (Fig. 2). Resistance of uninfected thymocytes to Friend MuLV had similarly been linked to Fv-4 mediated expression of an MuLV gp70-related antigen (Ikeda and Odaka 1984). These findings suggested that Akvr-1^R and Fv-4^R might represent a defective endogenous provirus(es) encoding this ecotropic MuLV-related envelope glycoprotein.

To determine if we could identify this putative defective provirus we analyzed the genome of resistant LC feral mice for recombinant phage clones containing ecotropic MuLV envelope related DNA. LC feral mice, like laboratory mice, contain 30-50 copies per haploid genome of MuLV related DNA sequences, none of which are highly homologous to the AKR ecotropic virus (Steffen et al. 1980). Most of these are silent genes or represent viral DNA defective for replication or noninfectious (xenotropic) for the natural host. To identify the putative Akvr-1 provirus admidst this high background "noise" of related sequences, we used a cloned 400 bp AKR ecotropic viral envelope specific DNA fragment (p E env) (Chan et al. 1980) to probe the DNA from a LC (Akvr-1^{RR}) wild mouse cell line. Under stringent hybridization conditions highly related sequences could not be detected in the feral mice DNA with this probe. However, under relaxed conditions capable of detecting sequences of $\leq$ 60% homology and using a number of restriction enzymes, we were able to detect multiple copies of ecotropic envelope-related sequences in the DNA from the resistant wild mouse cells. The sizes of the DNA fragments were different from those of the corresonding ecotropic MuLV fragments in the genome of AKR inbred mice. To isolate one or more of these bands which might represent the Akvr-1 resistance allele we made a genomic library of Akvr-1^{RR} wild mouse DNA, screened about 600,000 plaques with the p E env probe and obtained hybridization with three lambda recombinant clones. These clones were propagated and their DNA was hybridized with AKR MuLV DNA probes specific for gag, pol, env and LTR regions. Two clones hybridized only with the p E env probe and not with gag, pol or LTR probes. One clone (RR 24) had, in addition to env, an LTR at the 3' end and an incomplete pol sequence at the 5' end but lacked gag- related sequences. This clone showed homology to the 400 bp ecotropic envelope specific sequences in a 0.7 kb Bam Hl fragment (designated RR 24-B). We subcloned this RR 24-B fragment and used it to probe cell lines of known resistance or susceptibility (Akvr-1^{RR} or Akvr-1^{SS}) to ecotropic MuLV infection. Resistant cells uniformly hybridized with this probe whereas susceptible cells failed to hybridize. To map the envelope gene in genomic DNA, high molecular weight DNA from LC^{RR} cells was digested with different restriction enzymes. The probe RR24-B hybridized preferentially in each digest to one fragment and only weakly to other related sequences. Most remarkably, the sizes of the internal restriction fragments as well as the host viral junction fragments appeared essentially identical to those independently found for the Fv-4 resistance gene (Kozak et al. 1984) as shown in Table 1. Restriction enzymes Bam Hl and Sma l cut Akvr-1^{R} and Fv-4^{R} DNA internally whereas Pst l, Xba l and Kpn l cut once internally and once in the flanking host genome. An Eco Rl site was not present in the Akvr-1/Fv-4 envelope sequence. Restriction sites for Pst l, Sma l and Kpn l mapped at the same LTR location in both Akvr-1^{R} and Fv-4^{R} DNA. This striking degree of restriction map correspondence strengthened the likelihood that these DNA fragments in feral mice from California and Japan did indeed represent the same gene and supported previous evidence of their identicality based on allelism in genetic crosses (O'Brien et al. 1983) and alike properties of virus restriction in vivo and in vitro (Rasheed and Gardner 1983; Odaka et al 1980). Restriction maps of the AKR ecotropic MuLV, the putative Akvr-1/Fv-4 resistance gene and location of the RR 24-B clone are shown in Fig. 4.

Further evidence that the unique 0.7 kb Bam Hl fragment detected with the RR 24-B probe represented the Akvr-1/Fv-4 resistance gene was provided by the co-segregation of these sequences with ecotropic MuLV resistance in genetic crosses between resistant LC wild mice and susceptible AKR and NIH Swiss mice. The 0.7 kb Bam 1 marker fragment was detected in spleen DNA or embryo fibroblast DNA derived from virus-resistant LC^{RR}, $(LC^{RR}$ x AKR)Fls and $(LC^{RR}$ x NIH Swiss)Fls. The same 0.7 kb marker was not detected in spleen or embryo fibroblast DNA from virus susceptible AKR and NIH Swiss mice nor in the susceptible wild mouse SC-1 cell line (Hartley and Rowe 1975). Kozak et al (1984) found the same correlation in BALB/c mice backcrossed with Mus molossinus to derive a strain partially congenic for Fv-4 resistance.

Finally, we partially sequenced the Akvr-1 associated proviral envelope and compared about 1.0 kb to that of the published AKR MuLV envelope and $Fv-4^R$ genes (Ikeda et al 1985). Virtually 100% sequence homology was noted between $Akvr-1^R$ and $Fv-4^R$ DNA and about 70% homology was noted with the AKR MuLV envelope DNA. These results confirm the identicality of the $Akvr-1^R$ and $Fv-4^R$ alleles.

The glycoprotein-receptor interaction that forms the genetic basis of the Akvr-1/Fv-4 restriction gene effect also constitutes the molecular basis of virus interference assays first used to classify virus subtypes in the avian leukosis and sarcoma complex (Vogt and Ishizaki 1966). In the chicken, a dominant gene (I^e) (Payne et al. 1971), now known to represent an endogenous provirus locus (Robinson et al 1981), similarly encodes an envelope gp70 which binds to and masks the cell receptor for subgroup E leukosis virus, preventing virus entry. In mice, separate receptors exist for different classes of MuLV (ecotropic, xenotropic, amphotropic, recombinant) (Rein 1982) and the receptor genes have been assigned to different chromosomes. All ecotropic MuLVs are of the same interference class (Sarma et al. 1967) and thus utilize a single cell receptor whose gene is located on chromosome 5 (Gazdar et al. 1977). Therefore, entry of all ecotropic MuLVs is blocked at this cell receptor level by action of the Fv-4 gene. The DBA inbred mouse strain was found to restrict recombinant (MCF) MuLV infection at the cell surface level (Bassin et al. 1982), presumably by the same mechanism as $Fv-4^R$ restricts ecotropic MuLV. Laboratory mice in North America and Europe apparently lack the Fv-4 resistance gene probably because of the relatively narrow genetic base from which they were derived (Morse 1978). However, the Fv-4 resistance gene was recently found in Mus cervicolor DNA (Kozak et al. 1984). Other Asian wild mice that also showed resistance to ecotropic MuLV (Friend virus) lacked this locus and thus, viral interference cannot account for resistance in all wild mice.

The remarkable conservation of the Fv-4^R gene and flanking DNA in feral mice as genetically different as those from California (M. domesticus) and Japan (M. molossinus and M. cervicolor) (Steffen et al. 1980) may possibly be explained on the basis that this gene performs a useful function, which very likely is protection against ecotropic MuLV infection endemic in both populations of wild mice. This conservation must have extended over at least 1-2 million years since divergence of the Mus molossinus and Mus cervicolor from a common ancestor (Sage 1981). In LC wild mice, ecotropic MuLV infection causes a high incidence of lymphoma and a fatal paralytic spongiform polioencephalopathy, both occuring after 1 year of age (Gardner 1978). Thus, in the final analysis, susceptibility or resistance to the oncogenic and nononcogenic retroviral diseases in aging LC wild mice probably depends mainly on inheritance of the Akvr-1/Fv-4 resistance gene which segregates in this outbred population. In a limited sample based on crosses of LC x AKR mice, the allele frequency of this gene in LC wild mice was 0.47 and the genotype frequencies did not vary significantly from expectations of the Hardy Weinberg equilibrium (Gardner et al. 1980). Thus, the probable frequency of LC mice carrying at least one Fv-4^R allele is 0.72 and these mice would be expected to be resistant to the ecotropic virus induced lymphoma and paralysis. However, because this locus fails to suppress the highly prevalent amphotropic MuLV these mice are still susceptible to lymphoma late in life. Genotyping of wild mice in nature with the RR24-B probe should predict which individual animals will be at risk to the spontaneous neurologic disease.

Similar restriction genes may possibly control retrovirus infection in species other than chickens and mice. Understanding the molecular nature of these genes and learning how to manipulate them in this murine model system may therefore conceivably find future clinical application in predicting those at risk and in genetically engineering resistance to retroviral diseases in other animal species including man.

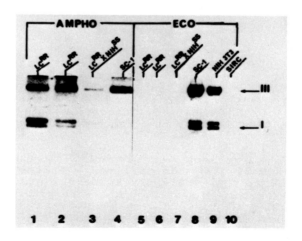

Fig. 1. Southern blot analysis of viral DNA intermediates from Hirt supernatents of different mouse cell lines infected with amphotropic or ecotropic MuLV. Lane 1-4: Cell lines infected

with amphotropic MuLV. Lane 5-10: Cell lines infected with ecotropic MuLV. Lane 1&5: LC^{RR} #30358; Lane 2&6: LC^{RR} #28633; Lane 3&7: (LC^{RR} x NIH Swiss^{SS})FI #2996; Lane 4&8: wild mouse^{SS} (SC-1); Lane 9: NIH 3T3^{SS}; lane 10: rabbit cornea (SIRC).

About 10^7 cells were infected with amphotropic or ecotropic virus at a multiplicity of infection of 0.8. After 24 hours, unintegrated viral DNA was extracted by the Hirt method. Southern blots containing proviral DNA were hybridized with nick translated ^{32}P-labelled 4070A amphotropic virus probe (lanes 1-4) or pE-env ecotropic envelope probe (lanes 5-10). Autoradiographs were exposed to Kodak XAR-5 film for 2-5 days. The proviral DNA detected consisted of linear (Form III) and circular (Form I) forms.

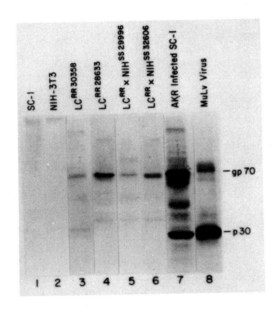

Fig. 2. Detection of ecotropic env-related proteins by Western blot. Lane 1: wild mouse^{SS} (SC-1 cells), Lane 2: NIH-3T3^{SS} cells, Lane 3: LC^{RR} #30358, Lane 4: LC^{RR} #28633, Lane 5: (LC^{RR} x NIH Swiss^{SS})F₁ #29996, Lane 6: (LC^{RR} x NIH Swiss^{SS})F₁ #32606, Lane 7: SC-1 cells chronically infected with AKR MuLV, Lane 8: Moloney MuLV. The blot has been reacted with goat anti AKR MuLV antiserum.

Ecotropic MuLV proteins were detected by the Western blot technique with slight modifications. Protein samples were separated on 10% SDS - polyacrylamide gel and transferred to nitrocellulose paper. Western blots were probed with goat AKR virus antibody. Blots were washed before incubating with ^{125}I labelled rabbit anti-goat immunoglobulin. Western blots were autoradiographed for 12 hours on Kodak XAR-5 film.

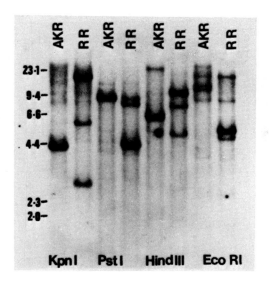

Fig. 3.   Detection of ecotropic MuLV env-related sequences in LC and AKR cellular DNA.

High molecular weight DNA from spleens of LC^{RR} or AKR mice were digested to completion by different restriction enzymes.   DNA digests were electrophoresed on 1% agaorse gels and transferred to nitrocellulose paper.   The blots were hybridized with ^{32}P-labelled 0.7 kb RR24-B DNA probe. Autoradiographs were exposed to Kodak XAR-5 film for 2-5 days.

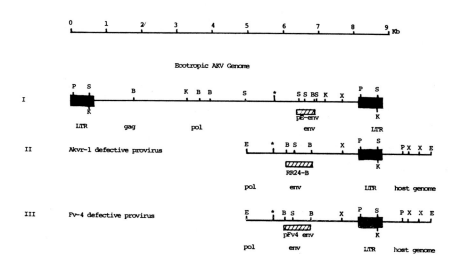

Fig. 4.   Comparison of Akvr-1 defective proviral genome with ecotropic AKV genome and Fv-4 proviral genome.   Positions of

restriction sites for EcoRI (E), Bam HI (B), Xba 1 (X), Pst I (P), Sma I (S) and Kpn 1 (K) are shown on the restriction maps. Locations of ecotropic MuLV envelope specific probe "p E env" in the AKV genome, Akvr-1 specific "RR-24B probe" in the Akvr-1 provirus and pFv4 env probe in the Fv-4 provirus are shown as hatched boxes. LTR regions are represented as closed boxes. The splice receptor sites are shown with asterisks.

TABLE 1

Ecotropic MuLV Envelope Related Fragments (Kb)

Restriction Enzyme	AKR	Akvr-1	Fv-4 (Kozak et al., 1984)
Bam HI	3	0.7	0.75
Pst I	8.2	4.2	4.1
Xba I	10.0	4.0	4.1
Hind III	6	9.4	9.3
Eco RI	5.0	5.3	5.2
Kpn I	4.0	17.0	17.3
Sst I	4.0	2.6	-
Pvu II	3.0	3.6	-

REFERENCES

Bassin RH, Ruscetti S, Aliqbal, Haapala DK, Rein A. (1982) Normal DBA/2 mouse cells synthesize a glycoprotein which interferes with MCF virus infection. Virol 123:139-151

Chan HW, Bryan T, Moore JL, Staal SP, Rowe WP, Martin MA. (1980) Identification of ecotropic proviral sequences in inbred mouse strains with a cloned subgenomic DNA fragment. PNAS 77:5779-5783.

Gardner MB. (1978) Type C viruses of wild mice: characterization and natural history of amphotropic, ecotropic, and xenotropic MuLV. Current Topics in Microbiology and Immunology. Vol. 79. pp. 216-256.

Gardner MB, Rasheed S, Pal BK, Estes, JD, O'Brien SJ. (1980) Akvr-1, a dominant murine leukemia virus restriction gene, is polymorphic in leukemia-prone wild mice. Proc Natl Acad Sci 77:531-535.

Gazdar AF, Oie H, Lalley P, Moss WW, Minna JD, Francke U. (1977) Identificaton of mouse chromosomes required for murine leukemia virus replication. Cell 11:949-956.

Hartley JW and Rowe WP (1975) Clonal cell lines from a fetal mouse embryo which lacks host-range restriction for murine leukemia viruses. Virol 65:128-134.

Ikeda H, Laigret F, Martin M, Repaske R. (1985) Characterization of a molecularly cloned retroviral sequence associated with Fv-4 resistance. J Virol 55:768-777.

Ikeda H and Odaka T. (1984) A cell membrane "gp70" associated with Fv-4 gene: immunological characterization, and tissue and strain distribution. Virol 133:65-76.

Kozak CA, Gromet NJ, Ikeda H, Buckler CE. (1984) A unique sequence related to the ecotropic murine leukemia viruses associated with the Fv-4 resistance gene. PNAS 81:834-837.

Morse HC, III (1978) Origins of inbred mice. Academic Press Inc., NY.

O'Brien SJ, Berman EJ, Estes JD, Gardner MB. (1983) Murine retroviral restriction genes Fv-4 and Akvr-1 are alleles of a single locus. J Virol 47:649-651.

Odaka T, Ikeda H and Akatsuka T (1980) Restricted expression of endogenous N-tropic XC-postivie leukemia virus in hybrids between G and AKR mice: An effect of the Fv-4^R gene. Int J Cancer 25:757-762.

Odaka T, Ikeda H, Yoshikura H, Moriwaki K and Suzuki S (1981) Fv-4: gene controlling resistance to NB-tropic Friend murine leukemia virus. Distribution in wild mice, introduction into genetic background of BALB/c mice, and mapping of chromosomes. J Nat Cancer Inst 67:1123-1127.

Payne LN, Rani PK, Weiss RA. (1971) A dominant epistatic gene which inhibits cellular susceptibility to RSV (RAV-0). J Gen Virol 131:455-462.

Pincus T, Hartley JW, Rowe WP. (1971) A major genetic locus affecting ecotropic and mink cell focus-inducing strains of Moloney murine leukemia viruses. I. Tissue culture studies of naturally occuring viruses. J Exp Med 133:1219-1233.

Rasheed S and Gardner MB. (1983) Resistance of fibroblasts and hematopoietic cells to ecotropic murine leukemia virus infection; an Akvr-1^R gene effect. Int J Cancer 31:491-496.

Rein A. (1982) Interference grouping of murine leukemia viruses: A distinct receptor for the MCF-recombinant viruses on mouse cells. Virol 120:251-257.

Robinson HL, Astrin SM, Senior AM, Salazar FH (1981) Host susceptibility to endogenous viruses: Defective, glycoprotein-expressing proviruses interfere with infections. J Virol 40:745-751

Sage RD. (1981) Wild mice. In: The Mouse in Biomedical Research. Vol 1, Chapt 4, pp 39-90. Ed. HL Foster, JD Small, JG Fox, Academic Press, NY.

Sarma PS, Cheong MP, Hartley JW, Huebner RJ. (1967) A viral interference test for mouse leukemia viruses. Virol 33:180-184.

Steffen DL, Bird S, Weinberg RG. (1980) Evidence for the asiatic origin of endogenous AKR-type murine leukemia proviruses. J Virol 35:824-835

Vogt PK and Ishizaki R (1966) Patterns of viral interference in the avian leukosis and sarcoma complex. Virol 30:368-374.

Retroviral Genes

Xenotropic and MCF Related Retroviral Genes in Wild Mice

C. A. Kozak and R. R. O'Neill

INTRODUCTION

The mouse leukemia viruses (MuLVs) of inbred mice are classically divided into host range subgroups based on their ability to exogenously
infect mouse cells and cells of other species. The ecotropic viruses
infect only mouse cells; the xenotropic viruses cannot infect mouse
cells but can infect cells of other species such as mink; and the poly-
tropic or mink cell focus-forming (MCF) viruses infect cells of both
mouse and non-mouse species. These host range differences are due to
differences in the major virion glycoprotein which is encoded by the
viral envelope (env) gene. Sequences homologous to the env genes of all
3 virus groups are present in the germline DNA of laboratory mice, and
these genes are inherited in a typical Mendelian fashion.

For the nonecotropic MuLVs, wild mice differ considerably from
laboratory mice in two respects. First, cells of many wild mice are
susceptible to infection by the xenotropic viruses which cannot repli-
cate in inbred mouse cells. Second, not all wild mice contain
sequences homologous to xenotropic and MCF proviral env genes, and
those that do are substantially different from inbred mice in the number of copies they inherit and in their chromosomal locations.

ENDOGENOUS VIRAL SEQUENCES IN WILD MICE

Southern blot hybridization with a cloned 455 base pair probe derived
from the amino terminal region of the xenotropic viral env gene has
demonstrated that there are more than 30 copies of related sequences in
the laboratory mouse genome (Hoggan et al. 1983). While this probe
does not react with ecotropic MuLVs, it cannot distinguish xenotropic
from MCF viruses. This distinction is an important one because of the
biological differences between xenotropic and MCF viruses. Xenotropic
viruses are not known to be pathogenic, but at least some of the integrated xenotropic viral copies are full-length and are readily induced
as infectious virus in a variety of cell types and by a variety of in-
ducers. In contrast, the MCF viruses can be leukemogenic, but are not
present as inducible viruses in cellular DNA. Instead, these viruses
are generated de novo in preleukemic tissues by recombination between
replicating ecotropic MuLVs and specific endogenous nonecotropic
sequences.

In order to distinguish these endogenous sequences, O'Neill and his
colleagues (Submitted) have derived smaller hybridization probes of ap-

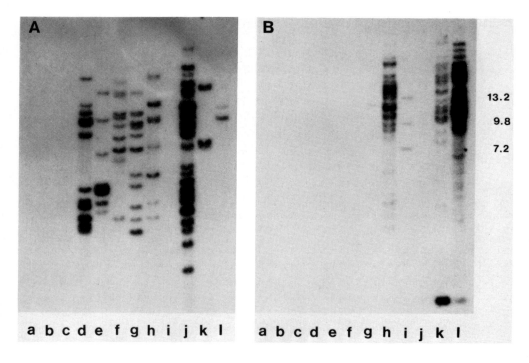

Fig.1. Southern blot analysis of mouse DNAs cleaved with HindIII and
hybridized with MCF-specific (Panel A) or xenotropic-specific (Panel B)
probes. HindIII does not cleave the xenotropic retroviral genome and
cleaves the MCF MuLV once. Therefore, HindIII generates provirus-cell
junction fragments of different sizes for each proviral integration.
DNAs were electrophoresed on 0.4% agarose gels, transferred onto nitrocellulose membranes and hybridized as described previously (Hoggan et
al. 1982) except that duplicate membranes were obtained by bidirec-
tional blotting. Kilobase size markers are indicated to the right. Lane
a, Mus caroli; lane b, M. cervicolor popaeus; lane c, M. hortulanus;
lane d, M.m. brevirostris; lane e, M.m. praetextus; lane f, M. spretus
(Morocco); lane g, M. musculus (NYD); lane h, M.m. musculus (Denmark);
lane i, size markers; lane j, M.m. domesticus (Haven's Farm); lane k,
M.m. castaneus; lane l, M.m. molossinus

proximately 100 base pairs from analogous regions in the MCF and
xenotropic env genes. Each probe is type-specific and thus, these
probes can simplify the analysis of endogenous xenotropic and MCF related sequences in the mouse germline.

Use of the MCF-specific env probe has shown that most of the 30 or more
nonecotropic env sequences present in inbred mice in fact resemble
progenitors of infectious MCF virus (O'Neill et al. Submitted). All
inbred mice tested have 20-30 copies of these genes and therefore, they
represent an important component of the inbred mouse genome. Among the

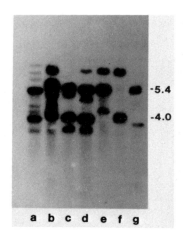

Fig. 2. Southern blot analysis of mouse DNAs cleaved with KpnI and hybridized with the MCF-specific probe. Kilobase size markers are indicated to the right. Lane a, BALB/c; lane b, M.m. musculus (Denmark);
lane c, M. musculus (NYD); lane d, M.m. brevirostris; lane e, M.
spretus (Morocco); lane f, M.m. castaneus; lane g, M.m. molossinus

wild mice, Asian mice such as Mus cervicolor and M. caroli lack these
sequences altogether and M.m. molossinus and M.m. castaneus have few
(2-3) copies (Fig.1, Table 1). Several of the European, American, and
African wild mice contain variable numbers of MCF-related env genes,
and copy numbers comparable to the inbred strains are found in some of
these DNAs. The size distribution of the HindIII env-reactive fragments
also differs among these mice further suggesting that proviral genes
are integrated into different chromosomal sites in these mice.

In order to investigate the relatedness of the viral sequences found in
wild mice and inbred strains, DNAs from strains with MCF-related env
genes were digested with restriction enzymes known to produce internal
fragments from infectious viral DNAs. Cleavage with PstI, KpnI, BglII,
and SacI reveals that the internal organization of most of the wild
mouse MCF proviral sequences resembles that observed in inbred mice
(Hoggan et al. 1982). Like laboratory mice, wild mice inherit more than
a single species of MCF-related proviral sequence. For example, KpnI
digestion recruits most of the env-reactive proviral genes of BALB/c
into major fragments of 4.0 and 5.4 kilobases. The six wild mice
examined contained one or both of these fragments along with a few
generally less intense fragments (Fig. 2).

Sequences related to xenotropic viruses are also present in all inbred
mice tested although the Swiss derived mice contain only a single copy
(O'Neill, et al. Submitted). Although 10 of the 14 wild mice tested do
not contain any xenotropic env sequences at all, three contained multiple copies (Fig. 1B, Table 1). Of these three, the Japanese mouse,
M.m. molossinus, is unique in that, like many laboratory strains, it
contains copies which can be induced as infectious virus (Kozak et al.
1984). Each of these three mice had a characteristic pattern of env-

Table 1

Mice	Susceptibility to Xenotropic MuLV	Number of Endogenous env-reactive fragments Xenotropic	MCF
M. platythrix	+	0	0
M. pahari	+	0	0
M. cookii	+	0	0
M. caroli	+	0	0
M. cervicolor	+	0	0
M. minutoides	+	NT	NT
M. hortulanus	+	0	0
M.m. brevirostris	+	0	>14
M.m. praetextus	+	0	8
M. spretus	+	0	10
M. musculus (NYD)	+	1	12
M.m. musculus (Denmark)	−	>20	8
M.m. domesticus (Haven's Farm)	+	0	>30
M.m. castaneus	NT	>15	3
M.m. molossinus	NT	>30	2
BALB/c	−	7	>15

NT = not tested

related fragments indicating a variation in provirus chromosomal locations in these mice.

SUSCEPTIBILITY TO EXOGENOUS XENOTROPIC MuLVs

In tests of 14 wild mouse populations, adult tail cultures of 11 were found to be susceptible to exogenous infection by a variety of xenotropic MuLVs (Table 1). The level of sensitivity was low with virus titers averaging 3 logs lower than titers of the same viruses on mink cells (Kozak 1985). However, these titers are at least 3 logs higher than the titers of these same viruses on laboratory mouse cells.

Two of the susceptible mice, M. spretus and M.m. praetextus were mated with laboratory mice. Cells from F_1 hybrids were as susceptible to virus infection as cells from the wild mouse parents indicating that susceptibility, not resistance, is inherited as a dominant trait. This suggests that the mechanism for resistance in inbred mice is not due to viral interference. Such an interference model has been used to explain the resistance to ecotropic virus in $Fv-4^r$ mice in which an endogenous ecotropic env glycoprotein interferes with exogenous infection (Ikeda et al. 1985). Inheritance of the Fv-4 mediated interference type of resistance is dominant rather than recessive.

F_1 hybrids from the spretus and praetextus crosses were intercrossed or backcrossed to resistant mice, and progeny were tested for virus sensitivity. The results were consistent with a single gene controlling susceptibility to xenotropic virus in both F_2 and backcross generations.

55 mice of 72 F_2 progeny (76%) were susceptible and 63 of 127 backcross mice (50%) were susceptible. This susceptibility gene, termed Sxv, was mapped to chromosome 1, 11 cM from Pep-3 with gene order: ln-Pep-3-Sxv-Bxv-1). The nature of Sxv is at present unknown, but several lines of evidence suggest that this gene may represent a wild mouse polymorphism of the MCF MuLV cell surface receptor (Kozak 1985).

CONCLUSIONS

The origin of retroviral genes remains obscure. However, this analysis raises the possibility that at least some of the diversity in endogenous retroviruses may be due to the wild mouse Sxv gene. The absence of endogenous xenotropic and MCF-related env sequences in some wild mice indicates that these MuLVs were introduced into the Mus germline during speciation. The simplest explanation for the acquisition of multiple retroviral copies involves infection of germline cells followed by chromosomal integration. For the mouse-tropic ecotropic virus, previous studies have documented the acquisition of new proviral insertions in viremic mice (Rowe and Kozak 1980). The identification of Sxv suggests that such reinfections may also occur for xenotropic MuLVs. Consistent with this possibility is the observed correlation between the early spontaneous production of infectious virus in M.m. molossinus and the large number of endogenous copies in this mouse (Kozak et al. 1984). Thus, since wild mouse cells are susceptible to infection by ecotropic, MCF and xenotropic MuLVs, a common mechanism of reinfection and reintegration may be responsible, at least in part, for the presence of multiple proviral genes in the mouse germline and account for the differences among mice in the number of copies they carry and their chromosomal organization in the mouse genome.

REFERENCES

Hoggan, MD, Buckler, CE, Sears, JF, Chan, HW, Rowe, WP and Martin, MA (1982) Internal organization of endogenous proviral DNAs of xenotropic murine leukemia viruses. J Virol 43;8-17

Hoggan, MD, Buckler, CE, Sears, JF, Rowe, WP, and Martin, MA (1983) Organization and stability of endogenous xenotropic murine leukemia virus proviral DNA in mouse genomes. J. Virol 45:473-477

Ikeda, H, Laigret, F, Martin, MA, and Repaske, R (1985) Characterization of a molecularly cloned retroviral sequence associated with Fv-4 resistance. J. Virol 55:768-777

Kozak, CA (1985) Susceptibility of wild mouse cells to exogenous infection with xenotropic leukemia viruses: control by a single dominant locus on chromosome 1. J. Virol 55:690-695

Kozak, CA, Hartley, JW, and Morse, HC, III (1984) Laboratory and wild-derived mice with multiple loci for production of xenotropic murine leukemia virus. J Virol 51: 77-80

O'Neill, RR, Khan, AS, Hoggan, MD, Hartley, JW, Martin, MA, and Repaske, R Specific hybridization probes demonstrate more MCF than xenotropic MuLV env related sequences in DNAs from inbred laboratory mice. J Virol Submitted

Rowe, WP and Kozak CA (1980) Germline insertion of AKR murine leukemia virus genomes in Akv-1 congenic mice. Proc Natl Acad Sci USA 77:4871-4874

Mammary Tumorigenesis in Feral Species of the Genus *Mus*

D. Gallahan, C. Escot, E. Hogg, and R. Callahan

INTRODUCTION

Spontaneous mammary tumorigenesis in mice is frequently associated with a chronic infection of the host mammary tissue by the mouse mammary tumor virus (MMTV). This was first recognized in inbred strains of M. musculus which had been selectively bred over several generations for a high incidence of mammary tumors (Weiss et al. 1982). The mechanism by which laboratory strains of MMTV induce mammary tumors in these mice is only beginning to be unraveled. MMTV, like other retroviruses, can act as an insertional mutagen on the cellular genome of the host. Two cellular genetic loci (designated int-1 and int-2), which are frequently occupied by an MMTV genome in mammary tumor cellular DNA, have been described (Nusse and Varmus 1982; Peters et al. 1983). The insertion of a viral genome at either locus leads to the activation of expression of a cellular gene within the affected locus (Dickson et al. 1984; Nusse et al. 1984). These two cellular loci are unrelated to each other and to the known proto-oncogenes (Nusse et al. 1984; Peters et al. 1984). Although direct evidence is lacking, it has been proposed that activation of int-1 or int-2 contributes to mammary tumor development. Two additional issues remain unresolved. First, what effect has inbreeding for high mammary tumor incidence had on the sensitivity of these mice to activation of the int loci by MMTV? Second, are there other as yet unidentified int loci which are at risk in MMTV-induced mammary tumorigenesis?

To approach these questions we have studied mammary tumorigenesis in pedigreed outbred colonies of feral species of the genus Mus. Earlier surveys of feral M. musculus domesticus demonstrated the existence of poorly infectious MMTV in milk and some mammary tumors (Andervont 1952). The incidence of mammary tumors in these feral mice was, in general, low, and tumor development occurred late in life (Andervont and Dunn 1962; Rongey et al. 1973). In the present report we summarize our observations on mammary tumor incidence in several species of Mus and our results showing that feral MMTV insertion frequently activates the int-1 locus in M. cervicolor popaeus mammary tumors and that a new int locus (designated int-3) is frequently occupied and activated by an MMTV genome in M. musculus musculus (Czech II) mammary tumors.

Mammary Tumor Incidence in Feral Species of Mus

Over the past several years we have established pedigreed breeding colonies of several species of Mus from different geographical regions of the world. The origins and characteristics of the colonies have been described (Marshall 1977; Callahan and Todaro 1978;

Arn et al. 1981) and are summarized in the Appendix. The colonies which have been monitored for mammary tumor development are indicated in Table 1. The mammary tumor incidence ranged from 0 to 48% with an average latency of 18 months. Histopathological examination of the tumors demonstrated that they were primarily mammary adenocarcinoma type A or type B (Dunn 1959). In addition, rare histopathological types (L, Y, and P) of mammary tumors were observed among the M. cervicolor popaeus (Tak) (Sass and Dunn 1979). The development of mammary tumors in feral mice is primarily pregnancy independent, although a significant number (40%) of M. cervicolor popaeus (TAK) mammary tumors were pregnancy dependent. The frequency of tumors in other tissues was, in general, low (ranging from 1.4 to 8%) and developed after a latency of 18-25 months of age.

Table 1. Mammary tumor incidence in breeding females of different Mus species

Species	Breeding Females	Mammary Tumors	Average Latency (Months)[a]	MMTV[b]
M. musculus musculus (Czech II)	209	24	18 (9-28)	+
M. spretus (Spain)	59	12	16 (9-28)	+
M. caroli	39	0	--	+
M. cervicolor cervicolor	122	7	19 (16-24)	+
M. cervicolor popaeus (TAK)	383	182	19 (6-38)	+
M. cervicolor popaeus (Chonburi and Saraburi)	137	3	19 (15-22)	+
M. cookii	87	4	13 (10-16)	+
M. pahari	78	0	--	-

[a] Numbers in the parenthesis show the range in months.
[b] The presence of MMTV was determined by either immunological assays, electron microscopy, or molecular hybridization to milk or tumor cellular DNA or RNA.

To determine whether there is a relationship between the spontaneous mammary tumors in these feral mice and MMTV, milk and tumor tissues were examined for the presence of viral proteins and, in some cases, viral particles. With the exception of M. pahari, all of the colonies contain milkborne MMTV. However, the virus is not ubiquitous among all breeding females in each colony. Similarly, not all of the mammary tumors contain MMTV. It was important to exclude the possibility that the feral milkborne virus resulted

356

from an interspecies transmission of MMTV from laboratory strains
of inbred mice to the feral mouse colonies. Using radioimmunoassays and immunoperoxidase assays for MMTV (C3H) and the M. cervicolor popaeus (TAK) milkborne virus (MC-MTV), it was possible to
show that the viral proteins expressed in milk and mammary tumors
of M. caroli, M. cervicolor, and M. cookii are immunologically distinguishable from laboratory strains of MMTV (Schlom et al. 1978;
Horan-Hand et al. 1980; Teramoto et al. 1980; Colcher et al. 1981).
Hybridization studies of normal tissues showed that the M. musculus
musculus (Czech II) mice lack endogenous MMTV genomes (Callahan et
al. 1982). However, recently we have obtained recombinant DNA
clones of an MMTV genome which was integrated into mammary tumor
DNA of these mice (Gallahan et al., manuscript in preparation). As
shown in Figure 1, a comparison of the position of EcoRl restriction sites clearly distinguishes the MMTV (Czech II) genome from
the genomes of laboratory strains of MMTV. The relatively low frequency of mammary tumors and long latency before tumor development
suggests to us that feral MMTV is poorly infectious. Two observations are consistent with this interpretation. First, we have been
unable to transmit the M. cervicolor popaeus MC-MTV to BALB/c mice
by foster nursing or injection of concentrated virus. Second, the
M. musculus musculus (Czech II) colony was derived from a single
breeding pair of mice, yet only a fraction of the breeding females
ever express MMTV in their milk. An alternative possibility is that

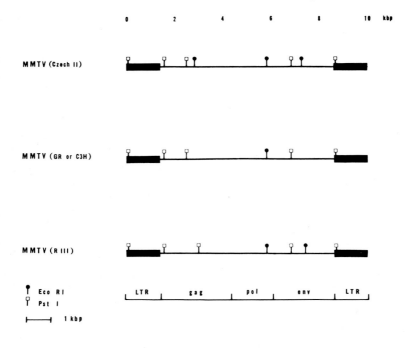

Fig. 1. Comparative restriction maps of infectious MMTV proviral
DNA.

within the feral population there are resistance genes that either attenuate or block virus infection.

Frequency of Feral MMTV Insertion into int Loci of Mammary Tumor DNA

Previous studies of MMTV-induced tumors in inbred strains of M. musculus have demonstrated the existence of two cellular genetic loci (designated int-1 and int-2), which are frequently occupied by an MMTV genome in tumor cellular DNA (Dickson et al. 1984; Nusse et al. 1984). To determine whether this is a general feature of MMTV-induced mammary tumors, these loci were examined in M. cervicolor popaeus (TAK) and M. musculus musculus (Czech II) tumor DNAs. The int loci in 20 DNAs from M. cervicolor popaeus (TAK) tumors and matching livers were compared by Southern blot analysis (Escot et al., manuscript in preparation). Tumor DNAs from 10 mice contained an altered int-1 locus while one tumor had an altered int-2 locus. The nongermline fragments, which are characteristic of the alteration detected by the int probes, were shown to be the result of the insertion of an MC-MTV genome within the int region of the cellular genome. Moreover, the MMTV-induced genetic alterations of the int-1 locus activated the expression of a 2.6-kb RNA species which is related to the C3H mouse strain int-1 transcribed region (Nusse et al. 1984).

Analysis of 16 M. musculus musculus (Czech II) tumor DNAs revealed no evidence for MMTV insertion into either the int-1 or int-2 loci (Gallahan et al., manuscript in preparation). However, five tumor DNAs appeared to contain common host-viral junction restriction fragments. Recombinant DNA clones containing these restriction fragments have been obtained. A subclone containing a unique host-flanking sequence detects a 8.6-kbp EcoRl fragment in normal liver cellular DNA. A similar examination of restricted virus-positive tumor cellular DNA revealed the presence of an additional 7.5-kbp or 7.0-kbp fragment in each of the five tumors with common host-viral junction or fragments. In each case the transcriptional orientation of the viral genome was in the same direction. MMTV insertion into this region of the cellular genome activates the expression of a 2.4-kbp species of mRNA which corresponds to cellular DNA sequences flanking the 5' end of an integrated viral genome. This species of RNA is not found in lactating mammary glands or tumors lacking viral insertions in this region of the cellular genome. Since this locus shares no detectable homology with int-1, int-2, or other known proto-oncogenes, we have designated it int-3. The chromosomal location of int-3 was established on chromosome 17 by restriction enzyme analysis of mouse/hamster somatic cell hybrids (Gallahan et al., manuscript in preparation). To further localize the position of int-3 on chromosome 17, 74 (C3H x Czech II) x Czech II backcross mice were examined. We have taken advantage of frequent restriction fragment length polymorphisms which exist between cellular genes in M. musculus musculus and laboratory inbred mouse strains (Robbins et al. 1984). Using this approach we have shown that the int-3 locus is located 11 cM distal to the MHC (H-2) locus.

It has been assumed that MMTV, after infection, is capable of integrating at random sites throughout the cellular genome (Weiss 1982). Indeed, this absence of specificity for integration sites appears to be substantiated by the large number of different endogenous proviral genomes (O'Brien 1984). A paradox arises when one inspects the frequency with which different strains of MMTV occupy one of the three _int_ loci in mammary tumor DNA (Table 2). Thus MMTV (C3H) and MC-MTV more frequently occupy the _int_-1 locus, MMTV (RIII) the _int_-2 locus, and MMTV (Czech II) the _int_-3 locus. Since different strains of mice were used in these experiments, it is not possible to evaluate the contribution of the genetic background of the mouse to this apparent specificity. With respect to the virus, it is known that MMTV (C3H) induces primarily pregnancy independent tumors, irrespective of the host mouse strain. Similarly, MMTV (RIII) and MMTV (GR) induce primarily pregnancy dependent tumors (Weiss et al. 1982). Beyond the fact that mammary tissue is the major site for MMTV infection, little is known about the identity of the primary cell types which are the target for MMTV infection in the developing mammary gland. Since insertion of an MMTV genome within a given _int_ locus is a selected event during mammary tumor development, it seems possible that different cell types will be at risk for the activation of different _int_ loci. The basis for the apparent specificity of different MMTV strains for a particular _int_ loci could be controlled by either: a) the availability of appropriate receptors on the cell surface for different MMTV strains; or b) the relative biological activity of the MMTV LTR in different cell types of developing mammary tissue.

Table 2.   Frequency of MMTV insertion into the _int_ loci[a]

int Locus	Virus	Mouse Strain	Incidence (%)
1	MMTV (C3H)	C3H	80
	MMTV (RIII)	(B6 x RIII)Fl	25
	MC-MTV	_M. cervicolor popaeus_ (TAK)	50
	MMTV (Czech II)	_M. musculus musculus_ (Czech II)	0
2	MMTV (C3H)	C3H	10
	MMTV (RIII)	(B6 x Rlll)Fl	50
	MC-MTV	_M. cervicolor popaeus_ (TAK)	5
	MMTV (Czech II)	_M. musculus musculus_ (Czech II)	0
3	MMTV (C3H)	C3H	0
	MMTV (RIII)	(B6 x Rlll)Fl	ND
	MC-MTV	_M. cervicolor popaeus_ (TAK)	0
	MMTV (Czech II)	_M. musculus musculus_ (Czech II)	33

[a] The frequency of MMTV insertion into the _int_-1 and _int_-2 loci of C3H and (B6 x RIII)Fl mice is from published data (Dickson et al. 1984; Nusse et al. 1984). MMTV insertion into the _int_ loci were examined in 20 _M. cervicolor popaeus_ and 16 _M. musculus musculus_ (Czech II) tumors. Insertion of MMTV into the _int_-3 locus in 17 C3H mammary tumors was examined. ND, not determined.

CONCLUSIONS

We were interested in determining whether the inbreeding program, which produced strains of mice with a high incidence of mammary tumors, affected the inbred mouse int loci in such a manner that the consequences of their activation were relevant only to these or closely related strains of mice. The results described here extend the previous findings by: a) demonstrating an association between MMTV-induced rearrangement or activation of the int-1 and int-2 loci and mammary tumor development in the distantly related feral species, M. cervicolor popaeus; b) the activation of these cellular genes in mammary tumors does not appear to be limited to highly infectious laboratory strains of MMTV; and c) the use of feral mice has led to the identification of a new int locus.

Not all of the M. cervicolor popaeus or M. musculus musculus (Czech II) mammary tumors contain insertions in the int-1, -2, or -3 loci. It is possible that some have occurred near the int loci but outside the regions defined by the restriction enzymes used in this study. In our view another possibility is that there are still other int loci which have not as yet been identified. Potential candidates could include other reported proto-oncogenes. Activation of the myc and ras proto-oncogene families by amplification or rearrangement has been implicated in the development of solid tumors of other tissues (Alitalo et al. 1983; Schwab et al. 1983). In other studies, transgenic mice containing recombinant c-myc linked to the MMTV LTR were found to have a high incidence of mammary tumors (Stewart et al. 1984). However, restriction enzyme analysis of the N-ras, K-ras, H-ras, N-myc, and c-myc oncogenes in M. cervicolor popaeus mammary tumor cellular DNA provided no evidence for rearrangements of these proto-oncogenes (Escot et al., manuscript in preparation). The availability of an increasing number of feral strains of MMTV possessing different biological and molecular properties coupled with a strain of mice lacking endogenous MMTV genomes should help to provide a resolution to this question. Direct evidence for the oncogenic potential of activated int loci is at present not available. However, the frequent association between their activation by different strains of MMTV and mammary tumor development in different species of mice, as well as the conservation of these loci in a distantly related species such as humans, promotes confidence in the view that int loci represent a new family of tumor-associated cellular genes.

REFERENCES

Alitalo K, Schwab MS, Lin CC, Varmus HE, Bishop JT (1983) Homogeneously staining chromosomal regions contain amplified copies of an abundantly expressed cellular oncogene (c-Myc) in malignant neuroendocrine cells from a human colon carcinoma. Proc Natl Acad Sci USA 80:1707-1711

Andervont HB (1952) Biological studies on the mammary tumor inciter in mice. Ann NY Acad Sci 54:1004-1011

Andervont HB, Dunn TB (1962) Occurrence of tumors in wild house mice. J Natl Cancer Inst 28:1153-1163

Arn K, D'Hoostelaere L, Gallahan D, Wax J, Potter M (1981) Mouse News Letter 64:62-64

Callahan R, Todaro G (1978) Four major endogenous retrovirus classes each genetically transmitted in various species of Mus. In: Morse III HC (ed) Origins of inbred mice, Academic Press, New York, p 689

Callahan R, Drohan W, Gallahan D, D'Hoostelaere L, Potter M (1982) Novel class of mouse mammary tumor virus-related DNA sequences found in all species of Mus, including mice lacking the virus proviral genome. Proc Natl Acad Sci USA 79:4113-4117

Colcher D, Horan-Hand P, Teramoto YA, Wunderlich D, Schlom J (1981) Use of monoclonal antibodies to define the diversity of mammary tumor viral gene products in virions and mammary tumors of the genus Mus. Cancer Res 41:1451-1459

Dickson C, Smith R, Brookes S, Peters G (1984) Tumorigenesis by mouse mammary tumor virus: Proviral activation of a cellular gene in the common integration region int-2. Cell 37:529-536

Dunn TB (1959) Morphology of mammary tumors in mice. In: Homburger F (ed) Physiopathology of cancer, 2nd ed, Hoeber, New York, p 38

Horan-Hand P, Teramoto YA, Callahan R, Schlom J (1980) Interspecies radioimmunoassay for the major internal protein of mammary tumor viruses. Virology 101:61-71

Marshall JT (1977) A synopsis of Asian species of Mus (Rodentia Muridae). Bull Am Museum Natl Hist 158:175-220

Nusse R, Varmus HE (1982) Many tumors induced by the mouse mammary tumor virus contain a provirus integrated in the same region of the host genome. Cell 31:99-109

Nusse R, Van Ooyen A, Cox D, Fung YKT, Varmus HE (1984) Mode of proviral activation of a putative mammary oncogene (int-1) on mouse chromosome 15. Nature 307:131-136

O'Brien SJ (1984) Genetic maps. Cold Spring Harbor Laboratory, Cold Spring Harbor, NY, p 357

Peters G, Brookes S, Smith R, Dickson C (1983) Tumorigenesis by mouse mammary tumor virus: Evidence for a common region for provirus integration in mammary tumors. Cell 33:369-377

Peters G, Kozak C, Dickson C (1984) Mouse mammary tumor virus integration regions int-1 and int-2 map on different mouse chromosomes. Mol Cell Biol 4:375-378

Robbins JM, Gallahan D, Hogg E, Kozak C, Callahan R (to be published) An endogenous mouse mammary tumor virus genome common in inbred mouse strains is located on chromosome 6. J Virol

Rongey RW, Hlavackova A, Lara S, Estes J, Gardner MB (1973) Type B and cRNA virus in breast tissue and milk of wild mice. J Natl Cancer Inst 50:1581-1589

Sass B, Dunn TB (1979) Classification of mouse mammary tumors in Dunn's miscellaneous group including recently reported types. J Natl Cancer Inst 62:1287-1293

Schlom J, Hand PH, Teramoto YA, Callahan R, Todaro G, Schidlovsky G (1978) Characterization of a new virus from Mus cervicolor immunologically related to the mouse mammary tumor virus. J Natl Cancer Inst 61:1509-1519

Schwab M, Alitalo K, Varmus HE, Bishop JM (1983) A cellular oncogene (c-Ki-ras) is amplified, overexpressed, and located within karyotic abnormalities in mouse adrenocortical tumor cells. Nature 303:497-701

Stewart TA, Pattengale PK, Leder P (1984) Spontaneous mammary adenocarcinomas in transgenic mice that carry and express MTV/myc fusion genes. Cell 38:627-637

Teramoto YA, Hand PH, Callahan R, Schlom J (1980) Detection of novel murine mammary tumor viruses by interspecies immunoassays. J Natl Cancer Inst 64:967-975

Weiss R, Teich N, Varmus H, Coffin J (1982) RNA tumor viruses. Molecular biology of tumor viruses. Cold Spring Harbor Laboratory, Cold Spring Harbor, NY

Endogenous MMTV Proviral Genomes in Feral
Mus musculus domesticus

R. Callahan, D. Gallahan, L. A. D'Hoostelaere, and M. Potter

INTRODUCTION

Retroviruses, unlike most viruses which are spread only as infectious agents, can also be transmitted within the germline of the
host (Weiss et al. 1982). In this situation, the viral genome is
passed from one generation to the next as a Mendelian genetic element within the cellular genome. The genetically transmitted viral
genomes are commonly referred to as endogenous retroviral genomes.
The mouse mammary tumor viruses are type B retroviruses which have
only been isolated from species of the genus Mus (Weiss et al.
1982). The inbred laboratory mouse strains have been shown to contain a limited number of endogenous MMTV genomes (Cohen and Varmus
1979; Morris et al. 1979; Groner and Hynes 1980). Recently, the
distribution of endogenous MMTV in several populations of feral Mus
species from different geographical regions of the world has been
examined (Cohen and Varmus 1979; Callahan et al. 1982). In these
studies using the Southern blot technique and stringent hybridization conditions, mice were identified that lacked endogenous MMTV
while other mice contained only a few copies of the viral genome.
In the present report, we have examined descendants of M. m. domesticus trapped at six locations in Maryland and Delaware for their
endogenous MMTV genotype. The purpose of this study was to assess
the extent of the genetic diversity of endogenous MMTV within these
populations. The geographical locations and characteristics of the
different mouse populations are described by D'Hoostelaere et al.
in this volume and are summarized in Table 1.

The proviral genome of MMTV from M. m. domesticus generally contains
a single EcoRl restriction site. Analysis of EcoRl-restricted
cellular DNA provides a means to estimate the number of copies of
endogenous MMTV. The size of the MMTV-related fragment is dependent
on the position of the EcoRl sites in the flanking cellular DNA.

Table 1. Origins of the Maryland and Delaware mice

Location	Designation	Founder Population	Number of Mice Examined
Lewes[a]	LW	2	4
Centreville[a]	CNV	4	10
Ridgely[b]	JDD	8	5
Haven's Farm[a]	HV	1 (pregnant)	6
Sanner's Farm[a]	SN	2	4
Tobacco Farm[b]	TBF		
chemical shed	CS	2	14
drying barn	DB	2	16
seed shed	SS	4	18
tool shed	TS	4	18

[a] These mice are being inbred.

[b] These mice are being bred in a semirandom fashion.

Thus, each complete endogenous MMTV genome yields two cosegregating EcoRl fragments. Figure 1 shows a composite of the different patterns of MMTV-related EcoRl restriction fragments observed in liver DNA from progeny of mice from the different trapping areas. Blots of EcoRl-restricted DNA from all of the mice examined were probed with MMTV LTR (long terminal repeat sequences), gag, pol, and env genes (data not shown). This type of analysis allowed us to determine the composition of each MMTV-related cellular DNA fragment. These results are summarized in Table 2.

Inspection of these data reveals a surprising diversity of endogenous MMTV sequences (a total of 17) which appear to segregate as different MMTV genes in mice from the six trapping areas. Although certain endogenous MMTV genomes (B, C, K, and P) appear in mice from geographically distant trapping areas, most populations are characterized by one or more unique endogenous MMTV genomes. The common endogenous MMTV (B, C, K, and P) probably represent relatively ancient MMTV integration events into the mouse germline and the subsequent migration patterns of the descendant progeny. At the tobacco farm there were also three endogenous MMTV genomes (A, F, and K) segregating in mice from two or more of the four buildings

364

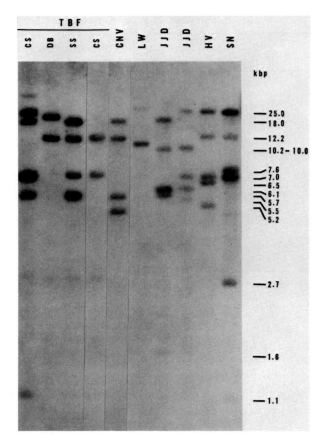

Fig. 1. EcoRl-restricted liver DNA from feral _M. m. domesticus_.
EcoRl-digested DNA was electrophoresed on agarose gels, blotted
onto nitrocellulose, and hybridized under stringent conditions
(Callahan et al. 1982) with ^{32}P-labeled MMTV proviral DNA,
representing the entire viral genome.

(Table 2). This suggests that there was a common founder population
for the tobacco farm.

Table 2. Distribution of endogenous MMTV sequences in feral M. m. domesticus

MMTV-related EcoRl fragments[a]	Cosegregating pair[b]	Complete MMTV genome[c]	Eastern Shore LWS	CNV	JJD	HVN	SNR	Western Shore CS	TPF DR	SS	TS
A 23 LGP/7.2 EL	+	+						+|		+|	
B 25 LGP/7.0 EL	+	+			+	+	+				+|
C 16.5 LGP/5.7 El	+	+		+|				+|			
D 20 LGPE	−	+							+		
E 10.5 LGPE	−	+	+								
F 30 LGP/1.2E	+	−			+			+|		+	+
G 18 LGP/5.7 PE	+	−			+			+|		+|	+
H 6.5 GP/5.5 PE	+	−				+					
I 6.1 PE/1.7 L	+	−			+						
J 26 PE	−	−	+								
K 12 L	−	−									
L 12 P	−	−		+|		+	+	+	+	+	+
M 10 P	−	−			+	+					
N 7.6 EL	−	−					+	+			
O 7.1 L	−	−					+	+			
P 5.5 L	−	−								+|	
Q 2.7 EL	−	−		+|						+|	
R Negative	−					+	+	+		+	+

a The numbers represent the size in kbp of the EcoRl fragment. The letters correspond to: (L), LTR; (G), gag; (P), pol; and (E), env genes of MMTV. Cosegregating fragments are separated by a slash (/).

b Endogenous MMTV genomes composed of two cosegregating EcoRl fragments.

c A complete endogenous MMTV genome is composed of cosegregating or individual EcoRl fragments which react with the LTR, pol, and env gene probes.

What are the possible explanations for the observed diversity of endogenous MMTV genomes? The most obvious is that MMTV frequently infects germ cells or early embryos. However, two additional observations make this scenario less likely as the only explanation for the diversity of endogenous MMTV genomes. Our experience (Gallahan et al. this volume) and that of Andervont (1952) is that MMTV from feral mice is poorly infectious. In addition, even in the C3H inbred mouse which is very sensitive to infection and contains a highly infectious strain of MMTV, there have been no new germline insertions of the MMTV genome in 60 years. A second possibility which cannot be excluded is that the extent of endogenous MMTV diversity is, in part, an experimental illusion. The effect of point mutations, which either create or remove EcoRl sites in the viral genome or flanking sequences, could create the appearance of diversity. Similarly, deletion of various portions of the endogenous viral genome would have the same effect. In the present study, two of the complete endogenous MMTV genomes (D and E) have lost the EcoRl site within the viral genome. In addition, 12 out of the 17 endogenous MMTV genomes contained deletions of viral genes. A third possibility is that endogenous MMTV genomes, like highly repetitive cellular DNA sequences, can move throughout the cellular genome by transposition (Burton et al. 1985). It is perhaps pertinent that at least one endogenous MMTV genome (mtv-8) from laboratory strains of inbred mice is inserted within a member of the BamHl family of repetitive sequences (Fanning et al. 1985). This particular BamHl repetitive element has been shown to have moved to new sites within the cellular genomes of two unrelated strains of mice (Robbins, to be published).

The high frequency of deleted endogenous MMTV genomes warrants further discussion. It is likely that many of the deletions represent genetic damage which has occurred subsequent to the integration of the viral genome. This could occur via recombination events or reflect an inherent genetic instability of hemizygous foreign DNA. However, there are at least two other contributing factors to consider. Recent studies which have examined retrovirus replication and integration have shown that deleted proviral DNA is frequently integrated into cellular DNA of the host. This seems to result from errors in replication at two levels.

MMTV env mRNA is the product of a splicing event which leads to the loss of gag and pol gene sequences. Majors and Varmus (1983) have shown that MMTV env mRNA can be reverse transcribed into proviral DNA, which is subsequently integrated into cellular DNA. Similarly, Wheeler et al. (1984) have shown that the mtv-6 locus in BALB/c mice probably represents the insertion of proviral DNA corresponding to an aberrantly spliced species of MMTV RNA. This proviral genome contains only the MMTV LTR and 5' leader sequences. The K, N, O, P, and Q endogenous MMTV genomes (Table 2) may represent similar instances where spliced MMTV RNA species have been converted to proviral DNA, which was integrated into the feral mouse germline. At another level, deleted circular proviral DNA molecules can arise by an inappropriate cleavage, signaled by a U-5 domain in the LTR (Olsen and Swanstrom 1984). Normally, circular proviral DNA contains two tandem LTR elements. Cleavage of this molecule prior to integration occurs at the junction of the U-5 region of the left-hand LTR and U-3 region of the right-hand LTR. In circular proviral DNA containing only one LTR, cleavage at the U-5 domain can result in molecules that have a large deletion extending into the gag gene. The I endogenous MMTV genome (Table 2) is a potential example of this phenomenon.

Examination of the endogenous MMTV genotypes (Table 3) of the progeny from the different trapping locations demonstrates that most of the viral genomes are still segregating in these mice. Indeed, three of the populations (HVN, SS, and TS) each contain mice which lack endogenous MMTV genomes. These results support our earlier conclusion that MMTV-negative mice are probably not rare and appear in natural breeding populations that contain a few (1 to 4) copies of nonallelic proviral genomes in their gene pool (Callahan et al. 1982). One consequence of viral integration into the germline (via infection or transposition) is that subsequent generations of mice will be hemizygous for a particular endogenous MMTV. Mice homozygous for a given endogenous MMTV would only be expected after inbreeding and only if the site of the viral integration did not alter an essential cellular gene. In five of the mouse populations (LWS, CNV, SNR, CS, and DB) one or more of the endogenous MMTV genomes was found in all of the progeny examined. In each case, with the exception of CNV, the founder population of the breeding stock was two mice. The CNV mice have been inbred for nine gener-

Table 3. Distribution of endogenous MMTV genotypes in feral M. m. domesticus

Trapping Location		Number of Mice	Genotypes[a]	Breeding Generation[b]
LWS		3/4	EJ	4-5
		1/4	E	
CNV		10/10	CKP	9
JJD		1/5	GIM	2-4
		1/5	BIM	
		1/5	BM	
		1/5	IM	
		1/5	I	
HVN		2/6	Negative	3-4
		1/6	BHKL	
		1/6	B, H	
		1/6	B	
		1/6	H	
SNR		3/4	BQNK	3
		1/4	BK	
TBF				
	CS	6/14	ACFK	4-5
		4/14	AK	
		3/14	ACK	
		1/14	KO	
	DB	8/16	DK	2-4
		8/16	K	
	SS	6/18	FK	4-6
		5/18	Negative	
		2/18	ABK	
		2/18	AFKP	
		1/18	AFP	
		1/18	AP	
		1/18	F	
	TS	10/18	K	3-4
		4/18	F	
		2/18	FK	
		2/18	Negative	

[a] Genotypes were assigned on the basis of the segregation of the MMTV-related EcoR1 restriction fragments listed in Table 2.

[b] Number of breeding generations in the laboratory.

ations and have been shown by genetic crosses to be homozygous for the C, K, and P endogenous MMTV genomes. We tentatively conclude the E, B, and K endogenous MMTV genomes are also probably fixed in the LWS, SNR, CS, and DB mice, respectively. Thus, potentially 5 of the 17 endogenous MMTV genomes detected in these mouse populations have occurred in neutral areas of the cellular genome.

CONCLUSIONS

In this report we have shown that feral M. m. domesticus from a limited geographical area contain a diverse array of endogenous MMTV genomes. The characteristic feature of each breeding population is the presence of one or more unique endogenous MMTV genomes. This seems to be independent of the relative proximity of the trapping locations as exemplified by the TBF mice. The diversity appears to be a function of the large number of sites in the cellular genome into which MMTV has integrated and to genetic alterations (point mutations and deletions) of endogenous MMTV subsequent to integration. At present, there is no evidence that endogenous MMTV provide functions which are essential to the development or survival of the individual. Indeed, MMTV-negative mice are probably relatively common in feral populations. Thus endogenous MMTV genomes represent nonessential cellular DNA which has the capacity to move to new sites in the germline via infection or transposition. Each insertion of a viral genome represents a potential mutagenic event which would be passed on to subsequent generations. Inheritable mutations of inbred mice have been described which result from the physical disruption of a cellular gene by a type C retroviral genome (Jenkins et al. 1981; Breindl et al. 1984). These considerations, coupled with the low copy number (1 to 4) of endogenous MMTV in individuals, suggest that they will be useful in: (a) population genetic studies of feral mice; (b) studies on the factors controlling the stability of nonessential cellular DNA; and (c) studies to determine the frequency of mutagenic insertion events in feral mice.

REFERENCES

Andervont HB (1952) Biological studies on the mammary tumor inciter in mice. Ann New York Acad Sci 54:1004-1011
Breindl TI, Harbers K, Jaenisch R (1984) Retrovirus-induced lethal mutation in the collagen I gene of mice is associated with an altered chromatin structure. Cell 38:9-16

370

Burton FH, Loeb DD, Chao SF, Hutchinson CK, Edgell MH (1985) Transposition of a member of the L1 major interspersed DNA family into the mouse beta globin gene locus. NAR 13:5071-5084

Callahan R, Drohan W, Gallahan D, D'Hoostelaere L, Potter M (1982) Novel class of mouse mammary tumor virus-related sequences found in all species of Mus, including mice lacking the virus proviral genome. Proc Natl Acad Sci USA 79:4113-4117

Cohen JC, Varmus HE (1979) Endogenous mammary tumor virus varies among wild mice and segregates during inbreeding. Nature 278:418-423

Fanning TG, Morris DW, Cardiff RD, Bradshaw HD (1985) Characterization of an endogenous retrovirus-repetitive DNA chimera in the mouse genome. J Virol 53:998-1000

Groner B, Hynes NE (1980) Number and location of mouse mammary tumor virus proviral DNA in mouse DNA of normal tissue and of mammary tumors. J Virol 33:1013-1025

Jenkins NA, Copeland NG, Taylor BA, Lee BK (1981) Dilute (d) coat color mutation of DBA/2J mice is associated with the site of integration of an ecotropic MuLV genome. Nature 293:370-374

Majors JE, Varmus HE (1983) Nucleotide sequencing of an apparent proviral copy of env in RNA defines determinants of the mouse mammary tumor virus env gene. J Virol 47:495-504

Morris VL, Kozak C, Cohen JC, Shank RR, Jolicoeur P, Ruddle F, Varmus HE (1979) Endogenous mouse mammary tumor virus is distributed among multiple mouse chromosomes. Virology 92:46-55

Olsen JC, Swanstrom R (1985) A new pathway in the generation of retrovirus DNA. J Virol 56:779-789

Robbins JM, Gallahan D, Hogg E, Kozak C, Callahan R (to be published) An endogenous mouse mammary tumor virus genome common in inbred mouse strains is located on chromosome 6. J Virol

Weiss R, Teich N, Varmus H, Coffin J (1982) RNA tumor viruses. Molecular biology of tumor viruses, Cold Spring Harbor Laboratory, Cold Spring Harbor, NY

Wheeler DA, Butel JS, Medina D, Cardiff RD, Hager GL (1983) Transcription of mouse mammary tumor virus: Identification of a candidate in RNA for the long terminal repeat gene product. J Virol 46:42-29

List of Wild Mouse Stocks and Sources

Listing of Stocks and Strains of Mice in the Genus *Mus* Derived from the Feral State

M. Potter

INTRODUCTION

The following is the first listing of stocks of mice whose origins
can be traced directly to a feral origin. Most of the strains
listed are of relatively recent origin, and no attempt has been made
to include strains that have been listed under the standard inbred
strains. Included in the list are species of mice that are included
in the Marshall classification of the genus Mus (Marshall 1977).
This classification subdivided the genus Mus into 4 subgenera:
Coelomys (mice of mountain forests), Pyromys (spiny mice), Nannomys
(African pygmy mice) and Mus (house and rice paddy mice). Each
subgenus contains multiple species (see also Marshall, this book).
It is not generally agreed that Coelomys, Pyromys and Nannomys are
part of the genus Mus (see Bonhomme, this book). Bonhomme proposes
these latter 3 groups of mice represent separate genera. Regardless
of the classification system, it appears that these species are more
closely related to Mus than to Rattus, however, the data are still
based on very restricted parameters. Because representative species
are available and have been included in a number of studies, they
are included in this listing, but it should be noted that further
analysis will be required to settle the relationship of Coelomys,
Pyromys and Nannomys to Mus. For example, the African murid rodents
are a highly complex group and only limited samples have been studied
by DNA hybridization and biochemical methods.

There is a general agreement that the genus Mus includes at least 9
species, all of which have a 2N chromosome number of 40 and a common
G-banding pattern (Table 1). The chromosomes in all of the species
are acrocentric, however M. dunni, whose karyotype differs the most,
has a small extra knob on the centromere (see Sharma, this book).
An exception to the 40 diploid chromosome number is found in a
growing number of feral populations of M. musculus. The late Alfred
Gropp and E. Capanna discovered many separate populations of M. m.
domesticus in Europe (e.g., M. m. poschiavinus) that had diploid
chromosome numbers of less than 40. These new karyotypes were the
consequence of centric translocations or Robertsonian (Rb) fusions.

Compilation of this listing went through many tedious steps, and I
am very grateful to Ms. Mary Millison for her expert assistance in
preparing the tables and making the many corrections and changes. I
thank Drs. Francois Bonhomme, Joe Nadeau and Verne Chapman for their
assistance in editing the text of this listing.

Rb chromosomes have subsequently been found in M. m. domesticus from a variety of locations (see Winking, Berry, Moriwaki et al., this book).

The two eastern European species known as Mus 4A (the Eastern Mediterranean short tailed mouse) and Mus 4B (the mound building mouse) are two distinct sibling species (see Bonhomme) that are parapatric in most of their range except in a restricted area where they interact sympatrically. These mice have a number of different names. M. 4A has also been called M. abbotti, M. spretoides or M. macedonicus, while M. 4B is also called M. hortulanus or M. spicilegus (see Bonhomme, this book). Marshall (this book) lists all of these species under M. spicilegus. This nomenclature will have to be settled in the future, hence it is advisable to refer to them provisionally as numbered taxa.

The nine distinct species in this classification do not hybridize naturally with any other, even though they may live sympatrically. In the laboratory hybrids of musculus with 4B, spretus or 4A can be produced, but the other species (Table 1) do not hybridize easily with musculus or with each other. Hybridization of M. caroli and M. musculus has been achieved very rarely (see Chapman, this book).

Mus musculus

M. musculus is a polytypic species with an extensive endemic range that extends over Asia and Europe. Four major races or subspecies are musculus, domesticus, bactrianus and castaneus (see Bonhomme, Moriwaki, this book). Several of these contain other varieties based on coat color, tail length and other morphological features (see Marshall, this book). None of the four races is a complete species but each through geographic separation over a period of time has diverged genetically from the others. Some may be in the process of developing into one or more species. The races probably intergrade with each other along the boundaries of their geographic range. In one area in Europe there is a true hybrid zone where M. m. domesticus and M. m. musculus interact (see Sage, this book). Marshall divides the races according to which side of the Himalayas they live: musculus occupies the northern sector, while castaneus, bactrianus and domesticus extend from east to west along the southern sector. Domesticus, the principal 'travelling mouse,' has survived trans-oceanic voyages throughout the centuries to spread from Europe to Africa, America and Australia.

The Japanese mouse, M. musculus molossinus, is probably a special example of intergrading that is applicable to other continental populations. Moriwaki and Yonekawa (this book) have made an extensive study of polymorphisms in Asian Mus musculus using a variety of cytogenetic (C-banding), biochemical and restriction fragment (mt-DNA) markers, and have demonstrated that M. m. molossinus is a hybrid resulting from the separate colonization of Japanese islands by M. m. castaneus from the south and M. m. musculus from the north.

The mice are listed in five categories:

   I.   Intentionally outcrossed stocks

      A.   Species that do not easily hybridize in the laboratory with M. musculus

      B.   Outcrossed stocks of mice and species that hybridize easily with laboratory mice

  II.   Sibmated stocks or developing inbred strains

 III.   Congenic stocks

A list of holders and their addresses is given:

Francois Bonhomme
Institut des Sciencs de L'Evolution
Universite Montpellier II
Place Eugene Bataillon
34060 Montpellier Cedex
France

Robert Callahan
Laboratory of Tumor Immunology
 and Biology, NCI
National Institutes of Health
Bethesda, MD 20892

Verne Chapman
Department of Molecular Biology
Roswell Park Memorial Institute
Buffalo, NY 14263

Muriel Davisson
Jackson Laboratory
Bar Harbor, ME 04609

Eva Eicher
Jackson Laboratory
Bar Harbor, ME 04609

K. Fischer-Lindahl
Howard Hughes Medical Institute
University of Texas HSCD
5323 Harry Hines Blvd.
Dallas, TX 75235

Murray Gardner
Department of Pathology
School of Medicine
University of California, Davis
Davis, CA 95616

Jean-Louis Guenet
Institut Pasteur
25 rue du Docteur Roux
F75015 Paris
France

Kazuo Moriwaki
National Institute of Genetics
Yata-1111 Mishima
Shizuoka-ken, 411
Japan

Joe Nadeau
The Jackson Laboratory
Bar Harbor, ME 04609

Michael Potter
Laboratory of Genetics, NCI
National Institutes of Health
Bethesda, MD 20892

Thomas Roderick
The Jackson Laboratory
Bar Harbor, ME 04609

T. Sharma
Banaras Hindu University
Cytogenetics Laboratory
Varanas-221.005, India

Lee Silver
Department of Molecular Biology
Princeton University
Princeton, NY 08544

Edward Wakeland
Pathology Department
University of Florida
College of Medicine
Box J-275, JHMHC
Gainesville, FL 32610

J. Barry Whitney, III
Medical College of Georgia
School of Medicine
Department of Cell and Molecular Biology
Augusta, Georgia 30912

Heinz Winking
Institute fur Pathologie
Medizinische Hochschule Lubeck
D-24 Lubeck 1
Ratzeburger Allee 160
West Germany

Table 1.   Species in the genus <u>Mus</u> that have 40 acrocentric chromosomes with a common G-banding pattern

Species	Geographic range	Hybridization to M. musculus domesticus	
M. musculus			
musculus	Northern Euro-asia	+[a]	+
castaneus	Southeast Asia, E. Indies, Philippines	+	?
bactrianus	S. of Himalayas from India to Near East	+	?
domesticus[b]	W. Europe N. Africa (worldwide)	+	+
hybrids[c] molossinus	Japan	+	?
M. spretus	S. France, Spain, N. Africa	+[a]	-
M. 4A[d]	E. Europe	+	-
M. 4B[d]	E. Europe	+	-
M. booduga	Pakistan, India, Burma	-	-
M. caroli	S.E. Asia, Ryukyu Islands to Indonesia	-	-
M. cervicolor	S.E. Asia	-	-
M. cookii	Mts. of Burma, Thailand, NW and central India	-	-
M. dunni	India	-	-

[a] ♂ F$_1$ hybrids may be sterile.
[b] See Marshall for discussion of varieties. Many varieties of M. domesticus carry varying numbers of Robertsonian metacentric chromosomes. The fundamental number of chromosomes remains the same.
[c] See Moriwaki, Yonekawa. <u>Molossinus</u> has genes from <u>musculus</u> and <u>castaneus</u>.
[d] See <u>Bonhomme</u>, Thaler for details.

I. STOCKS OF MICE THAT DO NOT EASILY HYBRIDIZE WITH LABURATORY MICE: INTENTIONALLY OUTCROSSED STOCKS
A. These are maintained by outcrossing.

Name	Origin	Year*	Breeding gen. in the lab	Latin name	Holder (year acquired)
Subgenus Pyromys					
SAXIa	India (Mysore)	1972	9	M. saxicola	Yosida to Sage to Potter ('81)
PTXa	India (Mysore)	-	3	M. saxicola	Yosida to Callahan to Bonhomme ('84)
Subgenus Coelomys					
PAHA-1b	Thailand (Tak Prov.)	1977		M. pahari	Marshall to Callahan ('77) to Potter ('81) 2 pairs
PAHA-2c	Thailand (Tak X Lampeng)	-	14	M. pahari	Callahan to Potter
PAHb	Thailand (Tak Prov.)	1977		M. pahari	Callahan to Bonhomme ('84)
Subgenus Nannomys					
MINU	Kenya (Nairobi near Kenyatta Univ.)	1981	12	M. minutoides	Aggundey to Potter, stock init. from 3 pairs
Subgenus Mus					
CARD	Thailand	1975	20	M. caroli	Marshall to Chapman
CAROd	Thailand (Chonburi)	1975	17	M. caroli owensi	Marshall to Potter
KARd	Thailand (Chonburi)	1981	11	M. caroli	Marshall to Chapman to Bonhomme
CERVe	Thailand (Chonburi)	1976		M. cervi. popaeus / M. cervicolor	Marshall to Callahan
CRV	Thailand	-	3	M. cervicolor	Potter to Bonhomme ('84)
CRPe	Thailand	-	4	M. cervi. popaeus	Potter to Bonhomme ('84)
COOK	Thailand (Loei)	1979	13	M. cookii	Marshall to Callahan to Potter ('79) 1 pair
COKf	Thailand	-	3	M. cookii	Potter to Bonhomme ('84)
-f	India	-		M. booduga	Sharma
-f	India	-		M. dunni	Sharma

* = year first isolated

Footnotes: a, SAXI and PTX are probably derived from the same original stock; b, PAHA-1 and PAX are derived from the same stock; c, PAHA-2 is a hybrid of TAK and Lampeng pahari mice; d, probably all derived from the same stock; e, CERV and CRP are M. cervicolor popaeus and are derived from the same stock; f, specimens may be obtained from Sharma.

B. Stocks of mice that hybridize with laboratory mice.
Mode of breeding not yet specified but in general is by
outcrossing in contrast to sibmating. The number of
generations bred in the laboratory is given.

M. musculus domesticus

Europe

Name	Origin	Year	Gen.	Special character-istics	Holder
DBP	Bulgaria (Pomorie)	1981	7	-	Bonhomme
DBV	Bulgaria (Vlas)	1984	5	-	Bonhomme
DDO	Denmark (Odis)	1985	2	-	Bonhomme
DFA	France (Annemasse)	1981	6	-	Bonhomme
DFC	France (Corsica)	1984	3	-	Bonhomme
DGD	Greece (Doirani)	1981	7	-	Bonhomme
DJO	Italy (Orcetto)	1984	4	-	Bonhomme
24BI	Italy (Binasco)	1982	7	2N=24S	Bonhomme
24CI	Italy (Cislago)	1985	2	2N=24N	Bonhomme
38CH	Italy (Chiarello)	1982	7	2N=38	Bonhomme
BEP	Spain (Palma de Majorca)	1981	8	-	Bonhomme
BEM	Spain (Menorca)	1981	6	-	Bonhomme
Posch-1	Italy (Tirano)	1981	11	-	Sage to Potter to Eicher
Posch-2	Switzerland (Zalende)	1981	8	-	Sage to Potter to Eicher

North America

Name	Origin	Year	Gen.	Special character-istics	Holder
CLA	Q.A. Co., MD	1976	21	-	Potter
WSA	Q.A. Co., MD	1976	19	-	Potter
WSB	Q.A. Co., MD	1976	19	-	Potter
JJD	Ridgely, MD	1981	8	-	Potter
Lewes	Delaware	1981	12	-	Potter
HAF	Davidsonville, MD	1982	12	-	Potter
SAF	Davidsonville, MD	1982	10	-	Potter
TFSS	U. Marlboro, MD	1982	9	-	Potter
TFCS	U. Marlboro, MD	1982	7	-	Potter
TFTS	U. Marlboro, MD	1982	7	-	Potter
TFDB	U. Marlboro, MD	1982	6	-	Potter
BQC	Bouquet Canyon, CA		6	-	Gardner to Rowe to Potter ('82)
	Lake Casitas RR	1981	-	$\frac{AKrr-1^{RR}}{Fv-4^{RR}}$	Gardner
	Lake Casitas, CA	1981	-		Gardner
	Lake Casitas, CA	1981	-		Gardner

Name	Origin	Year	Gen.	Special character- istics	Holder

M. musculus domesticus (cont.)

Africa

Name	Origin	Year	Gen.	Special characteristics	Holder
DMA	Morocco (Azrou)	1985	1	-	Sage to Chapman to Bonhomme
BREV	Morocco (Azrou)	1979	12	-	Sage to Potter
Praetextus	Egypt	1981	-	-	Sage to Chapman
ABUR	Egypt (Abu Rawash)	1981	8	-	Hoogstraal to Potter
A.M.P./Pas	Tunisia (Monastir)	1981	-	multi-meta-centrics 2N=22	Bonhomme to Guenet to Winking
22MO	Tunisia (Monastir)	1982	7	-	Bonhomme
BZO	Algeria (Orah)	1981	8	-	Bonhomme
BNC	Egypt (Cairo)	1981	8	-	Bonhomme
PRAE	Morocco (Erfoud)	1978	13	-	Sage to Potter

Middle East

Name	Origin	Year	Gen.	Special characteristics	Holder
Praetextus	Jerusalem	1981	-	-	Sage to Chapman
BIA/b	Israel (Afula)	1981	8	$Amy-1^b$	Bonhomme
BIB/a	Israel (Sede Boger)	1982	9	$Amy-1^{a/b}$	Bonhomme
BIB/c	Israel (Sede Boger)	1982	9	$Amy-1^b$	Bonhomme
BIK/g	Israel (Kefar Galim)	1982	9	$Amy-1^g$	Bonhomme

Oceania

Name	Origin	Year	Gen.	Special characteristics	Holder
DOT	Tahiti	1983	7	-	Bonhomme

Name	Origin	Year	Gen.	Special characteristics	Holder

M. musculus musculus

Europe

Name	Origin	Year	Gen.	Special characteristics	Holder
CZECH-I	Czech. (Studenec.)	1978	18	-	Kral to Sage to Potter
CZECH-II	Czech. (Bratislava)	1981	16	MMTV-	Kminiack to Sage to Potter
MAI	Austria (Illmitz)	1981	10	-	Bonhomme
MBB	Bulgaria (Bania)	1984	5	-	Bonhomme
MBK	Bulgaria (Kranevo)	1984	6	-	Bonhomme
MBS	Bulgaria (Sokolovo)	1984	4	-	Bonhomme
MBT	Bulgaria (General Tochevo)	1980	12	-	Bonhomme
MDL	Denmark (Losning)	1985	1	-	Bonhomme
MDJ	Denmark, Jutland (Skive, Viborg, Vejrumbro)	1973	20	-	Nielsen to Chapman
MDS	Denmark (Skive)	1985	1	-	Chapman to Bonhomme
MPW	Poland (Warsawa)	1984	6	-	Bonhomme
MYL	Yugoslavia (Ljubljana)	1981	9	-	Bonhomme to Chapman
Belgrade	Yugoslavia	1981	-	-	Sage to Chapman
BRNO	Czechoslovakia	1981	-	-	Sage to Chapman
PWD	Czechoslavakia	1984	F3	-	Forejt to Chapman
PWK	Czechoslovakia	1984	F4	-	Forejt to Chapman
VEJ	Denmark (Vejrumbro)	1973	12	-	Nielsen to Chapman to Potter

M. musculus castaneus

Asia

Name	Origin	Year	Gen.	Special characteristics	Holder
CAS	Thailand	1975	20		Marshall to Chapman
CAS	Thailand, Indonesia	1979	16	-	Bonhomme
CAST	Thailand	1976	17	2 pairs	Marshall to Callahan to Potter

Name	Origin	Year	Gen.	Special char- acteristics	Holder

Mus 4B (M. hortulanus, M. spicilegus)

Europe

Name	Origin	Year	Gen.	Special characteristics	Holder
ZBN	Bulgaria (No. Bulg.)	1980	11	4B	Bonhomme to Chapman
ZRU	Ukrania	1984	3	4B	Bonhomme
ZYD	Yugoslavia	1985	1	4B	Sage to Chapman to Bonhomme
ZYP	Yugoslavia	1985	1	4B	Sage to Chapman to Bonhomme
HORT-P	Yugoslavia (Pancevo, Serbia)	1979	9	M. hortulanus (mound building mouse)	Kataranovski to Sage to Potter ('81) 3 pairs
HORT-P	Yugoslavia, Pancevo	1981	9	M. hortulanus	Sage to Chapman 6 pairs
HORT-H	Austria (Halbturn)	1981	9	M. hortulanus (mound building mouse)	Sage to Potter 1 pair
HORT-D	Yugoslavia (Debeljica)	1981	?	M. hortulanus	Sage to Chapman 1 pair

Mus 4A (M. abbotti, M. macedonicus or M. spretoides)

Europe

Name	Origin	Year	Gen.	Special characteristics	Holder
XBJ	Bulgaria (Jitarovo)	1985	2	4A	Bonhomme
XBS	Bulgaria (Slantchev Briag)	1984	4	4A	Bonhomme to Chapman

M. m. molossinus

Molossinus (M. m. molossinus is a natural hybrid that carries genes from M. m. castaneus and M. m. musculus)

Name	Origin	Year	Gen.	Special characteristics	Holder
MOL	Japan (Misima)	1983	6	2B	Moriwaki to Bonhomme
MOA	Japan	-	-	-	Kondo
MOM	Japan	-	-	-	to Moriwaki
MOLO	Japan (Fukuoka)	1967	19	-	Hamajima to Potter 2 pairs

Name	Origin	Year	Gen.	Special characteristics	Holder

Mus spretus

Europe

Name	Origin	Year	Gen.	Special characteristics	Holder
SEI	Spain (Ibiza)	1981	-	-	Bonhomme
SET	Spain (Tarracena)	1983	-	-	Bonhomme
SEG	Spain (Granada)	1978	16	-	Bonhomme
SPRET		1978	-	-	Bonhomme to Chapman
SFM	France (Montpellier)	1982	9	-	Bonhomme
SPRET-1	Spain (Puerto Real)	1978	13	-	Sage to Potter
SPRET-1	Spain	1979	-	-	Sage to Chapman

Africa

Name	Origin	Year	Gen.	Special characteristics	Holder
SMA	Morocco (Azrou)	1984	3	-	Sage to Potter to Bonhomme
SPRET-2	Morocco (Azrou)	1981	13	-	Sage to Potter
STF	Tunisia (Fonduk Djedid)	1984	5	-	Bonhomme

Artificial natural hybrids of spretus and musculus

Name	Origin	Year	Gen.	Special characteristics	Holder
ADGR	France	1978	8	$Amy\text{-}1^d$	Bonhomme
AE	France	1978	11	$Amy\text{-}1^e$	Bonhomme
AD	France	1978	11	$Amy\text{-}1^d$	Bonhomme
AF	France	1978	15	$Amy\text{-}1^f$	Bonhomme
LBL	France	1978	-	$Ldh\text{-}2^l$	Bonhomme to Chapman to Jax

Wild-inbred hybrids

Name	Origin	Year	Gen.	Special characteristics	Holder
1D2	Israel + C57BL/6	1980	10	$Id\text{-}2^{50}$	Bonhomme to Jax
1PO	Greece + C57BL/6	1979	13	$Sod\text{-}1^{20}$	Bonhomme to Chapman to Jax
38IB	Spain + C57BL/6	1983	8	2N=38	Bonhomme to Winking to Jax
LBP	Peru + C57BL/6	1980	10	$Ldh\text{-}2^b$	Peters to Bonhomme
LBT	Tunisia + C57BL/6	1979	11	$Ldh\text{-}2^t$	Bonhomme to Chapman

II. SIBMATED OR STOCKS OF DEVELOPING INBRED STRAINS DERIVED
     DIRECTLY FROM WILD MICE

Name	Origin	Year	Filial gen.	Special characteristics	Holder
				Mus caroli	
CAR	Thailand	1981	7	-	Chapman to Eicher
				M. musculus domesticus	
	Europe				
BFM/2	France (Montpellier)	1976	30	-	Bonhomme to Guenet
BFM/1	France (Montpellier)	1976	27	-	Bonhomme
WLA76	France (Issus, Toulouse)	1976	27	Tame; prolific	Guenet
WLA	France (Lozere nr. Palaiseau)	1982	6	Poor breeders	Guenet
WGQ	France (LeMesnil, St. Denis, Chilly Mazarin)	1981	8	Breeds well	Guenet
Posch-1	Italy (Tirano)	1982	F8	-	Potter to Eicher
Posch-2	Switzerland (Zalende)	1982	F8		Potter to Eicher
SK/CAM	England (Skokholm Is., Pembroke-shire)	1962	42		Berry to Wallace to Eicher to Davisson ('84)
SK/CamRk	England (Skokholm Is.)	1962	19 30		Berry to Wallace at F19 to Roderick ('71)
	North America				
Casitas	Lk. Casitas, CA	1981	8	-	Gardner
PAC	Philadelphia, PA	1974	18	-	Conner to Chapman
MOR2/CV	Ohio	1968	43	-	Bruell to Chapman
WSA	Q.A. Co., MD	1976	17	Prolific	Potter
WSB	Q.A. Co., MD	1976	17	Prolific	Potter
CLA	Q.A. Co., MD	1976	21	Prolific	Potter
Lewes	Lewes, DE	1980	9	Prolific	Potter
SF/CAM/Ei	Berkeley, CA	1959	36	-	Barnawell to Wallace to Eicher to Davisson ('84)

II. SIBMATED OR STOCKS OF DEVELOPING INBRED STRAINS DERIVED DIRECTLY FROM WILD MICE (cont.)

Name	Origin	Year	Filial gen.	Special characteristics	Holder

M. musculus domesticus (cont.)

South America

Name	Origin	Year	Filial gen.	Special characteristics	Holder
PERA/Rk	Peru	-	50	See MNL 40:20-22 ('70)	Atteck to Wallace at F24 to Roderick ('71)
PERUA/CAM/Ei	-	-	40	-	Roderick to Eicher to Davisson ('84)

M. musculus musculus

Name	Origin	Year	Filial gen.	Special characteristics	Holder
PWK/PAS	Prague	?	35	Hybrid; sterility	Ivanyi and Forejt to Bonhomme to Guenet
MDS	Denmark, Skive	1973	8	-	Nielsen to Chapman
PWD	Czechoslovakia	1984	3	-	Forejt to Chapman
PWK	Czechoslovakia	1984	4	-	Forejt to Chapman
CZI-0	Czech. (Studenec)	1978	11	Ochre belly; ♂ BALB/c hybrids are sterile	Potter
CZECH-II	Czech. (Bratislava)	1978	5	MMTV⁻	Potter
SKIVE	Denmark	1975	6	-	Chapman to Potter
SKIVE	Denmark	1979	15	-	Chapman to Eicher

Mus spretus

Name	Origin	Year	Filial gen.	Special characteristics	Holder
SPE/11	Spain (Granada)	1978	5	-	Bonhomme
SPE/1	Spain (Granada)	1978	30	-	Bonhomme and Thaler to Guenet
SPRET-1	Spain (Puerto Real)	1983	10	-	Potter to Eicher
SPRET-2	Morocco (Azrou)	1983	5	-	Potter to Eicher

II. SIBMATED OR STOCKS OF DEVELOPING INBRED STRAINS DERIVED DIRECTLY FROM WILD MICE (cont.)

Name	Origin	Year	Filial gen.	Special characteristics	Holder
M. musculus castaneus					
CAST/Ei	-	-	34	-	Roderick to Eicher to Davisson ('85)
CASA/Rk	-	-	32	-	Marshall to Chapman to Roderick ('71)
M. musculus molossinus					
MOLG/Dn-HC2	-	-	11	-	Potter to Roderick ('69) to Eicher to Davidsson ('82)
MOLF/Ei	-	-	39	-	Potter to Roderick to Eicher to Davisson ('85)
MOLC/Rk	-	-	45	From ♂ 539 and ♀ from cage 603; also called MOL-3-I	Hamajima to Potter to Roderick ('69)
MOLD/Rk	-	-	50	Same as MOLC; also called MOL-3-III	Hamajima to Potter to Roderick ('69)
MOLE/Rk	-	-	48	From MOLD/Rk white spotting at F33	Roderick

III. CONGENIC STOCKS

List of Congenic Mice

Name	Marker gene	Origin of marker gene	Inbred background	N - Number backcrosses	Holders
129-t 0	t 0	Paris	129/Sv	25	Silver
129-t w5	t w5	New York	129/Sv	24	Silver
129-t w18	t w18	tw5	129/Sv	26	Silver
129-Tt h18	t h18	t0	129/Sv	12	Silver
129-Tt Orl	Tt Orl	Orleans, France	129/Sv	11	Silver
C3H-$\underline{T}$/$\underline{t}^0$	$\underline{Ttf}$/$\underline{t}^0$+	Paris, France	C3H/HeSn	N7F?N1F1	Nadeau
C3H-$\underline{T}$/$\underline{t}^{w32}$	$\underline{Ttf}$/$\underline{t}^{w32}$+	Clinton, MT	C3H/HeSn	N7F?N2F1	Nadeau
C3H-$\underline{T}$/$\underline{t}^{w5}$	$\underline{Ttf}$/$\underline{t}^{w5}$+	New York	C3H/HeSn	N7F?N3F1	Nadeau
C3H-$\underline{T}$/$\underline{t}^{w18}$	$\underline{Ttf}$/$\underline{t}^{w18}$+	tw5, Storrs, CT	C3H/HeSn	N7F?N1F1	Nadeau
C3H-$\underline{T}$/$\underline{t}^{w71}$	$\underline{Ttf}$/$\underline{t}^{w71}$+	S. Jutland, Denmark	C3H/HeSn	N7F?N2F2	Nadeau
C3H-$\underline{T}$/$\underline{t}^{w8}$	$\underline{Ttf}$/$\underline{t}^{w8}$+	Rumford, VA	C3H/HeSn	N7F?N1F4	Nadeau
C3H-$\underline{T}$/$\underline{t}^{w1}$	$\underline{Ttf}$/$\underline{t}^{w1}$+	New York	C3H/HeSn	N7F?N1F2	Nadeau
C3H-$\underline{T}$/$\underline{t}^{w12}$	$\underline{Ttf}$/$\underline{t}^{w12}$+	Oakland, CA	C3H/HeSn	N7F?N2F3	Nadeau
C3H-$\underline{T}$/$\underline{t}^{w75}$	$\underline{Ttf}$/$\underline{t}^{w75}$+	Jena, E. Germany	C3H/HeSn	N7F?N2F1	Nadeau
TT6/GnLe	$\underline{Ttf}$/$\underline{t}^6$+	Edinburgh, Scotland	C57BL/10Gn	F56	Nadeau

III. CONGENIC STOCKS (cont.) - Strains held by H. Winking

Name	Marker	Origin of marker chromosome	Back-ground
Rb(1.3)1Bnr	Rb(1.3)	Switzerland	undef.
Rb(1.10)10Bnr	Rb(1.10)	Switzerland	C57BL
Rb(1.18)10Rma	Rb(1.18)	Italy	C57BL
Rb(2.16)3Mpl	Rb(2.16)	Tunisia	undef.
Rb(2.17)11Rma	Rb(2.17)	Italy	undef.
Rb(2.18)6Rma	Rb(2.18)	Italy	undef.
Rb(3.8)3Rma	Rb(3.8)	Italy	undef.
Rb(4.6)2Bnr	Rb(4.6)	Switzerland	undef.
Rb(4.12)9Bnr	Rb(4.12)	Switzerland	C57BL
RB(4.15)4Rma	Rb(4.15)	Italy	C57BL
Rb(4.17)13Lub	Rb(4.17)	Italy	undef.
Rb(5.13)70Lub	Rb(5.13)	Italy	undef.
Rb(5.15)3Bnr	Rb(5.15)	Switzerland	undef.
Rb(5.17)7Rma	Rb(5.17)	Italy	undef.
Rb(6.7)13Rma	Rb(6.7)	Italy	undef.
Rb(6.12)3Sic	Rb(6.12)	Yugoslavia	undef.
Rb(6.13)3Rma	Rb(6.13)	Italy	C57BL
Rb(7.18)9Lub	Rb(7.18)	Italy	C57BL
Rb(8.12)5Bnr	Rb(8.12)	Switzerland	C57BL
Rb(8.14)16Rma	Rb(8.14)	Italy	undef.
Rb(8.17)38Lub	Rb(8.17)	Yugoslavia	undef.
Rb(8.17)6Sic	Rb(8.17)	Italy	undef.
Rb(9.14)6Bnr	Rb(9.14)	Switzerland	undef.
Rb(9.16)9Rma	Rb(9.16)	Italy	undef.
Rb(10.11)8Bnr	Rb(10.11)	Switzerland	undef.
Rb(10.11)5Rma	Rb(10.11)	Italy	C57BL
Rb(11.13)4Bnr	Rb(11.13)	Switzerland	undef.
Rb(13.15)10Mpl	Rb(13.15)	Tunisia	undef.
RB(13.16)1Mpl	Rb(13.16)	Ibiza	undef.
Rb(15.17)64Lub	Rb(15.17)	Greece	undef.
Rb(16.17)8Lub	Rb(16.17)	Italy	undef.
Rb(16.17)7Bnr	Rb(16.17)	Switzerland	C57BL
Rb(16.17)32Lub	Rb(16.17)	Yugoslavia	undef.
Rb(16.17)54 Lub	Rb(16.17)	Italy	undef.
Is(HSR)1Lub	HSR	Switzerland	undef.

III. CONGENIC STOCKS (cont.) - Strains held by J. B. Whitney

Name	Marker gene	Origin of marker	Inbred background	$\underline{N}$ - Number of backcrosses
Hbb^{spretus}	Hbb and non-albino	M. spretus	SPRET-1	7
Hbb^d	Hbb^d-like	Peru		12
Hbb^{unique}	Hbb unique	Is/CAM		6
Hbb^{unique}	Hbb unique	M. m. castaneus	CAST	13
Hba^j	Hba^j or Hba^{w1}	M. spretus	SPRET-1	7
Hba^k	Hba^k or Hba^{w2}	Centreville Light	CLA	2
Hba^l	Hba^l or Hba^{w3}	M. m. musculus Skive	Skive	6
Hba^n	Hba^n or Hba^{w4}	M. m. musculus Czech I or II		10
Hba^p	Hba^p or Hba^{w5}	M. m. domesticus brevirostris	BREV	10
Hba^b	Hba^b-like	Is/CAM		10
Hba^i	Hba^i	M. m. molossinus	MOLO	-

III. CONGENIC STOCKS (cont.) - Strains held by K. Fischer-Lindahl

Strain	Marker gene	Origin of marker	Inbred background	N - Number of backcrosses
NZB.Mtf$^\alpha$ (ANN)[b]	Mtf$^\alpha$	A.CA/Ibm	NZB/Bom	20
B6.Mtf$^\beta$ (NMB)[b]	Mtf$^\beta$	NMRI/Bom	C57BL/6JIbm	17
B6.Mtf$^\gamma$	Mtf$^\gamma$	WLA76	C57BL/6JIbm	11
D2.Mtf$^\gamma$	Mtf$^\gamma$	WLA76 (Toulouse/ Guenet)	DBA/2JIbm	9
B10.MilP	Mtf^P	M. m. domesticus (Pavia/Winking)	C57BL/10ScSn	5
B6.Mtf$^\delta$	Mtf$^\delta$	SUB-SHH	C57BL/6JIbm	6
BALB.Mtf$^\delta$	Mtf$^\delta$	SUB-SHH (Shanghai/ Moriwaki)	BALB/cJIbm	4
B10.B2m^{w1}	B2m^{w1}	SPRET-1/Pt	C57BL/10ScSn	6
B10.B2m^{w2}	B2m^{w2}	BREV/Pt	C57BL/10ScSn	5
BALB.B2m^{w3}	B2m^{w3}	bactrianus Lahore/Moriwaki	BALB/cJIbm	6
B.B.B2m^{w4}	B2m^{w4}	bactrianus Lahore/Moriwaki	BALB.B/OlaBii	6
B.B.B2m^{w5}	B2m^{w5}	bactrianus Lahore/Moriwaki	BALB.B/OlaBii	2
B6.CAS3	Hmt-b	domesticus - Isle of May/triggs	C57BL/6JIbm	8
B10.CAS3	Hmt-b	CAS (CAS3)	C57BL/10ScSn	6
C3H.CAS3	Hmt-b	CAS (CAS3)	C3H/HeJIbm	8
B10.CAS4	Hmt-b	CAS (CAS3)	C57BL/10ScSn	8
C3H.CAS4	Hmt-b	CAS (CAS4)	C3H/HeJIbm	6

III. CONGENIC STOCKS (cont.) - Strains held by K. Fischer-Lindahl

Strain	Marker gene	Origin of marker	Inbred background	N - Number of backcrosses
B10.BAC2	Hmt-b	M. m. bactrianus Lahore/Moriwaki	C57BL/10ScSn	6
B10.MilII	Hmt-b	M. m. domesticus MiIano/Winking	C57BL/10ScSn	5
B10.MilB	Hmt-b	M. m. domesticus MiIano/Winking	C57BL/10ScSn	6
B10.MilPᶜ	Hmt-b	M. m. domesticus /Winking	C57BL/10ScSn	5
B10.SPA1	Hmt-c	SPRET-1	C57BL/10ScSn	6
B10.SPA2	Hmt-c	SPRET-1	C57BL/10ScSn	5
B10.SPE	Hmt-c	SPE-1 (Sp3)	C57BL/10ScSn	2
B10.BAC1	Hmt-d	M. m. bactrianus Lahore/Moriwaki	C57BL/10ScSn	9

III. CONGENIC STOCKS (cont.) - Strains held by V. Chapman

Name	Marker gene (chr)	Origin of marker gene	Inbred background	N*
Ego, Es-1a	Ego,Es-1a (8)	YBR	C57BL/6J	16
GusA	GusA (5)	A/J	C57BL/6J	15
(Trfa),Bgld	(Trfa),Bgld (9)	CBA	C57BL/6J	13
GusW5	GusW5 (5)	MOR-domesticus	C57BL/6J	14
GusC1	GusC1 (5)	Castaneus	C57BL/6J	7
GusH	GusH (5)	C3H/HeHa	C57BL/6J	1
Agsm	Agsm (X)	Molossinus	C3H/HeHa	10
Pgk-1a,Agsm	Pgk-1a,Agsm (X)	Denmark	C3H/HeHa	10
GusW12	GusW12 (5)	Denmark	C57BL/6J	11
GusN	GusN (5)	PAC-M. domesticus	C57BL/6J	12
GusCs	GusCs (5)	Castaneus	C57BL/6J	16
GusW16	GusW16 (5)	Denmark	C57BL/6J	13
GusW17	GusW17 (5)	Denmark	C57BL/6J	12
GusW18	GusW18 (5)	M. domesticus- E. Aurora	C57BL/6J	11
GusS	GusS (5)	M. spretus	C57BL/6J	9
GusS	GusS (5)	M. spretus- Nielsen	C57BL/6J	11
Hprta,Pgk-1a, Agsm	Hprta,Pgk-1a, AgsM (X)	M. castaneus- M. m. Denmark recom.	C3H/HeHa	9
GusW26	GusW26 (5)	Hungarian	C57BL/6J	10
GusW28	GusW28 (5)	Belgrade	C57BL/6J	10
Hprta,Pgk-1a	Hprta,Pgk-1a (X)	Congenic-Hprta, Pgk-aa,Agsm	C57BL/6J	4
Hprta,Pgk-1a, Mdx	Hprta,Pgk-1a, Mdx (X)	M. castaneus- M. m. Denmark	C57BL/6J	4
GusHo	GusHo (5)	M. hortulanus	C57BL/6J	3
Hprta	Hprta (X)	M. spretus	C57BL/6J	5

*Number of backcrosses

III. CONGENIC STOCKS (cont.) - Strains held by M. Davissson
      Robertsonian chromosome stocks that have some feral background[1]

Strain or stock designation	Robertsonian chr carried	Filial gen.	Origin of feral part of genome
1. Named inbred or nearly inbred strains			
RBA/Dn	Rb(4.12)9Bnr	29	Mutten, Switzerland
RBB/Dn	Rb(1.10)10Bnr	41	Bondo, Switzerland
RBD/Dn	Rb(5.15)3Bnr	66	Valle Poschiavo, Switz.
	Rb(11.13)4Bnr		Valle Poschiavo, Switz.
	Rb(16.17)7Bnr		Valle Poschiavo, Switz.
RBE/DN	Rb(1.3)1Bnr	39	Valle Poschiavo, Switz.
	Rb(4.6)2Bnr		Valle Poschiavo, Switz.
	Rb(8.12)5Bnr		Valle Poschiavo, Switz.
	Rb(9.14)6Bnr		Valle Poschiavo, Switz.
RBF/Dn	Rb(1.3)1Bnr	67	Valle Poschiavo, Switz.
	Rb(8.12)5Bnr		Valle Poschiavo, Switz.
	Rb(9.14)6Bnr		Valle Poschiavo, Switz.
RBG/Dn	Rb(3.8)2Rma	18	Abruzzi, Italy
	Rb(4.15)4Rma		Abruzzi, Italy
	Rb(10.11)5Rma		Abruzzi, Italy
2. Inbred or nearly inbred unnamed Robertsonian strains			
Rb(1.3)1Bnr	Rb1Bnr	50	Valle Poschiavo, Switz.
Rb(4.6)2Bnr	Rb2Bnr	60	Valle Poschiavo, Switz.
Rb(11.13)4Bnr	Rb4Bnr	53	Valle Poschiavo, Switz.
Rb(16.17)7Bnr	Rb7Bnr	44	Valle Poschiavo, Switz.
Rb(1.7)1Rma	Rb1Rma	24	Abruzzi, Central Italy
Rb(3.8)2Rma	Rb2Rma	15	Abruzzi, Central Italy
Rb(4.15)4Rma	Rb4Rma	24	Abruzzi, Central Italy
Rb(10.11)5Rma	Rb5Rma	25	Abruzzi, Central Italy
Rb(2.18)6Rma	Rb6Rma	24	Abruzzi, Central Italy
Rb(5.17)7Rma	Rb7Rma	24	Abruzzi, Central Italy
Rb(12.14)8Rma, Rb(2.18)6Rma	Rb8Rma Rb6Rma	19	Abruzzi, Central Italy

[1] These strains have varying amounts of feral background. Most of
those carrying Rb1-7Bnr have been brother x sister bred starting
with F1 hybrids between a feral mouse and a Swiss strain by Gropp
and Winking. The remaining stocks have been crossed several times
to laboratory strains, but the regions around the centromeres can
be expected to be of feral origin.

III. CONGENIC STOCKS (cont.) - Strains held by M. Davisson (cont.)

Strain or stock designation	Robertsonian chr carried	Filial gen.	Origin of feral part of genome
2. Inbred or nearly inbred unnamed Robertsonian strains (cont.)			
Rb(2.17)11Rma	Rb11Rma	14	Molise, Central Italy
Rb(4.11)12Rma	Rb12Rma	22	Molise, Central Italy
Rb(6.7)13Rma	Rb13Rma	26	Molise, Central Italy
Rb(5.15)15Rma	Rb15Rma	27	Molise, Central Italy
Rb(10.12)17Rma	Rb17Rma	6	Molise, Central Italy
Rb(1.3)1Lub	Rb1Lub	17	Orobie, Northern Italy
Rb(2.8)2Lub,	Rb2Lub	21	Orobie, Northern Italy
Rb(7.18)9Lub	Rb9Lub		
Rb(5.15)4Lub	Rb4Lub	16	Orobie, Northern Italy
Rb(10.12)5Lub	Rb5Lub	16	Orobie, Northern Italy
Rb(11.13)6Lub	Rb6Lub	17	Orobie, Northern Italy
Rb(16.17)8Lub	Rb8Lub	13	Orobie, Northern Italy
Rb(7.18)9Lub	Rb9Lub	19	Orobie, Northern Italy
Rb(3.9)12Lub	Rb12Lub	20	Ancerano, Central Italy
Rb(1.2)18Lub	Rb18Lub	20	Lipari, Southern Italy
Rb(5.14)21Lub	Rb21Lub	19	Lipari, Southern Italy
Rb(8.12)22Lub	Rb22Lub	21	Lipari, Southern Italy
Rb(10.15)23Lub	Rb23Lub	29	Lipari, Southern Italy
Rb(6.16)24Lub	Rb24Lub	24	Lipari, Southern Italy

3. Robertsonian chromosomes being placed on inbred backgrounds

	Backcross gen.	
BALB/cByJ-Rb(8.12)5Bnr	4	Valle Poschiavo, Switz.
C57BL/6J -Rb(1.3)1Lub	5	Orobie, Northern Italy
C57BL/6J -Rb(2.8)2Lub	3	Orobie, Northern Italy
C57BL/6J -Rb(2.17)11Rma	4	Molise, Central Italy
C57BL/6J -Rb(6.7)13Rma	2	Molise, Central Italy
C57BL/6J -Rb(8.14)16Rma	5	Molise, Central Italy
C57BL/6J -Rb(10.12)5Lub	3	Molise, Central Italy

III.   CONGENIC STOCKS (cont.) - Strains held by K. Moriwaki

Name	Marker gene	Origin of marker	Inbred background	N = number of backcrosses
B10.MOL-YNG	H-2^{wm9}	M. Mol-Yng Yonaguni Is., Japan	B10	N15F18
B10.MOL-OKB	H-2^{wm8}	M. Mol-Okb Okinoerabu Is., Japan	B10	N13F23
B10.MOL-MSM	H-2^{wm5}	M. Mol-Msm Mishima, Japan (1979)	B10	N12F7
B10.MOL-TEN2	H-2^{wm2}	M. Mol-Ten2 Teine, Hokkaido, Japan		N11F22
B10.MOL-TEN1	H-2^{wm1}	M. Mol-Ten1 Teine, Hokkaido, Japan		N12F23